Obstetrics and Gynecology Advances

nova
Medicine & Health
New York

Obstetrics and Gynecology Advances

A Closer Look at Pregnancy and Childbirth
Louise J. Salgado (Editor)
2022. ISBN: 978-1-68507-658-0 (Hardcover)

Cancer and Pregnancy: A Practical Approach for the Gynecologist
Elisa Picardo, MD, Marco Mitidieri, MD and Saverio Danese, MD (Editors)
2021. ISBN: 978-1-53619-844-7 (Hardcover)
2021. ISBN: 978-1-53619-928-4 (eBook)

Hyaluronic Acid – Role in Pregnancy and Novel Applications in the Gestational Period
Vittorio Unfer (Editor)
2021. ISBN: 978-1-53619-743-3 (Softcover)
2021. ISBN: 978-1-53619-873-7 (eBook)

Uterine Fibroids: From Diagnosis to Treatment
Marco Mitidieri, MD, Saverio Danese, MD and Elisa Picardo, MD (Editors)
2021. ISBN: 978-1-53619-184-4 (Softcover)
2021. ISBN: 978-1-53619-284-1 (eBook)

The Thin Pink Line: Regulating Reproduction
Carol Lynn Curchoe Burton, PhD (Author)
2021. ISBN: 978-1-53619-150-9 (Softcover)
2021. ISBN: 978-1-53619-191-2 (eBook)

Fertility Preservation in Gynecological Cancer: Current Management and Novel Insights
Simone Garzon, MD (Editor)
Antonio Simone Laganà, MD, PhD (Editor)
2021. ISBN: 978-1-53619-179-0978 (Hardcover)
2021. ISBN: 978-1-53619-217-9 (eBook)

More information about this series can be found at
https://novapublishers.com/product-category/series/obstetrics-and-gynecology-advances/

Louise J. Salgado
Editor

A Closer Look at Pregnancy and Childbirth

nova
Medicine & Health
New York

Library of Congress Cataloging-in-Publication Data

ISBN: 978-1-68507-658-0

Published by Nova Science Publishers, Inc. † New York

Contents

Preface

This volume includes nine chapters that detail treatment options for health problems associated with pregnancy and childbirth. Chapter one gives an overview of the various technologies and techniques that can be used for prenatal diagnosis. Chapter two collects the latest evidence on treatment for tubal ectopic pregnancy and highlights the impact that drugs and surgical techniques used for this purpose may have. Chapter three discusses the problem of human childbirth and the rise of caesarean sections from the viewpoint of evolutionary anthropology. Chapter four collects the latest evidence on treatment for non-tubal ectopic pregnancy. Chapter five proposes a risk score model for venous thromboembolism prophylaxis for caesarean sections that balances clinical risks and cost-effectiveness. Chapter six establishes a differential protocol for placenta praevia based on a model of risk factors to enable food outcomes in caesarean section. Chapter seven provides a detailed analysis of the various therapeutic options available for ectopic tubal and non-tubal pregnancy, and their indications, contraindications and special considerations during the COVID-19 pandemic and patients affected with this disease. Chapter eight addresses the impact of ectopic pregnancy and the effects of treatments on patients' fertility. Finally, chapter nine addresses the course of ectopic pregnancy from diagnosis to treatment.

Chapter 1 - Prenatal diagnosis is that branch of medicine, and in particular of obstetrics, which applies and studies the techniques that reveal the normality or the presence of various types of pathologies in the fetus. All prenatal diagnostic techniques are performed during pregnancy and can be invasive or not. Invasive tests involve the analysis of the karyotype of fetal cells obtained through different types of samples. The aim is to highlight the possible presence of chromosomal diseases at the fetal level but also genetic diseases such as thalassemia, cystic fibrosis, hemophilia, spina bifida, albinism, and muscular dystrophy. Karyotype by the amniotic fluid is the most used technique today for invasive prenatal diagnosis. Amniotic fluid is collected by amniocentesis. Fetal cells suspended in the collected liquid allow to reconstruct the chromosomal map (or karyotype) of the fetus. However, genetic tests are not able to recognize the physical or psychological characteristics of the unborn child given by the interaction between several genes and the environment. Other types of more or less complex analyses are possible on the amniotic fluid, and it is also possible to preserve the amniotic stem cells (ASC). Another technique involves taking fetal cells from the chorionic villi by means of villocentesis or chorionic villus sampling (CVS). Also in this case, the cells are cultured to highlight their normality, but these are cells taken from outside the gestational chamber (chorionic villi). In both cases, the karyotype can be performed by traditional technique or by the comparative genomic hybridization (CGH) technique on micro-array (array-CGH), which, given the greater sensitivity, allows to highlight a greater number of chromosomal anomalies. Those described above are two invasive techniques (the liquid is taken by puncture in both cases), but there are also noninvasive procedures. The development of ultrasound, for example, has made it possible to develop some highly sensitive diagnostic techniques in the first trimester, such as the combined test or bi-test + nuchal translucency (NT), the "quadruple" test and, recently, the sex chromosome anomalies test (single "device" registered by the Ministry of Health) in the second trimester, all based on the ultrasound measurement of anatomic and functional parameters of the fetus and on the result of blood chemistry tests. These tests are screening tests, so they do not give a certain answer but have a very accurate statistical value that can lead to diagnostic tests. The methods of prenatal diagnosis can also include ultrasound of the second trimester of pregnancy (also called "morphological ultrasound") which can highlight any fetal malformations or abnormalities and fetal echocardiography which analyzes (always by ultrasound) the heart of the fetus not only anatomically but also from a dynamic-functional point of view. This technique cannot detect genetic diseases. A new technique developed by a group of researchers financially supported by the National Institute of Health (NIH) uses ultrasound to monitor the placenta and possible altered fetal blood flow in early pregnancy. Recently, an extremely sensitive test for the most common aneuploidies has been proposed that searches for and analyzes the fetal fraction, i.e., the percentage of cell-free fetal deoxy-ribonucleic acid (cffDNA) that circulates in the maternal plasma, commonly known as "noninvasive prenatal test" (NIPT). NIPT is based on the count of fragments of the chromosomes of interest (21 in the case of Down syndrome) present in the maternal blood. Although not included in the diagnostic but probabilistic tests, the test is the most accurate available so far, with values that are higher than 99.99% sensitivity for trisomy

21 (T21) and less than 0.2% of false-positive rate (FPR). Currently, in Italy, there are three types of new generation NIPT. The distinction of these tests made on a technological basis, takes into consideration two parameters: 1) the method used for sequencing/alignment of sequences; and 2) the method of counting the amount of DNA, since it is possible to detect chromosomal aneuploidies depending on the amount of DNA detected. Based on the first parameter, it is possible to distinguish between those tests that use a massive parallel sequencing (MPS), that is the whole genome shotgun sequencing, and those that use targeted sequencing. On the basis of the second parameter, instead, the authors distinguish between the tests that perform the counting of all the sequences produced and those that instead perform a count of certain single-nucleotide polymorphisms (SNP). The tests that use the MPS method combined with the count of all the sequences are: 1) Fetal-DNA Test, entirely performed at the Altamedica Laboratories (Rome, Italy), is a NIPT that involves the analysis of cffDNA circulating on maternal blood, using Thermo Fisher Scientific NGS technology in synergy with the digital polymerase chain reaction (dPCR) amplification technique (the entire workflow is European conformity [CE]/in vitro diagnostic [IVD] validated with a proprietary Bio-informatics); 2) Aurora, performed by Illumina Incorporated (Inc.) laboratories, United States of America (US) and distributed in Italy by Sorgente Genetica limited liability company (LLC); 3) IONA test, performed in Premaitha certified laboratories (Manchester, United Kingdom [UK]), is CE-IVD certified by one of the numerous "notified companies" exclusively for the preparation of the library and is distributed by Labospace LLC (Italy); 4) Genetic (G)-test, performed at the Tor Vergata University of Rome and distributed by the Bio-science Institute of the San Marino Republic (SMR) 5) Materni-T21 Plus, performed by Sequenom (US), and Prenatest, performed by Lifecodexx (Germany); 6) Prenatal-Safe, performed by Genoma Group (Italy), detects the most common fetal aneuploidies using the latest generation Illumina sequencing platforms; 7) Tranquility, performed in Europe by Genoma Swiss Biotechnology (Switzerland); 8) Vera Prenatal Test, performed by Ames Instrumental Poly-diagnostic Center (Italy), partner of Verinata-Illumina (US) which performs the Verify test (similar to the Vera Prenatal Test), is CE/IVD certified on the complete workflow: from cffDNA extraction, library preparation, and sequencing to reporting; 9) Vera Plus (–), performed by Ames Instrumental Poly-diagnostic Center (Naples, Italy), detects aneuploidies and structural alterations affecting each chromosome of the fetal karyotype, even if these investigations are not recognized by international scientific societies; and 10) Nativa, performed by Bio-Rep LLC

company of the Sapio Group (Italy), which performs the VeriSeq NIPT Solution version 2 (v2) test by Illumina Inc. technologies, is CE/IVD certified on the complete workflow: from cffDNA extraction, library preparation, and sequencing to reporting. The test that uses targeted sequencing coupled with the enumeration of certain SNP is Panorama, performed by Natera (US) and marketed in Italy by Genetic-lab. The test using Affimetryx Array technology (no sequencing) is Harmony Prenatal Test, performed by Ariosa (US) and Toma (Italy), marketed in Italy by Archimed, Synlab, Cam, and Toma (also through Matherna). There are also tests being tested in numerous laboratories. In particular, the Pavia hospital, the Sant'Anna hospital in Turin, through a new immune-fluorescence test proposed by Vanadis and distributed by Perkin Elmer, and other private centers. For the choice between these tests, it is good to rely on the advice of a specialist physician, who is also able to explain the differences between these tests (a geneticist or, alternatively, a gynecologist). Since these are absolutely advanced technologies, they are available at a high price, so the economic factor has its weight. However, these tests are not the same in terms of versatility and result, therefore it is possible to choose according to other parameters as well, for example the cases of validation reported by scientific publications, which however can provide other useful information among the following: 1) the false-negative rate (FNR) and the FPR; 2) the timing for the test result; 3) the reliability of the test at the first sampling (or conversely, the incidence of the need for re-sampling); 4) if, in addition to the main trisomies (chromosomes 13, 18, and 21), the authors search on the sex chromosomes and on other pairs of chromosomes, although such investigations are not recognized by international scientific societies; 5) if the test gives the possibility to analyze also possible chromosomal micro-deletions, even if these investigations are not recognized by the international scientific societies; 6) if a sample from the father is also required for testing; 7) various services offered by those who market the test, such as genetic counseling, the free offer of an invasive procedure in the case of a test with a pathological result (classic karyotype, and array-CGH), the guarantees offered in the event of discordant results, etc.; and 8) then there are more technical parameters on which it is possible to base the choice: certain tests accurately measure the cffDNA, although some tests do not report this data. Tests that make use of the targeted sequencing method need to measure this parameter, since it is used to calculate a statistic risk, which consists of the test result. The tests that involve the MPS method, on the other hand, do not need to quantify the fetal fraction, since they use the number of fetal sequences actually evaluated as a limiting parameter. However, it is a good idea that this parameter is measured. Finally, certain pregnancies have particular conditions for which some tests cannot be taken into consideration, for example twin pregnancies, or cases in which the pregnancy is following an egg donation. It is important to note that, in fact, there is no civil liability for the clinician in the event that he prescribes a prenatal screening test aimed at ascertaining the risk for fetal trisomy. In fact, since it is a screening test, and not a diagnosis one, the result is not sure by definition. In fact, in the available tests it is always well reported, in explicit and reiterated form, in the informed consents that the result, to be considered "diagnostic," must be validated both in the case of positivity and negativity through an invasive prenatal diagnosis (villocentesis or amniocentesis). Therefore, failure to perform the diagnostic confirmation test totally decriminalizes the physician from responsibility for a screening that does not adhere to the diagnosis. However, it is essential that the physician has correctly informed the parents of the difference between screening (fallible) and diagnosis (safe) and that they have signed the acceptance of the limits of screening in the informed consent. In fact, the current jurisprudence has focused the responsibility of the physician performing the prenatal diagnosis tests, not on the diagnostic correctness of the test or on the nonobservance of the deontological rules (different types of tests recognized as more or less valid). Rather, it requires that the complaints are well founded, both as regards the violation of the law (articles 1218 and 2236 of the civil code), and above all with reference to the information obligations on the potential of the indicated test, so that these obligations are incumbent on the health care professional by virtue of the contract stipulated with the patient, as the responsibility for failure to provide information by the physician about more effective prenatal diagnostic tests (see: Supreme Court of Cassation [Cass. Civ.], Section III, sentence May 11th, 2009, no. 10741; Cass. Civ., III, sentence January 10th-October 2nd, 2012, no. 16754; and Cass. Civ., III, sentence November 27th, 2015, n. 24220). With regard to the CE-IVD marking, relating to IVD devices, this literally states that "the devices can be placed on the market and/or put into service only if they meet the requirements set out in the Community directive" (98/79/European Community [EC]). This was then modified, for formal clarifications, by 2007/47/EC. Recently, European Union (EU) Regulation 2017/746 of the European Parliament and of the Council of April 5th, 2017, relating to IVD medical devices, progressively repeals Directive 98/79/EC (still in force today) and decision 2010/227/EU of the Commission, and completely replaces them by 2023. The tests used must therefore meet the prescribed requirements. Virtually all the tests available today adhere to the full "declaration of conformity," an internal document or, better, drawn up by an external private faculty called "Notified Organism," which certifies, under its own responsibility, that a specific test or diagnostic step complies with the provisions of Community directive 98/79 at point 2 reference annex 8. Exactly where this directive states: "the manufacturer or his representative (Notified Organism) draws up, for devices intended for performance evaluation, a declaration containing the information referred to in point 2 and ensure that the relevant provisions of this Directive are met." The European directives are valid for all IVD tests and, obviously, they do not make any specific mention of prenatal diagnosis screening tests, therefore, the declarations of conformity must not cover the entire work-flow, but only specific parts of it, such as the preparation of "libraries," or the software used (Illumina Inc.). Nevertheless, some laboratories, even if not requested, are now commissioning, to the chosen Notified Organism, the certification of the entire work-flow producing, in the final document, the various certifications of the subsequent analytical steps.

Chapter 2 - Ectopic pregnancy is defined as a pregnancy implanted at a place other than the endometrial line of the uterine body, mostly the fallopian tube (96%). In these days, EP remains the leading cause of early pregnancy related death. Diagnosis of this condition is usually made via transvaginal ultrasound. Serial serum beta-human chorionic gonadotrophin (β-hCG) measurement may help to differentiate normal from abnormal pregnancies and rise suspicion of an ectopic pregnancy. Choosing between expectant, medical or surgical treatment is based on clinical characteristics, medical conditions, radiologic and laboratory findings as well as patient-informed choice based on discussion of each approach. In this chapter, the authors' aim is to collect the latest evidence on treatment for tubal ectopic pregnancy, as well as to highlight the impact that drugs and surgical techniques used for this purpose may have. Expectant management is restricted to a limited number of patients who must be asymptomatic, be aware of the clinical implications and have a serum β-hCG concentration below 1500 mIU/mL. Although surgical approach is the prop of treatment, medical therapy has shown similar success rates in selected patients. The main pharmacologic agent used for ectopic pregnancy treatment is metothrexate (MTX), a drug which inhibits dihydrofolate reductase, leading to the inhibition of DNA synthesis, repair, and cellular replication. MTX is usually administered intramuscularly at a single dose of 50mg/m2. The candidates to this line of treatment are those patients who are hemodynamically stable, have serum β-hCG concentration below 5000 mIU/mL, do not present fetal cardiac activity on the ultrasound scan and do not have any contraindications for the use of this drug. Some other drugs have been proposed to be used in combination with MTX-based therapy such as mifepristone - a progesterone antagonist - and gefitinib, a selective inhibitor of the tyrosine kinase domain of epidermal growth factor receptor. However, none of these drugs have managed to oust MTX as treatment of choice. Patients who meet the inclusion criteria to receive medical treatment are generally candidates to surgery. Emergency surgical treatment is indicated for patients with hemodynamic instability or evidence of an ongoing ruptured ectopic mass. In stable or asymptomatic women, surgery is necessary in heterotopic pregnancies, if medical treatment is contraindicated or follow-up cannot be achieved or if the patient has a concurrent abnormality that may be solved in the same procedure. Laparoscopic approach is preferable. Salpingectomy should be performed in women with severe tubal damage, significant bleeding and in cases of desired fertility with a healthy contralateral tube. Salpingostomy is technically more difficult and needs serial β-hCG measurements but it should be performed in cases of previous contralateral salpingectomy or tubal damage and reproductive wish.

Chapter 3 - Caesarean sections (CS) are one of the most frequently performed surgeries in women of reproductive age. Currently, the average global rate of CS is about 21.1%, the prevalence however, differs markedly between different countries but also between different social strata within a country. Although Caesarean sections are lifesaving procedures which helped to reduce maternal and new-born mortality rates, the worldwide rising rates of C-sections however, are subject to growing concern. The main argument to perform caesarean sections is to reduce maternal and new-born mortality, because human childbirth is still a dangerous experience for many women. Consequently, caesarean sections are nearly exclusively seen from an obstetrical or public health perspective. From the viewpoint of evolutionary anthropology however, the authors have to ask: why is human childbirth so painful and dangerous making caesarean sections necessary? This is completely uncommon in nature. Therefore, in the present review the problem of human childbirth and the consequently rising rates of caesarean sections are discussed from the viewpoint of evolutionary anthropology.

Chapter 4 - Ectopic pregnancy (EP) is defined as a pregnancy implanted at a place other than the endometrial line of the uterine body, mostly the fallopian tube (96%). However, EP can have other locations such as the ovary (3%), interstitial/cornual (2-3%), abdominal (1%), c-section scar (<1%) and cervical (<1%). In these days, EP remains the leading cause of early pregnancy related death. Diagnosis of this condition is usually made via transvaginal ultrasound (TVUS). Serial serum beta-human chorionic gonadotropin (bHCG) measurement may help to differentiate normal from abnormal pregnancies and rise suspicion of an EP. Non-tubal ectopic pregnancies (NTE) are a very rare entity. Their heterogeneous clinical presentation, diagnostic difficulties and absence of gold-standard treatments cause high rates of morbidity and mortality compared to tubal ectopic pregnancies. In this chapter, the authors' aim is to collect the latest evidence on treatment for non-tubal EP. Ovarian ectopic pregnancy accounts for cases where embryonic implantation occurs within the ovary. Even though cases are rare, its incidence is increasing due to assisted reproduction techniques. Diagnosis is a challenge, with most of cases being misdiagnosed as corpus luteum, tubal ectopic pregnancy or ovarian tumors. Therefore, patients usuallydebut with intraperitoneal hemorrhage and laparoscopic partial or total oophorectomy is the management of choice. Methotrexate (MTX) may be an option in high-risk patients or persistent residual trophoblast. Interstitial pregnancies implant in the proximal tubal segment that lies within the muscularuterine wall. Insertion on the round ligament is the characteristic anatomic finding. Regarding its low incidence, no clear criteria for medical treatment have been assessed and surgical management is based on cornual resection. Abdominal pregnancy is implanted within the peritoneal cavity. Diagnosis is usually sonographic and drugs such as MTX have had minimal success on its treatment, so surgery is always the first option once this entity is confirmed. C-section scar pregnancies are located in the myometrium at the site of a previous uterine c-section. Cases have risen lately and they are supposed to increase slowly. Optimal management is still unknown. Expectant, medical, and surgical approaches have been used. Surgical approach either using hysteroscopy, laparoscopy, suction curettage or open surgery has the highest success rate and lowest complication rates. Clinical and sonographicfeatures, gestational age at diagnosis, complication rates, desire of the patient and the physician's experience should be considered when choosing between treatments. Cervical pregnancy involves implantation in the cervical canal. It seems like its incidence has been rising lately due to ART. Diagnosis is based on symptoms and TVUS. Because of its oddity, there are no clear criteria for medical treatment, although MTX is usually the first-line therapy.

Chapter 5 - The relative risk of venous thromboembolism (VTE) in pregnancy is increased four-to six-fold and is further increased postpartum particularly after caesarean section. VTE, although rare, is a major cause of maternal mortality and morbidity in developed countries. Recommendations for VTE prophylaxis from authoritative guideline for women undergoing caesarean delivery differed significantly. The Royal College of Obstetricians and Gynaecologists (RCOG) and the Council of the Society of Obstetric Medicine Australia and New Zealand (SOMANZ) recommend pharmacological prophylaxis by low molecular weight heparin (LMWH) for all the women undergoing emergency caesarean sections and in women with risk factors undergoing elective caesarean sections. The American College of Chest Physicians (ACCP) is less stringent and recommends pharmacological prophylaxis in post caesarean section patients having one major or two or more minor risk factors. The American College of Obstetricians and Gynecologists (ACOG) guidelines, in contrast, recommends postpartum pharmacological prophylaxis for only a small group of particularly high-risk women with thrombophilia or prior VTE event. There is a lack of standardization among the international guidelines, and the recommendations are largely based on expert opinion rather than from randomised controlled trials or meta-analyses. Giving pharmacological prophylaxis to a large proportion of women undergoing caesarean delivery would lead to significant financial costs and also increase in bleeding complications. The authors have developed a modified risk score model adapted from the RCOG guidelines of VTE prophylaxis for caesarean section in Chinese women. The authors' risk score model resulted in around 12.7% of women undergoing caesarean section requiring mechanical prophylaxis and around 3.3% women required additional pharmacological prophylaxis in the authors' cohort. In contrast, applying the RCOG guidelines to the authors' cohort, 75.6% women would receive LMWH compared with no women under the ACOG guidelines, while all would require mechanical thromboprophylaxis. There was no VTE in the authors' cohort. The authors' risk score model appears to be a more reasonable recommendation, balancing clinical risks and cost-effectiveness. Local VTE prophylaxis guideline for women undergoing caesarean section is recommended based on the incidence of VTE in that locality. This guideline should be safe, easy to apply, rational and financially practical.

Chapter 6 - Placenta praevia is known to be one of the leading causes of severe postpartum haemorrhage (PPH). Many risk factors have been associated with severe bleeding during caesarean section (CS) for placenta praevia. However, the importance of individual factors in predicting pregnancy outcome remains controversial. Various predictive models to identify high risk cases for severe haemorrhage have been proposed in the literature. However, some of these models have been difficult to apply in practice as they require sophisticated ultrasound parameters, while other models involve a tedious scoring system. The authors have recently proposed a simple model based on three simple parameters, namely the presence of significant antepartum haemorrhage (APH) from the history, and anterior or posterior placenta and major or minor praevia from ultrasound findings, and found that it could predict up to 96.2% of all severe PPH. More importantly, the absence of APH, a posterior minor praevia, was associated with a negative predictive value (NPV) of 99.1% of severe PPH, implying that such cases could be treated as 'normal' low risk CSs. Various conservative surgical treatment modalities have been proposed for the management of severe haemorrhage during CS for placenta praevia, including intrauterine balloon tamponade systems, intrauterine gauge packing, various compression sutures, radiological uterine artery ligation or a combination of these methods. There is now emerging evidence that prophylactic use of balloon tamponade may reduce the incidence of severe PPH in placenta praevia. The establishment of a differential protocol for placenta praevia based on a simple model of risks factors and meticulous planning to prepare for contingency measures are essential elements conducive to good outcomes in CS for placenta praevia.

Chapter 7 - Ectopic pregnancy is defined as an incorrect implantation of pregnancy implanted at a place other than the endometrial line of the uterine body, mostly the fallopian tube (96%). In these days, EP remains the leading cause of early pregnancy related death. Diagnosis of this condition is usually made via transvaginal ultrasound. Serial serum beta-human chorionic gonadotrophin (β-hCG) measurement may help to differentiate normal from abnormal pregnancies and rise suspicion of an ectopic pregnancy. In earlier years, ectopic pregnancy was treated only by radical surgery, and a broad therapeutic armamentarium only became available in the late 20th century. This led directly to advances in diagnostic methods, specifically the advent of new techniques that allow uncomplicated ectopic pregnancy to be readily diagnosed with a high sensitivity and specificity. At the beginning of the COVID-19 pandemic, questions concerning the best surgical approach for the treatment of an ectopic pregnancy aroused. During the first months, some international societies priorized open surgery to laparoscopy (LPS) because of the unknown effects of using pneumoperitoneum in an infected patient. Little was known, about the best surgical option in cases of EP. Nowadays, there is no scientific evidence supporting viral transmission through aerosol particles during LPS surgery. LPS indications remain unchanged. However, some authors recommend additional safety measures such as smoke evacuation or minimizing energy device. The authors provide a detailed analysis of the various therapeutic options available for ectopic tubal and non-tubal pregnancy, and their indications, contraindications and special considerations during COVID-19 pandemic and patients affected with this disease. In this chapter, the authors' aim is to collect the latest evidence on treatment for tubal EP, focusing on the impact that drugs, expectant management and surgical techniques used for this purpose may have on contagion, morbidity and secondary effects derived from SARS-CoV-2.

Chapter 8 - Ectopic pregnancy (EP) is defined as a pregnancy implanted at a place other than the endometrial line of the uterine body, mostly the fallopian tube (96%). However, EP can have other locations such as the ovary (3%), interstitial/cornual (2-3%), abdominal (1%), c-section scar (<1%) and cervical (<1%). These days, EP remains the leading cause of early pregnancy related death. Choosing between expectant, medical or surgical treatment is based on clinical characteristics, medical conditions, radiologic and laboratory findings as well as patient-informed choice based on discussion of each approach. In this chapter, the authors' aim is to address the impact of EP and these treatments on patients 'fertility. Loss of fertility after an episode of tubal ectopic pregnancy (TEP) is obviously related to tubal lesions and, in some cases, tubal occlusion. There is no clinical trial data available regarding post-treatment fertility after expectant management. However, authors have not found statistically significant differences when comparing this treatment line to others as far as subsequent intrauterine pregnancy is concerned. As for methotrexate therapy, data suggests it does not affect fertility markers used in the authors' daily practice, although conclusions are taken from small, observational studies. Further investigation concerning relevant fertility outcomes, like intrauterine pregnancy or live-birth rates, are needed. When it comes to new drugs such as mifepristone, gefitinib or vinorelbine, data is extremely limited. However, only gefitinib appears to cause a significant impairment of female fertility due to its ovarian toxicity. Surgical approach is usually addressed laparoscopically and it can be conservative (salpingotomy) or radical (salpingectomy). There is a meta-analysis which concludes there is no reason to believe salpingectomy harms fertility, although the authors should be cautious with the results. There are two RCTs showing no difference in the outcomes between salpingectomy and salpingostomy for subsequent intrauterine pregnancy, while there are sixteen cohort studies which indicate that salpingectomy is approximately 50% less likely to result in a subsequent intrauterine pregnancy than it is with salpingostomy. However, surgical management should be individualized in each case. Non-tubal ectopic pregnancy (NTEP) is a heterogeneous set of clinical presentations, so singling every case out will be crucial. This means it is very hard to determine an overall impact of treatment on the authors' patients 'fertility.

Chapter 9 - Ectopic pregnancy (EP) is defined as the implantation of a fertilized ovum anywhere outside of the endometrial cavity and constitutes 1% of all pregnancies. Most common etiology is delayed transport of the fertilized ovum through the fallopian tube. EP mostly occurs in a fallopian tube (95-98%) and is rarely seen in ovaries, hysterectomy scar, cervical region, and abdomen. Risk factors in ectopic pregnancy include previous ectopic pregnancy, history of pelvic (particularly fallopian tube surgery) or abdominal surgery, and pelvic inflammatory disease. Most common symptoms include abdominal pain and/or abnormal vaginal bleeding and menstrual delay. EP is diagnosed easily and promptly by a detailed pelvic examination, β-hCG test, and transvaginal ultrasound. There are two important notions to address in EP patients: prompt intervention following a rapid and accurate diagnosis and preservation of fertility. EP accounts for 4 - 10% of all pregnancy-related deaths. In the treatment of EP, laparoscopic techniques are used in the diagnosis and treatment to provide a correct and rapid intervention and conservative treatments (dilation and curettage [D & C] and methotrexate) can be used to preserve fertility. Surgical treatment is performed in patients that are hemodynamically unstable, suspected of tubal rupture, contraindicated to methotrexate treatment, or who do not respond to methotrexate therapy.

Chapter 1

Prenatal Diagnosis: Indications and Techniques

Ciro Comparetto[1,*] and Franco Borruto[2]
[1]Department of Obstetrics and Gynecology, San Paolo Private Clinic, Pistoia, Italy
[2]Professor of Obstetrics and Gynecology, Principality of Monaco

Abstract

Prenatal diagnosis is that branch of medicine, and in particular of obstetrics, which applies and studies the techniques that reveal the normality or the presence of various types of pathologies in the fetus. All prenatal diagnostic techniques are performed during pregnancy and can be invasive or not. Invasive tests involve the analysis of the karyotype of fetal cells obtained through different types of samples. The aim is to highlight the possible presence of chromosomal diseases at the fetal level but also genetic diseases such as thalassemia, cystic fibrosis, hemophilia, spina bifida, albinism, and muscular dystrophy. Karyotype by the amniotic fluid is the most used technique today for invasive prenatal diagnosis. Amniotic fluid is collected by amniocentesis. Fetal cells suspended in the collected liquid allow to reconstruct the chromosomal map (or karyotype) of the fetus. However, genetic tests are not able to recognize the physical or psychological characteristics of the unborn child given by the interaction between several genes and the environment. Other types of more or less complex analyses are possible on the amniotic fluid, and it is also possible to preserve the amniotic stem cells (ASC). Another technique involves taking fetal cells from the chorionic villi by means of villocentesis or chorionic villus sampling (CVS). Also in this case, the cells are cultured to highlight their

---

* Corresponding Author's E-mail: cicomp@tin.it.

In: A Closer Look at Pregnancy and Childbirth
Editor: Louise J. Salgado
ISBN: 978-1-68507-658-0

normality, but these are cells taken from outside the gestational chamber (chorionic villi). In both cases, the karyotype can be performed by traditional technique or by the comparative genomic hybridization (CGH) technique on micro-array (array-CGH), which, given the greater sensitivity, allows to highlight a greater number of chromosomal anomalies. Those described above are two invasive techniques (the liquid is taken by puncture in both cases), but there are also noninvasive procedures. The development of ultrasound, for example, has made it possible to develop some highly sensitive diagnostic techniques in the first trimester, such as the combined test or bi-test + nuchal translucency (NT), the "quadruple" test and, recently, the sex chromosome anomalies test (single "device" registered by the Ministry of Health) in the second trimester, all based on the ultrasound measurement of anatomic and functional parameters of the fetus and on the result of blood chemistry tests. These tests are screening tests, so they do not give a certain answer but have a very accurate statistical value that can lead to diagnostic tests. The methods of prenatal diagnosis can also include ultrasound of the second trimester of pregnancy (also called "morphological ultrasound") which can highlight any fetal malformations or abnormalities and fetal echocardiography which analyzes (always by ultrasound) the heart of the fetus not only anatomically but also from a dynamic-functional point of view. This technique cannot detect genetic diseases. A new technique developed by a group of researchers financially supported by the National Institute of Health (NIH) uses ultrasound to monitor the placenta and possible altered fetal blood flow in early pregnancy. Recently, an extremely sensitive test for the most common aneuploidies has been proposed that searches for and analyzes the fetal fraction, i.e., the percentage of cell-free fetal deoxy-ribonucleic acid (cffDNA) that circulates in the maternal plasma, commonly known as "noninvasive prenatal test" (NIPT). NIPT is based on the count of fragments of the chromosomes of interest (21 in the case of Down syndrome) present in the maternal blood. Although not included in the diagnostic but probabilistic tests, the test is the most accurate available so far, with values that are higher than 99.99% sensitivity for trisomy 21 (T21) and less than 0.2% of false-positive rate (FPR). Currently, in Italy, there are three types of new generation NIPT. The distinction of these tests made on a technological basis, takes into consideration two parameters: 1) the method used for sequencing/alignment of sequences; and 2) the method of counting the amount of DNA, since it is possible to detect chromosomal aneuploidies depending on the amount of DNA detected. Based on the first parameter, it is possible to distinguish between those tests that use a massive parallel sequencing (MPS), that is the whole genome shotgun sequencing, and those that use targeted sequencing. On the basis of the second parameter, instead, we distinguish between the tests that perform the counting of all the sequences produced and those that instead perform a count of certain single-nucleotide polymorphisms (SNP). The tests that use the MPS method combined with the count of all the sequences are: 1) Fetal-DNA Test, entirely performed at the Altamedica Laboratories (Rome, Italy), is a NIPT that involves the analysis of cffDNA circulating on maternal blood, using Thermo Fisher Scientific NGS technology in synergy with the digital polymerase chain reaction (dPCR) amplification technique (the entire workflow is European conformity [CE]/in vitro diagnostic [IVD] validated with a proprietary Bio-informatics); 2) Aurora, performed by Illumina Incorporated (Inc.) laboratories, United States of America (US) and distributed in Italy by Sorgente Genetica limited liability company (LLC); 3) IONA test, performed in Premaitha certified laboratories (Manchester, United Kingdom [UK]), is CE-IVD certified by one of the numerous "notified companies" exclusively for the preparation of the library and is distributed by Labospace LLC (Italy); 4) Genetic (G)-test, performed at the Tor Vergata University of Rome and distributed by the Bio-science Institute of the San Marino Republic (SMR); 5) Materni-T21 Plus, performed by Sequenom (US), and Prenatest, performed by Lifecodexx (Germany); 6) Prenatal-Safe, performed by Genoma Group (Italy), detects the most common fetal aneuploidies using the latest generation Illumina sequencing platforms; 7) Tranquility, performed in Europe by Genoma Swiss Biotechnology (Switzerland); 8) Vera Prenatal Test, performed by Ames Instrumental Poly-diagnostic Center (Italy), partner of Verinata-Illumina (US) which performs the Verify test (similar to the Vera Prenatal Test), is CE/IVD certified on the complete workflow: from cffDNA extraction, library preparation, and sequencing to reporting; 9) Vera Plus (+), performed by Ames Instrumental Poly-diagnostic Center (Naples, Italy), detects aneuploidies and structural alterations affecting each chromosome of the fetal karyotype, even if these investigations are not recognized by international scientific societies; and 10) Nativa, performed by Bio-Rep LLC company of the Sapio Group (Italy), which performs the VeriSeq NIPT Solution version 2 (v2) test by Illumina Inc. technologies, is CE/IVD certified on the complete workflow: from cffDNA extraction, library preparation, and sequencing to reporting. The test that uses targeted sequencing coupled with the enumeration of certain SNP is Panorama, performed by Natera (US) and marketed in Italy by Genetic-lab. The test using Affimetrix Array technology (no sequencing) is Harmony Prenatal Test, performed by Ariosa (US) and Toma (Italy), marketed in Italy by Archimed, Synlab, Cam, and Toma (also through Matherna). There are also tests being tested in numerous laboratories. In particular, the Pavia hospital, the Sant'Anna hospital in Turin, through a new immune-fluorescence test proposed by Vanadis and distributed by Perkin Elmer, and other private centers. For the choice between these tests, it is good to rely on the advice of a specialist physician, who is also able to explain the differences between these tests (a geneticist or, alternatively, a gynecologist). Since these are absolutely advanced technologies, they are available at a high price, so the economic factor has its weight. However, these tests are not the same in terms of versatility and result, therefore it is possible to choose according to other parameters as well, for example the cases of validation reported by scientific publications, which however can provide other useful information among the following: 1) the false-negative rate (FNR) and the FPR; 2) the timing for the test result; 3) the reliability of the test at the first sampling (or conversely, the incidence of the need for re-sampling); 4) if, in addition to the main trisomies (chromosomes 13, 18, and 21), we search on the sex chromosomes and on other pairs of chromosomes, although such investigations are not recognized by international scientific societies; 5) if the test gives the possibility to analyze also possible chromosomal micro-deletions, even if these investigations are not recognized by the international scientific societies; 6) if a sample from the father is also required for testing; 7) various services offered by those who market the test, such as genetic counseling, the free offer of an invasive procedure in the case of a test with a pathological result (classic karyotype, and array-CGH), the guarantees offered in the event of discordant results, etc.; and 8) then there are more technical parameters on which it is possible to base the choice: certain tests accurately measure the cffDNA, although some tests do not report this data. Tests that make use of the targeted sequencing method need to measure this parameter, since it is used to calculate a statistic risk, which consists of the test result. The tests that involve the MPS method, on the other hand, do not need to quantify the fetal fraction, since they use the number of fetal sequences actually evaluated as a limiting parameter. However, it is a good idea that this parameter is measured. Finally, certain pregnancies have particular conditions for which some tests cannot be taken into consideration, for example twin pregnancies, or cases in which the pregnancy is following an egg donation. It is important to note that, in fact, there is no civil liability for the clinician in the event that he prescribes a prenatal screening test aimed at ascertaining the risk for fetal trisomy. In fact, since it is a screening test, and not a diagnosis one, the result is not sure by definition. In fact, in the available tests it is always well reported, in explicit and reiterated form, in the informed consents, that the result, to be considered "diagnostic," must be validated both in the case of positivity and negativity through an invasive prenatal diagnosis (villocentesis or amniocentesis). Therefore, failure to perform the diagnostic confirmation test totally decriminalizes the physician from responsibility for a screening that does not adhere to the diagnosis. However, it is essential that the physician has correctly informed the parents of the difference between screening (fallible) and diagnosis (safe) and that they have signed the acceptance of the limits of screening in the informed consent.

In fact, the current jurisprudence has focused the responsibility of the physician performing the prenatal diagnosis tests, not on the diagnostic correctness of the test or on the nonobservance of the deontological rules (different types of tests recognized as more or less valid). Rather, it requires that the complaints are well founded, both as regards the violation of the law (articles 1218 and 2236 of the civil code), and above all with reference to the information obligations on the potential of the indicated test, so that these obligations are incumbent on the health care professional by virtue of the contract stipulated with the patient, as the responsibility for failure to provide information by the physician about more effective prenatal diagnostic tests (see: Supreme Court of Cassation [Cass. Civ.], Section III, sentence May 11th, 2009, no. 10741; Cass. Civ., III, sentence January 10th-October 2nd, 2012, no. 16754; and Cass. Civ., III, sentence November 27th, 2015, n. 24220). With regard to the CE-IVD marking, relating to IVD devices, this literally states that "the devices can be placed on the market and/or put into service only if they meet the requirements set out in the Community directive" (98/79/European Community [EC]). This was then modified, for formal clarifications, by 2007/47/EC. Recently, European Union (EU) Regulation 2017/746 of the European Parliament and of the Council of April 5th, 2017, relating to IVD medical devices, progressively repeals Directive 98/79/EC (still in force today) and decision 2010/227/EU of the Commission, and completely replaces them by 2023. The tests used must therefore meet the prescribed requirements. Virtually all the tests available today adhere to the full "declaration of conformity," an internal document or, better, drawn up by an external private faculty called "Notified Organism," which certifies, under its own responsibility, that a specific test or diagnostic step complies with the provisions of Community directive 98/79 at point 2 reference annex 8. Exactly where this directive states: "the manufacturer or his representative (Notified Organism) draws up, for devices intended for performance evaluation, a declaration containing the information referred to in point 2 and ensure that the relevant provisions of this Directive are met." The European directives are valid for all IVD tests and, obviously, they do not make any specific mention of prenatal diagnosis screening tests, therefore, the declarations of conformity must not cover the entire work-flow, but only specific parts of it, such as the preparation of "libraries," or the software used (Illumina Inc.). Nevertheless, some laboratories, even if not requested, are now commissioning, to the chosen Notified Organism, the certification of the entire work-flow producing, in the final document, the various certifications of the subsequent analytical steps.

Keywords: prenatal diagnosis, prenatal screening, prenatal testing, chromosomal aneuploidies, ultrasound, cell-free fetal DNA, genome sequencing, amniocentesis, chorionic villus sampling, counseling

Introduction

Medical care and the clinical chemistry laboratory's role in it have changed remarkably over the last 60 years [1]. In the modern history of reproductive medicine, with particular emphasis on the past years since the establishment of the National Institute of Child Health and Human Development (NICHD), five examples of how fundamental and clinical research have contributed to patient care and, in turn, received stimulus from them are: fertility regulation and reproductive endocrinology, prematurity and the initiation of parturition, antenatal testing of fetal maturity, antenatal diagnosis, and neonatal intensive care [2]. Routine obstetric screening for all patients should include a Papanicolaou (Pap) smear, urine analysis and urine culture, complete blood count, blood type, Rhesus (Rh) factor, and direct Coombs' test. Patients should also be screened for syphilis, rubella, gonorrhea, and diabetes. For patients at high risk for certain conditions, additional studies of value include obstetric ultrasound, serum alpha-fetoprotein (α-FP) level and screening for sickle cell anemia (SCA), herpes, hepatitis B, Chlamydia, and Human Immunodeficiency Virus (HIV) [3].

In the last four decades, perinatal medicine has made tremendous advances in scientific knowledge and in the successful application of this knowledge toward understanding the fetal aspects of pregnancy. Evaluation of the health of the fetus and screening for birth defects has become an important part of prenatal care [4]. The assessment of fetal health has occupied our professional attention for many years. As the development of technologies for prenatal diagnostic techniques has progressed, applications of such technologies have aided in the overall assessment of fetal well-being. Fetal heart-rate (FHR) monitoring remains the main form of fetal assessment for high-risk pregnancies (Figure 1). The additional assessments afforded by the analysis of ST and T-wave changes of the fetal electrocardiogram (ECG) hold promise for improving the predictive value of FHR assessments. Ultrasound has been invaluable for the assessment of fetal anatomy, and the use of Doppler ultrasound has given insight into fetal cardiovascular responses to such conditions as intrauterine growth restriction (IUGR) and fetal anemia caused by red blood cell alloimmunization. As prenatal diagnostic techniques evolve, their application to the assessment of fetal well-being offers insight into pathophysiological mechanisms of fetal disease, innovative tools to assess fetal health, and fertile ground for future investigation [5].

Knowledge of human genetics has increased dramatically in the past few decades. The genetic basis of disease and the response to therapy is rapidly being elucidated and may soon become a part of routine medical practice [6]. Genetic testing may be applied in a variety of clinical situations, including preconception counseling, prenatal diagnosis, and postnatal determination of genetic predisposition to disease. Cystic fibrosis, Huntington's disease, and cancer are three diseases for which genetic testing has become a reality, and they are exemplary of the clinical and ethical dilemmas that arise with this type of testing [7]. Possibilities for treating or, ideally, avoiding hereditary diseases have increased enormously with the rapid and radical developments in the field of molecular biology. The cost-benefit ratio of providing genetic services is extremely favorable, and prevention is often far cheaper than treatment. Genetic counseling is particularly important because of the psychological impact of knowledge of genetic risk and the difficult decisions that often face individuals identified as being at risk [8]. Currently, advances in molecular technology involving recombinant deoxy-ribonucleic acid (DNA) have led to dramatic breakthroughs in genetic diseases, cancer research, and identification of foreign DNA. Of particular interest is the impact these tools have made and will make on the clinical laboratory. Specific examples of available applications include carrier detection and prenatal diagnosis in cystic fibrosis, hemophilia, and SCA [9].

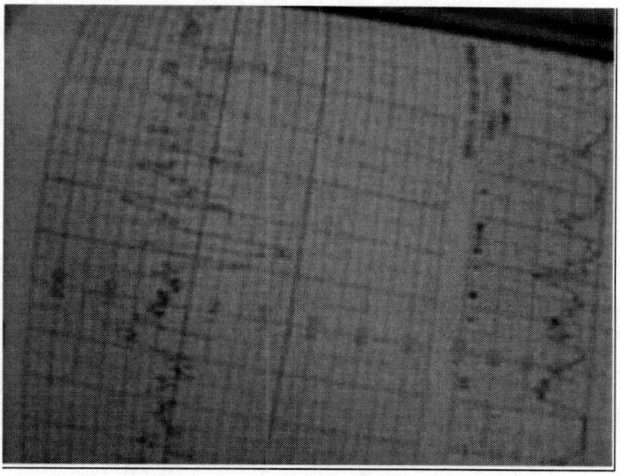

Figure 1. Cardiotocography (CTG) for fetal heart-rate (FHR) monitoring.

Historical Notes

Screening for inherited disease is a preventative health measure that started in the 1960s with the development of programs for the detection of phenilketonuria (PKU) in newborns and that has had a major impact on reducing the burden of disease. Developments in technology have led to the availability of large-scale testing for an increasing number of both acquired and genetic disorders [10]. Prenatal diagnosis is a sub-field of clinical genetics and gynecology that exemplifies the effective integration of theoretical and clinical medicine. Milestones in its history include the development of cytogenetic, molecular genetic, and molecular cytogenetic methods as well as advances in ultrasonography. The latter technique not only improves the safety of invasive procedures, but also enables earlier and more reliable diagnosis of congenital malformations. Invasive prenatal diagnosis is most commonly performed to assess the embryonal/fetal chromosome set. An increasing number of monogenic diseases can be diagnosed prenatally by either genetic or biochemical testing, depending on the particular disease being sought. Polygenic and multi-factorial diseases cannot be reliably diagnosed by genetic testing at present, although a number of malformations can be ascertained prenatally by ultrasonography [11]. Interest in cytogenetics may be traced to the development of the chromosomal theory of inheritance that emerged from efforts to provide the basis for Darwin's theory "On the origin of species by means of natural selection." Despite their fundamental place in biology, chromosomes and genetics had little impact on medical practice until the 1960s. In 1959, 63 years after the death of John Langdon Down, Jérôme Lejeune discovered trisomy 21 (T21) as the genetic reason for Down syndrome. The discovery that a chromosomal defect caused Down syndrome was the spark responsible for the emergence of medical genetics as a clinical discipline. Prenatal diagnosis of trisomies, biochemical disorders, and neural tube defects (NTD) became possible and hence the proliferation of genetic counseling clinics. Maternal serum screening for NTD and Down syndrome followed, taking the new discipline into social medicine. Safe amniocentesis needed ultrasound, and ultrasound soon found other applications in obstetrics, including scanning for fetal malformations. Progress in medical genetics demanded a gene map, and cytogeneticists initiated the mapping workshops that led to the Human Genome Project (HGP) and the complete sequence of the human genome. As a result, conventional karyotyping has been augmented by molecular cytogenetics, and molecular karyotyping has been achieved by micro-arrays. Genetic diagnosis at the level of the DNA sequence is with us at last. It has been a remarkable journey from disease phenotype to karyotype to genotype, and it has taken almost 60 years. The mission now is to ensure that the recent advances such as prenatal screening, micro-arrays, and noninvasive prenatal diagnosis (NIPD) are available to the patients. History shows that it is by increased use that costs are reduced and better methods discovered. Chromosome research has been behind the major advances in this field, and it will continue to be the key to future progress, not least in our appreciation of chromosomal variation and its importance as a mechanism in Darwinian evolution [12].

The collection of fetal genetic materials is required for the prenatal diagnosis of fetal genetic diseases. The conventional methods for sampling fetal genetic materials, such as amniocentesis and chorionic villus sampling (CVS), are invasive in nature and are associated with a risk of fetal miscarriage. The history of amniocentesis and CVS indicates that women have played various roles in the developmental and diffusion stages of both procedures. Effective policies regarding the impact of prenatal diagnosis on women can be shaped on the basis of lessons learned from that history [13]. For decades, scientists had been pursuing studies with goals to develop noninvasive methods for prenatal diagnosis. First trimester screening, combining maternal age, maternal serum parameters, and ultrasound findings, emerged in the 1990s with a detection rate (DR) of around 90-95% and a false-positive rate (FPR) of around 5%, also looking for T13 and T18. With the development of high-resolution ultrasound, around 50% of fetal anomalies are now detected in the first trimester [14]. Fetal face was the main concern of researchers who developed three-dimensional (3D) ultrasound. 3D ultrasound beginnings date back to 1973. Parallel concerns of researchers from different parts of the world have led to a constantly changing the equipment and software. 3D images of the fetal face were obtained since 1986, but those that are available on the ultrasound devices sold today dates from 1992, and the four-dimensional (4D) since 1996. Techniques such as volume rendering and multi-planar volume rendering led to the development of 3D ultrasound. Late 2000 revealed study fetal face by multi-plane 3D ultrasound, through the acquisition of volume and its processing. Study of fetal profile by this method provides new data on the jaw, naso-maxillo-mandibular angle, even a diagram of the fetal profile or of dimensions of the fetal face, or nasal bone length. Fetal profile analyzed by 16 parameters measured by 3D ultrasound, with the creation of a craniofacial index variable is useful in assessing normal and abnormal fetal face. Today, the bones of fetal face (nose, jaw, bone palace, and those of the orbit) can be studied in dynamics, from 12-14 gestational weeks. The best ultrasound images can be obtained after 21 gestational weeks, when fetal size and its ratio with amniotic fluid are optimal for the acquisition of fetal volume [15].

The discovery of quantitative and qualitative differences of the circulating DNA (cirDNA) between healthy and diseased individuals inclined researchers to investigate these molecules as potential biomarkers for noninvasive diagnosis and prognosis of various pathologies. However, except for some prenatal tests, cirDNA analyses have not been readily translated to clinical practice due to a lack of knowledge regarding its composition, function, and biological and evolutionary origins. To fully grasp the nature of cirDNA and the extracellular vesicles and protein complexes with which it is associated, it is necessary to probe the early and badly neglected work that contributed to the discovery and development of these concepts. cirDNA enters target cells and provokes a myriad of gene regulatory effects associated with the messaging functions of various natures, disease progression, somatic genome variation, and trans-generational inheritance. This challenges the traditional views on each of the former topics. All of these discoveries can be traced directly back to the iconic works of Darwin, Lamarck, and their followers. The history of cirDNA is rich in information that should be considered in clinical practice, when designing new experiments, and should be very useful for generating an empirically up-to-date view of cirDNA and extracellular vesicles. Furthermore, it will invite many flights of speculation and stimulate further inquiry into its biological and evolutionary origins [16]. In 1997, the existence of fetal-derived cell-free DNA molecules in plasma of pregnant women was first demonstrated. This finding provided a new source of fetal genetic material that could be obtained safely through the collection of a maternal blood sample and provided a new avenue for the development of NIPD. Now, 25 years later, the diagnostic potential of fetal cirDNA analysis has been realized. Fruitful research efforts have resulted in the clinical implementation of noninvasive prenatal testing (NIPT) based on maternal plasma DNA analysis and included tests for fetal sex assessment, fetal Rh blood group D antigen (RhD) genotyping, and fetal chromosomal aneuploidy detection. Most recently, research groups have succeeded in decoding the entire fetal genome from maternal plasma DNA analysis which paved the way for the achievement of NIPD of many single-gene diseases. A paradigm shift in the practice of prenatal diagnosis has begun [17]. NIPT for T21, T13, and T18 is a highly efficient screening method and has been applied as a first-line or a contingent screening approach all over the world since 2012, in some countries without a systematic screening program. Concomitant with the rise in technology, the possibility of screening for other genetic conditions by analysis of cell-free fetal DNA (cffDNA), such as sex chromosome anomalies, rare autosomal anomalies, and micro-deletions and duplications, is offered by different providers to an often not preselected population of pregnant women. Most of the research in the field is done by commercial providers, and some of the tests are on the market without validated data on test performance. This raises difficulties in the counseling process and makes it nearly impossible to obtain informed consent. In parallel with the advent of new screening technologies, an expansion of diagnostic methods has begun to be applied after invasive procedures. The karyotype has been the gold standard for decades. Chromosomal micro-array analyses (CMA) able to detect deletions and duplications on a submicroscopic level have replaced the conventional karyotyping in many countries. Sequencing methods such as whole-exome sequencing (WES) and whole-genome sequencing (WGS) tremendously amplify the diagnostic yield in fetuses with ultrasound anomalies [11].

Genetic Screening

Overview

Genetic screening is used to identify individuals who have genetic variations or mutations that are associated with a particular disorder. Genetic screening may be useful to plan for periodic evaluation, implementation of preventive strategies, or initiation of therapeutic interventions. Current practice is to offer genetic screening for certain diseases during the preconception encounter or, more commonly, as part of early prenatal care [18]. During the course of the last decades, there has been extensive discussion on the role of genetics and genomics in global healthcare, with major diagnostic advances regularly announced, such as WES to identify and classify de novo, autosomal, and X-linked mutations in people with severe intellectual disability, and WGS for prenatal diagnosis of chromosomal anomalies, in the differential diagnosis of acute neonatal disorders, and in devising improved treatment protocols. There are, however, a number of basic issues that need to be addressed if advances of this nature are to be more widely translated in terms of healthcare [19].

Genetic screening utilizes analytical approaches adapted for high throughput to identify carrier and affected individuals in a targeted population. Current approaches to genetic screening include carrier screening, prenatal screening, and newborn screening to identify infants who would benefit from early treatment. Other approaches are reproductive genetic screening to assist reproductive decision making, and family history assessment to identify individuals who would benefit from additional prevention measures. Although the traditional goal of screening is to identify early disease or risk in order to implement preventive therapy, genetic screening has always included an atypical element, i.e., information relevant to reproductive decisions. New technologies offer increasingly comprehensive identification of genetic conditions and susceptibilities. Tests based on these technologies are generating a different approach to screening that seeks to inform individuals about all of their genetic traits and susceptibilities for purposes that incorporate rapid diagnosis, family planning, and expediting of research, as well as the traditional screening goal of improving prevention. Use of these tests in population screening will increase the challenges already encountered in genetic screening programs, including false-positive and ambiguous test results, over-diagnosis, and incidental findings. Whether this approach is desirable requires further empiric research, but it also requires careful deliberation on the part of all concerned, including genomic researchers, clinicians, public health officials, health care payers, and especially those who will be the recipients of this novel screening approach [20].

Carrier Screening

Carrier screening aims to identify asymptomatic hetero-zygotes of heritable disorders and has a vital, ever-changing role in its application to the prenatal detection of disease. An explosion of new technologies for the identification of single-gene disorders challenges our ability to evaluate each individual test prior to its introduction into the private and public sectors. The efficacy of carrier screening is dependent on several factors including the validity of the test, the incidence of disease within the community, and as many genetic disorders segregate along ethnic and racial lines, which populations should be offered testing. The difficulties in evaluating prenatal screening programs are highlighted by the recent conflicting recommendations from the American College of Medical Genetics and Genomics (ACMG) and the American College of Obstetricians and Gynecologists (ACOG) over several single-gene disorders. In addition, changes in the recommendation for universal versus risk-based screening for ethnically segregated disorders remain controversial. These conflicts have major impacts in the provision of genetic counseling in the prenatal outpatient setting [21]. Many genetic disorders are detectable in the prenatal period, and the capacity to identify them has increased remarkably as molecular genetic testing techniques continue to improve and become incorporated into clinical practice. Prenatal genetic screening and diagnostic testing can identify many disorders that will require specialized newborn care and follow-up. Over the last two decades, there have been important changes in the breadth and depth of prenatal screening and diagnostic procedures. Carrier screening for selected genetic disorders is now offered routinely to pregnant women or those contemplating pregnancy. Newly developed strategies for first-trimester screening for fetal chromosome abnormalities have improved the DR for these disorders, while maintaining a low screen-positive rate. The ACOG and the ACMG now recommend that invasive prenatal diagnostic testing be made available to all pregnant women, regardless of age or prenatal screening results, and prenatal ultrasound findings of unknown clinical significance require that pediatricians provide appropriate follow-up in the newborn period and beyond. Prenatal genetic screening and diagnostic tests are changing rapidly, and results of these tests may impact the postnatal evaluation and treatment strategies for pediatric care [22].

Prenatal Screening

The indications for prenatal genetic testing vary widely, including follow-up of an anomaly found by routine ultrasound or maternal aneuploidy screening, a family history of genetic disease, advanced maternal or paternal age, or evaluation of a low-risk pregnancy due to parental concern. The interpretation of genetic variants identified in the prenatal period poses unique challenges due to the lack of ability for deep phenotyping as well as the option to make critical decisions regarding pregnancy continuation and perinatal management [23]. Improved testing procedures now allow prenatal screening for a wide range of congenital defects, including cystic fibrosis and muscular dystrophy. An emerging technique also allows diagnosis of congenital anomalies during the preimplantation stage of in vitro fertilization (IVF). Thus, clinicians need an established criterion to use as a guide when counseling parents about what prenatal testing is possible, feasible, and desirable. For example, there are limits to prenatal testing for conditions like mutations in the breast cancer gene because affected individuals do not necessary develop the condition and a cure may be found by the time the condition develops. It is even questionable if parents should be given this information until the child reaches an appropriate age. One approach to development of guidelines is to classify congenital abnormalities according to severity, age of onset, and type (structural-functional versus mental). This system reveals anomalies that are clearly lethal, lead to moderate or severe disability with little or no prospect of improvement or cure, are characterized by early onset, and/or involve obvious mental retardation. This approach is particularly relevant in cases of T21, and progressively invasive screening techniques are available to detect this most common pattern of malformation in humans [24].

Newborn Screening

Newborn screening should serve as a model for all genetic screening, with more than 50 years of experience and numerous lessons learned. As with all genetic screening, there are policy concerns in newborn screening regarding which disorders and technologies should be selected, and how centralized or decentralized the process to set policy should be. The need to share experiences and develop databases transcends all other policy considerations in genetic screening. The future will see population-based screening for adult-onset disorders. However, there needs to be extensive research to define predictive risk for various ethnocultural groups and to determine effective interventions. Ethical concerns regarding the timing of population screening, as well as the scope of use of information, will need to be resolved if genomic medicine will achieve its promise of a predictive, preventive, and personalized medicine [25]. The pediatrician who cares for a child with a birth defect or genetic disorder may be in the best position to alert the family to the possibility of a recurrence of the same or similar problems in future offspring. The family may wish to know about and may benefit from methods that convert probability statements about recurrence risks into more precise knowledge about a specific abnormality in the fetus. The pediatrician also may be called on to discuss abnormal prenatal test results as a way of understanding the risks and complications that the newborn infant may face. Along with the increase in knowledge brought about by the sequencing of the human genome, there has been an increase in the technical capabilities for diagnosing many chromosome abnormalities, genetic disorders, and isolated birth defects in the prenatal period [26]. Family history captures the collective influence of shared genetic susceptibility, shared environmental factors, and common behaviors within families. Throughout the reproductive continuum, pediatricians, obstetricians, family practitioners, genetic counselors, and other clinicians can work with families to elicit relevant family history information and factor it into risk-assessment calculations and, when appropriate, decision-making. Current screening tools have focused on understanding the risk for single-gene disorders, chromosomal conditions, and teratogen exposures during the preconception, prenatal, and inter-conception periods. More research and data are needed to understand how family history influences risk for a wide variety of complex birth outcomes such as preterm birth, stillbirth, and many birth defects. With a better understanding of the impact of family history on many adverse birth outcomes, tools for the collection of a broader set of pertinent family history information must be developed [27]. Developments in mutation analysis have led to significant benefits for patients with inherited metabolic disorders and their families. This is particularly the case where new methodologies have prevented the need for invasive tissue biopsies or have allowed carrier detection or first-trimester prenatal testing to be undertaken. Whereas in the past it may have only been possible to identify specific "common" mutations, the availability of techniques, such as automated sequencing, and novel technologies including mutation scanning techniques, multiplex ligation dependent probe amplification, and array technologies, have vastly improved the diagnostic efficiency of molecular testing [28].

Ethnicity and Population-based Screening

The aim of screening is to improve individual health through an early detection of diseases at a stage where the prognosis of disease could be significantly better. However, this kind of intervention is costly and it's necessary to respect criteria in selection of targeted diseases and screening tests [29]. The aim of carrier testing is to identify carrier couples at risk of having offspring with a serious genetic (autosomal recessive) disorder. Carrier couples are offered genetic consultation where their reproductive options, including prenatal diagnosis, are explained. The Ashkenazi Jewish population is at increased risk for several recessively inherited disorders (Tay-Sachs disease, cystic fibrosis, Canavan disease, Gaucher disease, familial dysautonomia, Niemann-Pick disease, Fanconi anemia, and Bloom syndrome). With the rapid identification of disease-causing genes in recent years, DNA-based assays are increasingly available for carrier detection. Approximately 5% of the world's population carries a mutation affecting the globin chains of the hemoglobin molecule. Among the most common of these disorders are the thalassemias. The global birth rate of affected infants is at least 2 per 1000 (in unscreened populations), with the greatest incidence in Southeast Asian, Indian, Mediterranean, and Middle Eastern ethnic groups. Carriers are detected by evaluation of red cell indices and morphology, followed by more sophisticated hematological testing and molecular analyses. The following issues need to be considered in the development of a carrier screening program:

1. test selection based on disease severity and test accuracy;
2. funding for testing and genetic counseling;
3. definition of the target population to be screened;
4. development of a public and professional education program;
5. informed consent for screening; and
6. awareness of community needs [30].

Screening ostensibly normal populations is appropriate in certain ethnic groups to determine heterozygosity for selected disorders: Blacks for SCA, Mediterranean people for beta-thalassemia (β-thalassemia), Southeast Asians and Filipinos for α-thalassemia, and Ashkenazi Jews and perhaps French-Canadians for Tay-Sachs disease. Cystic fibrosis screening through the assessment of delta-F508 (δ-F508) mutations should be offered to relatives of an individual having δ-F508 cystic fibrosis. Irrespective of the extent of screening programs for Mendelian traits, the mutant allele will remain in the general population because by far the greatest genetic load lies in clinically normal hetero-zygotes, affected contributing far less to the load despite the obvious clinical effect [31].

The Ashkenazi Jewish community is a unique and ideal population in which to provide multiple disease screening because detection rates are high (>95%) by testing a limited number of mutations. The residual risk that remains is very low. In addition, the lessons learned from carrier screening in this community indicate that only through genetic counseling and education can screening in the general population gain wide acceptance and provide maximum benefit [32]. Multiple-option prenatal carrier testing in the Ashkenazi Jewish community for genetic disorders has been readily accepted in this prenatal, health-oriented, and knowledgeable population. Counseling of screens concerning the nature (severity, treatability, etc.), inheritance, and frequencies of each disorder is essential for informed test choices and future reproductive decision making. Studies identified issues of education, confidentiality, post-test anxiety, and self-esteem that must be continuously addressed in the Ashkenazi population. However, an important value of these studies is that they provide a framework for the development of mass carrier screening programs in the general population or in specific segments of the population with similar demographic characteristics and in more diverse prenatal populations [33].

Various studies have shown that high consanguinity can be a contributing factor to the high incidence of some rare autosomal recessive diseases [34]. Consanguineous marriages are associated with many problems, although the prevailing opinion is that the advantages outweigh the disadvantages. This explains why the custom is still extremely prevalent, particularly in Arab countries, India, and small isolated communities. Among Israeli Arabs there has been a reduction in the rate of such marriages, although it is still sufficiently high to cause medical problems. Among Israeli Jews, the rate has always been much lower. Future goals are to expand the educational programs aimed at the Israeli Arab community and to promote the uptake of genetic counseling and prenatal testing where available in order to reduce the health problems even further [35]. Israeli society is a complex one, ethnically, religiously, and culturally diverse, comprised of Jews of many ethnic backgrounds, as well as Christian and Moslem Arabs, Druze, and Bedouins. Multiple founder mutations have been documented in these various ethnic populations, often down to the level of specific villages or tribes. Although carrier screening and prenatal diagnostic testing are well established in the general population, the rejection of pregnancy termination by many religious communities often prevents participation in testing. Culturally appropriate genetic programs have been initiated in religious Jewish and non-Jewish communities in an attempt to overcome cultural barriers and reduce the frequency of severe genetic diseases nationwide. Ongoing research in order to identify specific genes will enable more conditions to be detectable early in pregnancy. We expect that the willingness of families to agree to termination of affected pregnancies will reduce the number of babies born with these conditions [36].

Prenatal Diagnosis

Overview

Screening for genetic abnormalities is an integral part of obstetrics. Prior to initiating screening, however, several prerequisites must be met:

1. capacity to alter clinical management;
2. cost-effectiveness;
3. reliable means (usually assays) of assessment; and
4. capacity to handle problems.

In all pregnancies one should determine in systematic fashion whether family history places a pregnant woman at increased risk over the background risk of 2-3% congenital anomalies [31]. Prenatal genetic diagnostic testing is intended to determine, with as much certainty as possible, whether a specific genetic disorder or condition is present in the fetus. In contrast, prenatal genetic screening is designed to assess whether a patient is at increased risk of having a fetus affected by a genetic disorder. Originally, prenatal genetic testing focused primarily on Down syndrome (T21), but now it is able to detect a broad range of genetic disorders. Although it is necessary to perform amniocentesis or CVS to definitively diagnose most genetic disorders, in some circumstances, fetal imaging with ultrasonography, echocardiography, or magnetic resonance imaging (MRI) may be diagnostic of a particular structural fetal abnormality that is suggestive of an underlying genetic condition. The objective of prenatal genetic testing is to detect health problems that could affect the woman, fetus, or newborn and provide the patient and her obstetrician-gynecologist or other obstetric care provider with enough information to allow a fully informed decision about pregnancy management. Prenatal genetic testing cannot identify all abnormalities or problems in a fetus, and any testing should be focused on the individual patient's risks, reproductive goals, and preferences. It is important that patients understand the benefits and limitations of all prenatal screening and diagnostic testing, including the conditions for which tests are available and the conditions that will not be detected by testing. It also is important that patients realize that there is a broad range of clinical presentations, or phenotypes, for many genetic disorders and that results of genetic testing cannot predict all outcomes. Prenatal genetic testing has many benefits, including reassuring patients when results are normal, identifying disorders for which prenatal treatment may provide benefit, optimizing neonatal outcomes by ensuring the appropriate location for delivery and the necessary personnel to care for affected infants, and allowing the opportunity for pregnancy termination [37, 38].

An abnormal chromosome complement (aneuploidy) contributes significantly to fetal loss during pregnancy, as well as to perinatal morbidity and mortality. The contribution of chromosomal abnormalities to fetal loss decreases as pregnancy continues with an estimated 50% of first-trimester spontaneous abortions due to chromosomal abnormalities, but only 5% of stillbirths (after 28 weeks) [39]. The purpose of prenatal screening for aneuploidy is to provide an assessment of the woman's risk of carrying a fetus with one of the more common fetal aneuploidies. This is in contrast to prenatal diagnostic testing for genetic disorders, in which the fetal chromosomes are evaluated for the presence or absence of abnormalities in chromosome number, deletions, and duplications, or the fetal DNA is evaluated for specific genetic disorders. The wide variety of screening test options, each offering varying levels of information and accuracy, has resulted in the need for complex counseling by the health care provider and complex decision making by the patient. No one screening test is superior to other screening tests in all test characteristics. Each test has relative advantages and disadvantages. It is important that obstetrician-gynecologists and other obstetric care providers be prepared to discuss not only the risk of aneuploidy but also the benefits, risks, and limitations of available screening tests. Screening for aneuploidy should be an informed patient choice, with an underlying foundation of shared decision making that fits the patient's clinical circumstances, values, interests, and goals [40, 41].

There are several methods of antenatal screening for aneuploidy. Most are aimed at the identification of women at increased risk of Down syndrome, the most common abnormal karyotype conferring a significant risk of serious long-term morbidity. Prenatal diagnosis of chromosomal disorders is generally offered to women who will be 35 years or older at the time of delivery or who have been determined via serum screening to be at risk similar to that of a woman older than 35 years. This age threshold was based on four major rationales that reflect considerations of resources and effectiveness. New information calls the 35-years threshold into question. Guidelines regarding use of prenatal diagnosis account for the preferences of the individual patient as well as for individual risk [42]. The process of genetic screening has evolved from a simple notation of maternal age to a complex algorithm incorporating age, maternal serum screening, and sonographic findings. The extent to which each of these variables should contribute to the overall screening result is much debated and deserves continued research. It is clear that maternal age provides useful information when used as part of this equation but should not represent the sole screening modality. The use of genetic screening in a general population should be examined in terms of cost-effectiveness without sacrificing patient preference and autonomy [43].

Traditional maternal-age-based screening has largely been replaced by programs based on biochemical markers in maternal serum in the second trimester of pregnancy. However, in recent years there has been a considerable drive towards earlier screening such that there are now a range of potential programs based on various combinations of maternal age, serum markers, and ultrasound findings. There is currently much debate as to which are the most effective methods of screening for aneuploidy [44]. The goal of screening both low- and high-risk obstetrics populations for chromosomally abnormal fetuses continues to be developed in many centers worldwide. Advances in the past years have been multi-focal in their approach: NTD, the development of new markers for aneuploidy, and moving screening into the first trimester [45].

Prenatal testing in early pregnancy is used to detect serious congenital fetal abnormalities, with a view to terminating the pregnancies in which they are found [46]. Prenatal diagnosis is now offered to the majority of pregnant women in Europe and the United States of America (US). Prenatal diagnostics has seen a rapid increase in the number of genetic disorders amenable to prenatal detection owing to advances in technology and research into the genetic etiology of many conditions [47]. Indeed, gene carriers can be identified before pregnancy in some cases [48]. Professional guidelines have been established covering both sampling procedures and diagnostic testing, and legislation is in place regarding termination of pregnancy and preimplantation genetic diagnosis (PGD). The close liaison of the various groups of professionals involved has led to well-developed prenatal diagnostic and screening services. These links have been the major contributory factor to the current state of prenatal diagnosis and have been of great benefit to patients undergoing prenatal testing [49].

Pretest and post-test counseling is an integral part of prenatal diagnosis. Timely referral, preferably prepregnancy, is important. There is more or less a consensus regarding offering prenatal diagnosis for lethal/chronic disabling or difficult/expensive to treat conditions. Ethical issues are already around regarding prenatal testing for disabilities like deafness and late-onset disorders [50]. Laboratory testing is only one facet of a screening program and consideration should be given to availability of testing to all individuals, education regarding the program, effectiveness of treatment, long-term benefits both for individuals and society, ethical issues, and cost-benefits [10].

Invasive Prenatal Diagnosis

Prenatal diagnosis of fetal chromosomal abnormalities is the most common indication for invasive prenatal testing. The prevalence of chromosomal abnormalities in clinically recognized early pregnancy loss is greater than 50%. Common fetal aneuploidies include Down syndrome (T21), Edward syndrome (T18), Patau syndrome (T13), Turner syndrome (45,X), Klinefelter syndrome (47,XXY), triple X syndrome (47,XXX), and 47,XYY syndrome. Fetuses with aneuploidy account for 6-11% of all stillbirths and neonatal deaths. Chromosomal abnormalities that are compatible with life but cause considerable morbidity occur in 0.65% of newborns, and structural chromosomal rearrangements that will eventually affect reproduction occur in 0.2% of newborns. Consequently, screening and diagnostic programs to detect the most common autosomal trisomies in live-born infants, including Down syndrome, are well established [51]. During pregnancy, fetal cells suitable for genetic testing can be obtained from amniotic fluid by amniocentesis, placental tissue by CVS, or fetal blood. As invasive diagnostic methods still have an important role to play in evaluating the fetus, one of the most important questions to address during genetic counseling is the procedure-related risk of these techniques. New developments have recently occurred in the laboratory techniques used in prenatal diagnosis. During genetic counseling, an individually-tailored risk assessment needs to be established before any invasive procedure. This should take into account all the factors modifying the specific risk for aneuploidy or other disorders of the fetus, as well as the actual procedure-related risks [52]. It has been shown that in NIPT there is a small chance of a false-positive or false-negative result. This is partly due to the fact that the cffDNA present in maternal plasma is derived from the cytotrophoblast of chorionic villi, which is not always representative for the fetal karyotype due to chromosomal mosaicism. Therefore, a positive NIPT result should always be confirmed with invasive testing, in order to investigate the fetal karyotype. However, since amniocentesis can only be safely performed after 15 weeks of gestation while NIPT can be done from the 10th week of gestation, this potentially means an unacceptable long waiting time for the prospective parents to receive a definitive result. Based on the experience with cytogenetic investigations in chorionic villi and the literature, CVS may be appropriate for confirmation of an abnormal NIPT result [53]. So, pregnant women identified as having an increased risk of a fetal genetic abnormality secondary to the process of established prenatal screening protocols (maternal serum ± imaging, high-risk cffDNA results, abnormal diagnostic fetal imaging, or a positive family history of an inherited condition) may require or request counseling about pregnancy risks and benefits of an invasive ultrasound-guided procedure to determine the etiology, diagnosis, and/or pathology for the possible fetal anomaly or anomalies. The health care provider should counsel the at-risk pregnant woman on the different levels of genetic fetal testing in order for her to have a clear understanding and expectation of the level of testing and type of results that are offered. As part of the informed consent process, the health care provider should review with the at-risk pregnant woman the risks and benefits of in utero genetic diagnostic techniques associated with fetal genetic testing options. During risk/benefit counseling, the health care provider should advise that the best estimate of the pregnancy loss rate related to:

1. amniocentesis is 0.5-1.0% (range 0.17-1.53%);
2. CVS is 0.5-1.0%; and
3. cordocentesis or percutaneous umbilical blood sampling is 1.3% for fetuses with no anomalies and 1.3-25% for fetuses with single or multiple anomalies or IUGR [54].

In 1991, concerns about the relative safety of these procedures arose after reports were published that described a possible association between CVS and birth defects in infants. Subsequent studies support the hypothesis that CVS can cause transverse limb deficiencies. Following CVS, rates of these defects, estimated to be 0.03-0.10% (1/3,000-1/1,000), generally have been increased over background rates. Rates and severity of limb deficiencies are associated with the timing of CVS; most of the birth defects reported after procedures that were performed at ≥70 days' gestation was limited to the fingers or toes. The risk for either digital or limb deficiency after CVS is only one of several important factors that must be considered in making complex and personal decisions about prenatal testing. For example, CVS is generally done earlier in pregnancy than amniocentesis and is particularly advantageous for detecting certain genetic conditions. When performed prior to the routine sampling window of 15 weeks, amniocentesis may increase the risk of talipes equinovarus, the highest risk being encountered prior to 13 weeks' gestation. The laboratory analysis of both procedures is reliable. CVS has a 1-2% incidence of confined placental mosaicism (CPM), requiring additional evaluation in some cases. Prospective parents considering the use of either CVS or amniocentesis should be counseled about the benefits and risks of these procedures. The counselor should also discuss both the mother's and father's risks for transmitting genetic abnormalities to the fetus [55, 56]. A major disadvantage of second-trimester amniocentesis is that the results are available relatively late in pregnancy (after 16 weeks' gestation). Earlier alternatives are CVS and early amniocentesis, which can be performed in the first trimester of pregnancy. Second-trimester amniocentesis increased the risk of pregnancy loss, but it was not possible to quantify this increase precisely from only one study, carried out more than 30 years ago. Early amniocentesis was not as safe as second-trimester amniocentesis, illustrated by increased pregnancy loss and congenital anomalies (talipes). The spread of both first-trimester screening for chromosomal abnormalities and the possibility to check for single-gene disorders at DNA-analysis has increased the request for CVS in the first trimester. In order to perform placental biopsy, two routes are possible: the trans-cervical (TC) and the trans-abdominal (TA). In early days, the TC technique was the most diffused, but since its introduction into clinical practice, the TA technique has become the approach of choice in detriment of the TC technique [57]. TC CVS compared with second-trimester amniocentesis may be associated with a higher risk of pregnancy loss, but results were quite heterogeneous. Diagnostic accuracy of different methods could not be assessed adequately because of incomplete karyotype data in most studies [58, 59].

Genetic mid-trimester amniocentesis is a common invasive procedure. The origin of the commonly quoted 0.5% rate of procedure-related pregnancy loss after amniocentesis is obscure and is in conflict with the only randomized prospective study that reported a procedure-related rate of loss of 1.0% The examination of experience with 68,119 amniocenteses from both controlled and uncontrolled studies provides a substantive basis for several conclusions:

1. contemporary amniocentesis with concurrent ultrasound guidance in controlled studies appears to be associated with a procedure-related rate of excess pregnancy loss of 0.6% (95% confidence interval [CI], 0.31-0.90); to determine the total rate of loss, this must be added to the reported natural rate of loss without amniocentesis among control patients of 1.08%;
2. the use of concurrent ultrasound guidance appears to reduce the number of punctures and the incidence of bloody fluid; concurrent ultrasound guidance was associated with a reduced rate of loss when all studies were compared, but not among controlled studies;

3. direct fetal needle trauma is rare, and rarely proved, but may occur more frequently than is reported because of a failure to diagnose and a failure of the consistent production of sequelae; and
4. this experience does not substantiate an increased rate of pregnancy loss if placental puncture is required [60].

Recent studies in Canada and the US have shown that CVS is both safe and accurate, with a fetal loss rate likely not slightly higher than that of amniocentesis but still at an acceptable level (1%). Although CVS may become the dominant prenatal diagnosis procedure, it is unlikely that it will completely replace amniocentesis. The two procedures are essentially complementary in the provision of prenatal diagnosis in the first and second trimesters [61]. When performed between 10- and 14-weeks' gestation, it is both safe and effective, with risks comparable to those of second-trimester amniocentesis. Cytogenetic results have been confirmed to be reliable and accurate. Earlier concerns about procedure-induced limb defects have been reduced with the accumulation of additional data, showing minimal to no risk when CVS is performed after 70 days of gestation. In experienced hands, it may be the procedure of choice for sampling multiple gestations. Secondary to the advantage of safe, early diagnosis, CVS appears to be the optimal choice for first-trimester testing [62]. In fact, CVS has been used as a successful and safe first-trimester prenatal diagnostic technique for over 35 years. Developed to avoid the medical and psychological complications of later prenatal diagnosis by amniocentesis, CVS rapidly has become a primary tool for the diagnosis of fetal chromosomal, molecular, and biochemical disorders. In addition, its development has led to an improved understanding of several biological processes, including CPM and uni-parental disomy (UPD) [63].

In most pregnancies, the chromosomal complement detected in the fetus is also present in the placenta. The detection of an identical chromosomal complement in both the fetus and its placenta has always been expected as both develop from the same zygote. However, in approximately 2% of viable pregnancies studied by CVS at 9 to 11 weeks of gestation, the cytogenetic abnormality, most often trisomy, is confined to the placenta. This phenomenon is known as CPM. It was first described by Kalousek and Dill in term placentas of infants born with unexplained IUGR. Contrary to generalized mosaicism, which is characterized by the presence of two or more karyotypically different cell lines within both the fetus and its placenta, CPM represents tissue specific chromosomal mosaicism affecting the placenta only. The diagnosis of CPM is most commonly made when, after the diagnosis of chromosomal mosaicism in a CVS sample, the second prenatal testing (amniotic fluid culture or fetal blood culture analysis) shows a normal diploid karyotype. Although CPM occurs in approximately 2% of cases requiring interpretation, and occasionally additional invasive testing, its finding adds additional information about perinatal outcome and can alert the practitioner to fetal genetic disorders [64]. This frequency is ten times greater than the level of mosaicism observed in newborn surveys and, thus, must reflect phenomenon other than true fetal mosaicism. Indeed, only 23% of mosaicism detected at CVS is confirmed in the fetus (2.3 per 1,000 CVS), which is much closer to the newborn rate (1 per 1,000). This indicates that most mosaicism encountered in CVS is unrelated to the fetal karyotype and as such is an inaccurate prediction of the fetal genotype, the purpose of prenatal diagnosis. Most of the mosaicism detected in CVS is due to CPM. Either as a result of error-prone cell division generating an excess of abnormal cells in extra-embryonic tissues or reduced selection against aneuploid cells in these tissues allowing their persistence, chorionic villi and placenta appear to show much higher levels of mosaicism than seen in fetuses. This explains the more frequent finding of multiple cell lines in CVS than in amniocentesis or live-born individuals. The discrepancy between levels of mosaicism present in chorionic villi and fetal tissues means that most instances of mosaicism detected in CVS are not associated with a fetal abnormality and should be evaluated by further prenatal testing, i.e., amniocentesis or fetal blood sampling. Because of the frequency of chromosomal mosaicism in CVS and its attendant need for further testing, a discussion of mosaicism should be included in counseling prior to CVS. The higher frequency of discrepant results in direct CVS preparation emphasizes the prudence of delaying decision-making until the results of the CVS culture have been obtained. Although the observation of mosaicism clearly complicates genetic counseling and decision-making, it does not appear to be associated with an adverse fetal outcome. Whereas most of the mosaicism observed in CVS is the result of CPM, other types of discrepancies also occur. Maternal cell contamination occurs in about 1% of cases, but is easily evaluated by examining the direct preparation and analyzing chromosome polymorphism. The incidence of pseudomosaicism in CVS cultures is unclear but probably low. Interestingly, CVS analysis has suggested that twinning may be a more common phenomenon at conception than reported at birth and that some discrepancies may reflect the non-viability of twins with abnormal karyotypes. CVS remains a viable alternative to amniocentesis for early prenatal diagnosis [65].

Usually, genetic diseases segregate in a stable, predictable fashion throughout a family. For many inherited disorders, a mutation at the DNA level has been characterized, and prenatal diagnosis is available. Based on the inheritance patterns of the disease and type of mutation, prenatal diagnosis is possible using direct or indirect methods of detection. Recently, however, the dogma of traditional Mendelian inheritance has been challenged by the discovery of new patterns of gene segregation and expression. Although direct mutation analysis is highly accurate, accuracy of indirect mutation analysis depends on the distance of the DNA marker to the disease locus. In the past decades, the discovery of new concepts, such as atypical inheritance patterns due to UPD and imprinting and triplet repeat disorders, have helped to increase understanding of the molecular basis of these unusual genetic disorders. Unstable DNA segments varying in size have been associated with both fragile X syndrome and myotonic dystrophy and can now be diagnosed by direct DNA analysis. UPD, the inheritance of both members of a chromosome pair from one parent, has been documented in autosomal and X-linked recessive diseases. Prenatal detection of UPD is a methodological challenge, and a positive testing result requires comprehensive considerations on the clinical consequences as well as ethical issues. Whereas prenatal testing for UPD in families which are prone to UPD formation (e.g., in case of chromosomal variants and imprinting disorders) is often embedded in genetic counseling, the incidental identification of UPD is often more difficult to manage. With the increasing application of high-resolution test systems enabling the identification of UPD, an increase in pregnancies with incidental detection of UPD can be expected. Imprinted genes, the expression of which is dependent on the parent of origin, are being increasingly identified, especially in syndromes with abnormalities of growth. Prenatal diagnosis using a single cell from a blastomere is rapidly becoming routine in clinical practice. Noninvasive procedures to obtain fetal DNA for molecular testing also are progressing very rapidly. With the completion of the HGP, resources now are available for developing new technologies, such as micro-arrays (DNA chips), for accurate, simultaneous, mutation detection. In the near future, the number of prenatally diagnosed disorders will expand as tests for unstable DNA, UPD, and imprinting become widely available. The next few decades hold the promise of many more advances in genetic testing, drug discovery, and therapy [66-68].

Emerging antenatal interventions and care delivery to the fetus require diagnostic support, including laboratory technologies, appropriate methodologies, establishment of special algorithms, and interpretative guidelines for clinical decision-making. Fetal diagnostic and therapeutic interventions vary in invasiveness and are associated with a spectrum of risks and benefits. Fetal laboratory assessments are well served by miniaturized diagnostic methods for blood analysis. Expedited turnaround times are mandatory to support invasive interventions such as cordocentesis and intrauterine transfusions. Health-associated reference intervals are required for fetal test interpretation. Fetal blood sampling (cordocentesis) is a well-accepted and widely practiced procedure by experienced perinatologists. Its simple and safe access to the fetal circulation has broadened the spectrum of congenital disorders diagnosed prenatally. Some fetal disease states can now be identified and treated earlier, directly, more quickly, and more effectively than before, resulting in improved patient care. Although cordocentesis has been embraced by the perinatal community, it is, by definition, a technique of obtaining a fetal blood sample. A prerequisite for the procedure to exert its full impact on perinatal care is a highly capable clinical laboratory. The facility must be aware of the commonly requested fetal serological, hematological, and serum chemistry studies, as well as their normal values. Efforts must be made to perform fetal blood studies rapidly and reliably on small specimens. Laboratory personnel should be familiar with the indications and pitfalls of these tests and those that are best referred to a specialty laboratory. A general understanding of the perinatologist's needs and concerns will lead to a cooperative working relationship between clinician and laboratory. In this manner, we will truly discover what can be learned from cordocentesis [69]. Cordocentesis has pioneered perinatal medicine in the last 30 years with the ability to obtain genetic information, to diagnose and to treat erythrocyte and platelet alloimmunization, to discover the presence of perinatal infections, and to determine the acid-base status of the fetus. Fetal blood sampling has also allowed the perinatologist a greater understanding of fetal physiology, such as thyroid-pituitary function. Cordocentesis has enabled obstetricians to have a better understanding of fetal thyroid development and function [70]. The volume of fetal blood to be retrieved and collection media for blood will be dictated by the indication for the procedure and thus the desired laboratory tests. These items and the preferred sampling site should be planned in advance by the operator. However, a flexible approach to fetal blood sampling should be maintained, anticipating the variability of fetal positions, cord insertions, and ultimate specimen volume. Teamwork among the perinatologist, sonographer, laboratory, and patient will continue to expand the role of fetal blood sampling in obstetrics (Figure 2) [71].

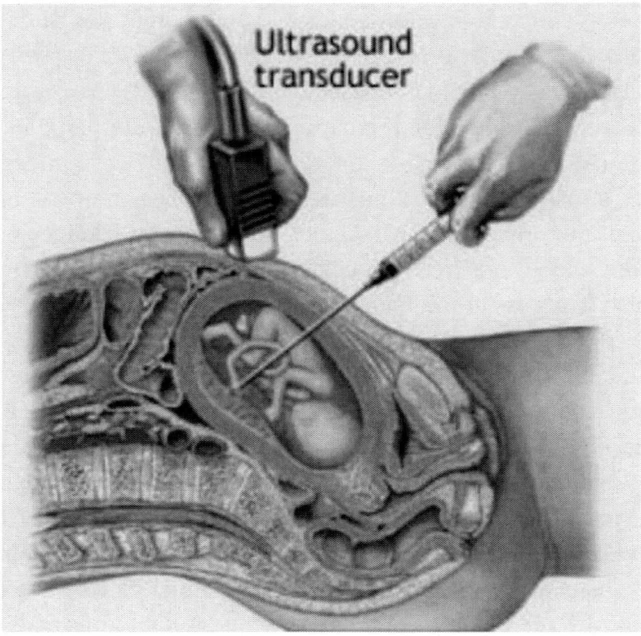

Figure 2. Ultrasound-guided fetal blood sampling (cordocentesis).

Ultrasonography has expanded the capabilities of perinatologists to examine, test, and treat the fetus. Amniocentesis and CVS are safe and widely available procedures, which can be used to diagnose a multitude of abnormalities through karyotype analysis and molecular studies. CVS allows earlier diagnosis, but both procedures can provide highly accurate results in the first half of pregnancy. Cordocentesis has fewer indications, but allows direct laboratory testing of fetal blood. Fetocentesis and fetal biopsy are reserved for limited indications, but can play a crucial role in the diagnosis of some conditions, which cannot be assessed less invasively. By providing guidance for all of these procedures, real-time ultrasonography has revolutionized prenatal diagnosis and therapy; it will continue to be a crucial component in evaluating and treating complicated pregnancies [72]. Fetal blood sampling by cordocentesis carries substantial risk and is therefore performed only when fetal health is impaired, or at risk. When the suspected pathology is not confirmed, however, normative fetal data can be collected. After birth, definitive assessment of prenatal environmental and/or drug exposures to the fetus can be retrospectively assessed by analysis of meconium, hair, and other alternative matrices. A rapidly advancing technology for fetal assessment is the use of fetal laboratory diagnostic techniques that use cffDNA collected from maternal plasma, and genetic analysis based on molecular counting techniques. Developmental changes in fetal biochemical and hematological parameters in health and disease are continually delineated by analysis of collective outcome-based experience. Noninvasive technologies for fetal evaluation are realizing the promise of lower risk yet robust diagnostics; examples include sampling and analysis of cffDNA from maternal blood, and analysis of fetal products accessible at maternal sites. Application of diagnostic technologies for non-medical purposes (e.g., sex selection) underscores the importance of ethical guidelines for new technology implementation [73]. In utero sampling of fetal skin, liver, and muscle may be required to diagnose before-birth disorders that cannot be diagnosed by analysis using chorionic villi or amniotic fluid. Nowadays, many of these conditions can be detected by DNA analysis, and the need for these procedures has decreased dramatically. First performed by fetoscopy, fetal tissue sampling is now most frequently done by inserting a biopsy needle under continuous ultrasonographic guidance [74]. Embryoscopy is a new technique that allows direct visualization of the embryo/fetus as early as the first trimester of pregnancy. A rigid fiber-optic endoscope is passed transcervically into the extracelomic cavity and is used to identify developmental milestones and diagnose structural anomalies. Using this technology has established the feasibility of access to the human embryonic circulation. Future applications for embryoscopy include direct targeted embryonic or fetal interventions, such as gene or stem cell therapy [75-77].

The modern obstetrics care includes NIPT such as first-trimester screening performed between 11- and 14-weeks' gestation and second-trimester screening performed between 15 and 20 weeks. In these screening tests, biochemical markers are measured in the maternal blood with or without ultrasound for fetal NT with reported accuracy of up to 90%. Invasive procedures, including amniocentesis or CVS, are used to achieve over 99% accuracy. During these procedures, direct fetal material is examined and, therefore, these tests are highly accurate with the caveat of a small risk for pregnancy loss. Now, other noninvasive highly accurate and risk-free tests can identify fetal material in the maternal blood. Fetal cells and fetal DNA/ribonucleic acid (RNA) provide fetal information but are hard to find in an overwhelming background of maternal cells and in the absence of specific fetal cell markers. The most experience has been accumulated with fetal Rh and fetal sex determination from maternal blood, with an accuracy of up to 100% by using gene sequences that are absent from maternal blood. Fetal cells, cffDNA/RNA, and fetal proteomics in combination with cutting edge technology are used to prenatally diagnose aneuploidies and single-gene disorders [78]. Currently, the techniques for amniocentesis and CVS tend to be described in local and national guidelines, but certain aspects, including the choice of instruments, is predominantly based upon the operator's personal preference. A survey of practice in the specialist United Kingdom (UK) centers revealed a wide variation of practice; therefore, standardizing any element of technique could potentially influence the safety of the procedure. Overall, the quality of evidence is not sufficient to change current clinical practice. In the absence of clear evidence, the operators should continue to use methods and technique modifications with which they are most familiar with. Any randomized controlled trials (RCT) of technique modifications that are performed to high standard with adequate safety outcomes and power to detect important clinical differences would be clearly welcome [79]. The rapid development of noninvasive serum analyte screening as well as molecular genetic and sonographic techniques to evaluate the fetus has altered our ability to both educate trainees as well as to maintain physician competence to perform invasive procedures. Simulation-based learning is being incorporated into medical training across a broad range of specialties, including obstetrics and gynecology. Prenatal diagnosis procedures will continue to be necessary for direct fetal assessment but on a much more limited scale. It is possible that all trainees will not be able to become competent in amniocentesis and other even fewer common procedures. Furthermore, experienced physicians may lose competence, given the lack of available procedures for skill retention. Innovative methods of skill acquisition and maintenance may be required in the near future. Although long-term assessments of efficacy are currently lacking, the introduction of comprehensive, simulation-based curricula has the potential to both educate trainees and help maintain physician competence [80-86].

Noninvasive Prenatal Diagnosis

Infant mortality is higher in the US than in many other industrialized nations; better access to early prenatal care may help reduce this mortality rate. Several common laboratory tests can significantly contribute to prenatal care. Prenatal diagnosis of chromosomal abnormalities and single-gene disorders can be accurately made by cytogenetic studies of samples obtained from invasive procedures, such as amniocentesis or CVS. Since these procedures are associated with an approximately 0.5-1% risk of miscarriage, the common approach is to perform noninvasive test to define an individual woman's risk of having a chromosomal abnormal pregnancy. Screening for chromosomal abnormalities has developed over the last decades. Prenatal screening can be performed in the late first trimester, the early second trimester, or in both. Screening test can be carried out biochemically, ultrasonographically, or by both modalities. A major goal of screening test is to achieve maximum accuracy and minimum harm at low cost. The integrated test for many years has met best those criteria [87]. Algorithms that combine ultrasound and serum markers in the first and second trimesters have been evaluated. Furthermore, the practice of using age cutoffs to determine whether women should be offered screening or invasive diagnostic testing has been challenged [88]. Identification of cell-free fetal nucleic acids (DNA and RNA) in maternal plasma and the recognition that they represent a useful source of fetal genetic material for prenatal diagnosis has led to intensive efforts to develop NIPT [89].

The advantage of noninvasive methods is that they provide an opportunity to make a genetic diagnosis without risk, and therefore are applicable for use in mass screening programs [90]. The failure of screening studies based on maternal age to reduce substantially the birth incidence of chromosomally abnormal babies has stimulated the search for new methods of screening. The two best approaches to screening for fetal chromosomal abnormalities are: maternal blood analysis and examination of the fetal anatomy by ultrasound. Maternal prenatal screening is essential in preventing pregnancy complications as well as preventing and/or predicting neonatal and infant medical issues after delivery that are due to certain communicable diseases. Maternal screenings should be performed at the first provider visit once pregnancy has been confirmed. Additional screenings vary based on the specific disease and on maternal risk factors. Methods of screenings involve measuring antigen or antibody titers, a combination of antigen/antibody titers, or by specialized genetic tests. Providers responsible for pregnant women should be able to identify which diseases they need to screen for and how to interpret the findings. Neonatal providers should be able to interpret the findings and they should also be able to manage neonates appropriately [91]. Maternal serum analyte screening is an integral component of contemporary antenatal care. Maternal serum screening is a well-understood technique that should be universally offered to pregnant women, regardless of their risk status. Measurement of maternal serum α-FP originated in the early 1970s as a means to screen for fetal NTD, a relatively common and devastating class of malformations. Since that time, assay methods have improved, interpretation has been refined, follow-up testing for NTD has advanced, and many other disease associations have been uncovered. It is a unique test, both in its clinical application and its laboratory implementation [92]. The past years have seen major challenges to existing maternal serum α-FP testing protocols for both NTD and chromosomal anomalies [93]. Early measurement of maternal serum hCG can permit estimation of the date of conception. Use of maternal serum α-FP in the second trimester provides the clinician with risk estimates for NTD and Down syndrome. Adding hCG and possibly unconjugated estradiol (UE3) to this screen can increase the number of Down syndrome cases identified without increasing the proportion of abnormal results [94]. Based on elevated maternal serum α-FP levels, 85% to 90% of NTD (e.g., anencephaly or spina bifida) can be detected. Using a combination of serum analytes (e.g., maternal serum α-FP, hCG, and UE3), 55% to 60% of fetal Down syndrome can be detected. Other strategies for Down syndrome screening have included the use of new markers such as dimeric inhibin-A and urinary β-core fragment of hCG, as well as first-trimester screening, particularly with pregnancy-associated plasma protein A (PAPP-A) and free β-hCG [95]. Increasing data have clearly shown the advantages of multiple markers, particularly β-hCG over α-FP alone. There continues to be considerable controversy over the best mathematics algorithm and which markers are best (e.g., β-hCG, UE3, and so forth). There seems to be a plateau of detection frequencies at about 65% to 70% with current methodologies. Further work needs to be done, however, including some new approaches, if there is to be substantial improvement of screening sensitivity. The combination of biochemical with biophysical parameters represents the next level of sophistication in the attempt to identify the highest proportion of abnormalities with the fewest false-positives [96].

The value of all NIPT must be viewed with the perspective of the consequences of invasive testing. Regarding second-trimester noninvasive testing, biochemical screening is more accurate in establishing risk than maternal age alone. As we will see after, one or more major ultrasound abnormalities, nuchal thickening, or a shortened humerus should raise concern for Down syndrome regardless of the patient's a priori risk based on age or biochemical markers. Isolated minor ultrasound markers should not be used in calculating risk in low-risk patients regarding Down syndrome, unless the biochemical profile already places the patient at risk or in a borderline risk zone. If the ultrasound finding is hyper-echoic bowel, problems other than aneuploidy may be the cause, including cystic fibrosis, infection, or hemorrhage, and these problems must be considered if hyper-echoic bowel is an isolated finding. Improved risk adjustment seems to be applicable to a priori high-risk patients with completely normal sonograms. Genetic sonograms with specific risk adjustment schemata may be used to adjust a priori risk (either maternal age or biochemical screening results) at centers in which this has proven to be accurate. The goal of second-trimester ultrasound screening is to identify at-risk fetuses better and offer invasive testing to a more selected group of patients. As the value of first-trimester screening has become more evident and practical, and if the risk of CVS becomes an acceptable norm, the patient population that reaches the second trimester of pregnancy will be selected. Therefore, second-trimester screening and invasive testing may be needed only in a minority of cases, and the practice standards of prenatal testing and sonography (including minor ultrasound markers) have changed entirely [97].

Maternal serum screening for NTD and fetal aneuploidy in the second trimester has been incorporated into obstetrical practice over the past three decades. Now, as a result of several multicenter trials, there is extensive evidence that effective screening for major chromosomal abnormalities can be provided in the first trimester of pregnancy. First-trimester screening between 11 and 14 weeks has been shown to be an effective and reliable screening test for Down syndrome and T18. Benefits of first-trimester screening include earlier identification of the pregnancy at risk for fetal aneuploidy and anatomic defects, in particular, cardiac anomalies, and the option of earlier diagnosis by CVS, if available [98]. Randomized studies have established that the risk of miscarriage from CVS in the first trimester is the same as for amniocentesis in the second trimester. Prospective studies have demonstrated that screening by a combination of fetal NT and maternal serum free β-hCG and PAPP-A can identify 90% of fetuses with T21 and other major chromosomal abnormalities for a FPR of 5%. This is superior to the 30% detection rate achieved by maternal age and 65% by second-trimester maternal serum biochemistry. A further improvement in the effectiveness of first-trimester screening has been achieved by a risk-orientated two-stage approach. In this, the patients are subdivided into a high-risk group, requiring invasive testing, a low-risk group, which can be reassured that an abnormality is unlikely, and an intermediate-risk group (risk of 1 in 101 to 1 in 1000), in which further assessment is performed by first-trimester ultrasound examination (for presence/absence of the nasal bone or presence/absence of tricuspid regurgitation or normal/abnormal Doppler velocity waveform in the ductus venosus), and CVS is performed if their adjusted risk becomes 1 in 100 or more [99]. Prospective studies in a total of 200,868 pregnancies, including 871 fetuses with T21, have demonstrated that increased NT can identify 76.8% of fetuses with T21, which represents a FPR of 4.2%. When fetal NT was combined with maternal serum free β-hCG and PAPP-A in prospective studies in a total of 44,613 pregnancies, including 215 fetuses with T21, the detection rate was 87.0% for a FPR of 5.0%. Studies from specialist centers with 15,822 pregnancies, which included 397 fetuses with T21, have demonstrated that the absence of the nasal bone can identify 69% of T21 fetuses, which represents a FPR of 1.4%. It has been estimated that first-trimester screening by a combination of sonography and maternal serum testing can identify 97% of T21 fetuses, which represents a FPR of 5%, or that the DR can be 91%, which represents a FPR of 0.5%. In addition to increased NT, important sonographic markers for chromosomal abnormalities include fetal growth restriction, tachycardia, abnormal flow in the ductus venosus, megacystis, exomphalos, and single umbilical artery [100].

Three screening and diagnostic modalities are of potential application in noninvasive first-trimester testing for fetal aneuploidy: ultrasound, maternal biochemical markers, and analysis of fetal cells retrieved from maternal sources. Sensitivities of the sonographic finding of NT thickness in combination with maternal age for T21, performed between 10 and 14 weeks of gestation in experienced hands, and maternal biochemical markers independently may be as high as 86% and 60%, respectively. Analysis of fetal cells retrieved from maternal sources, although more complex, may offer definitive NIPD [101]. As we have seen before, combined screening for T21 based on maternal age, fetal NT, and the serum markers free β-hCG and PAPP-A results in a detection rate of about 90% for a FPR of 3-5%. With the addition of further ultrasound markers, the FPR can be roughly halved. Screening based on cffDNA identifies about 99% of the affected fetuses for a FPR of 0.1%. However, there is a test failure rate of about 2%. The ideal combination between combined and cffDNA screening is still under discussion. Currently, a contingent screening policy seems most favorable where combined screening is offered for everyone and cffDNA analysis only for those with a borderline risk result after combined screening. Significant advances in screening for T21 have been made over the past two decades. Contemporary screening policies can detect for more than 95% of affected fetuses for FPR of less than 3% [102].

First-trimester combined screening (sonographic NT combined with serum markers PAPP-A and the free β-hCG) has superseded second-trimester serum screening (α-FP, total hCG, and UE3 with or without inhibin-A) as a screening paradigm for the detection of T21. This move is attributed to the recognition of superior detection rates, lower FPR, and earlier results associated with the former strategy. Septated cystic hygroma has been recognized as a distinct entity which confers a high risk of aneuploidy and structural malformations. Most pregnant women prefer screening in the first rather than in the second trimester. Further advances in screening performance are achievable by combining the results of first- and second-trimester screenings in a sequential manner, with much interest generated by programs that only include second-trimester testing contingent upon first-trimester results. Screening strategies for aneuploidy continue to evolve, with the most recent evidence favoring a contingent sequential approach [103]. Counseling regarding the options for aneuploidy risk assessment is complicated and requires thorough confrontation with the patient. Second-trimester serum risk assessment has been the gold standard because of widespread availability, low cost, and vast experience with counseling and performance. With the advent of first-trimester techniques, controversy has arisen as there are advocates for the different recently available approaches. Clearly, implementation of first-trimester risk assessment requires special training and meticulous quality control standards for NT and laboratory measurements, access to CVS, and also appropriate counseling regarding risk assessment options. This process was well established by the Fetal Medical Foundation (FMF) several years ago and is widely accepted internationally [104]. It is apparent that there is no ideal biochemical screening available to either ensure fetal well-being or reliably predict fetal compromise. The trend in modern obstetric management is toward an array of biophysical tests of fetal well-being. Biochemical screening in early gestation is used to assess future fetal-placental status and to predict risk for later pregnancy complications. Combinations of these biochemical and biophysical modalities have achieved the greatest predictive success in assessing fetal and placental well-being [105].

Up to 5% of babies are born with a congenital abnormality. Findings from studies on the association between fetal malformations and chromosomal abnormalities indicate that a high percentage of fetuses with an abnormal karyotype can be detected by ultrasound (Figure 3) [106]. Ultrasound is a readily available, noninvasive, and safe means of evaluating fetal health, determining gestational age, and assessing the intrauterine environment. It is an indispensable tool for the practice of obstetrics. The routine ultrasound examination is a beginning. It is a diagnostic test, yielding results that must be interpreted and integrated in a knowledgeable way. As it is true for physical examination, the ultrasound study is most helpful when performed in a consistent and reproducible fashion, carefully documenting the pertinent positive and negative findings that are important in clinical decision making.

The information gained from routine obstetric ultrasound may provide reassurance, guide therapy, or identify a pathological condition that merits further investigation. It is always informative [107]. Screening for fetal anomalies by an ultrasound scan was introduced in many maternity units in the UK in the late 1970s and has become routine in most since then although there is little uniformity as to how the scan is performed and when it is offered [108]. Several diagnoses are possible to identify by ultrasound examination of the fetus, including cystic fibrosis, skeletal dysplasias, kidney diseases, cardiac disease, and central nervous system (CNS) disorders [109]. In the past years, improved ultrasonographic quality has allowed the imaging of more and more subtle anomalies. As we have said before, the combination of ultrasonographic and maternal blood test results (e.g., serum α-FP level) is a satisfactory screening method for commonplace anomalies such as Down syndrome or spina bifida [110].

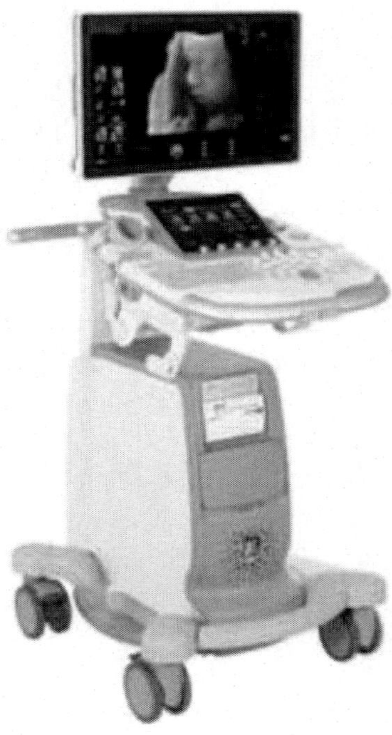

Figure 3. Ultrasound machine.

Screening tests for T21 have gradually become more refined and now involve complex statistical models that combine demographic, biophysical, and biochemical parameters to produce individualized risk estimates for pregnant women. An understanding of the evolution of the principles, methods, and statistical techniques applied to Down syndrome screening is valuable as these processes can be transferred to other, more prevalent, adverse pregnancy outcomes. First-trimester ultrasound forms the foundation of this process [111]. Ultrasound and biochemical screening are complementary screening tests that each have limitations and advantages. The last several years have seen variable progress in the evolution of these techniques, which has resulted in an appropriate role for each to achieve a cost-effective, highly sensitive, and specific screening approach that has allowed couples the most comfort in detecting problems during pregnancy, as well as a high degree of confidence that normal results are accurate [112].

Results from ultrasound in low-risk pregnant women are significant when routine screening is performed on a large population because the anomalies are rare. Professionals expect from routine ultrasound objective information that cannot usually be obtained by clinical procedures. Parents seek reassurance about the absence of fetal congenital anomalies and overall fetal health. Therefore, Europeans view routine ultrasound as a part of obstetric care, capable of filling important gaps by delivering much key information for improving obstetric practice. Fetal anomalies screening requires higher education and qualifications than obstetric ultrasound. The health insurance systems support ultrasound screening and allow its spread in most European countries; approximately 98% of pregnant women are examined by ultrasound and, frequently, two to three times (usually once per trimester). DR of congenital anomalies is about 28% in geographical areas (private practice and hospitals), and 60% to 80% in ultrasound labs. Routine ultrasound screening policy has not proved to result in an immoderate use of ultrasound; on the contrary, chaotic use of routine ultrasound can lead to an unproductive and excessive number of scans. New trends in fetal anomalies screening, such as the early detection of fetal defects and chromosomal anomalies, bring more arguments for routine screening. Effectiveness should increase by enhancing education and training and the systematic referral for fetal anomalies screening to accredited laboratories [113]. The value of ultrasound examinations depends heavily on the preparation of the personnel carrying out the examination and the technical capabilities of the equipment they use. Only well-organized regional or national programs are able to provide high level, cost-effective care based on certification of quality. Such certification must include the training of professionals, the definition of competence levels, accreditation of laboratories, and the establishment of professional protocols. Together, these factors can guarantee the standard of care and provide legal protection for practitioners. It is worth carrying out routine screening in each pregnancy because the majority of abnormalities occur in pregnancies with low risk. Abnormalities detected on screening cases and the examination of high-risk groups should be referred to higher level centers. Here, appropriate technical background and qualified personnel are present to provide cost-effective care. At the same time, necessary invasive interventions can also be performed. A minimum of three screening tests should be performed during pregnancy. The first should be performed at the fetal age of 10-14 weeks to detect abnormalities and pathological conditions in early pregnancy. The second one has to be performed between the fetal ages of 18 and 22 weeks to assess detailed fetal anatomy and rate of development. The third should be performed between the fetal age of 30 and 34 weeks to assess fetal anatomy, rate of development, placentation, and circulation. It is worth considering a fourth screening at approximately 36-38 weeks to assess the intrauterine condition of the fetus and determine the appropriate method of delivery. Finally, besides improving the standard of living, education, and hygienic conditions in developing countries, developed countries also have to help improve the standard of pregnancy care. Within this context, the dissemination of diagnostic ultrasound must be given special emphasis [114].

Prenatal ultrasound may reduce perinatal mortality, primarily through elective abortions for congenital anomalies, but does not appear to lower live birth rates. Although ultrasound has no proven effect on neonatal morbidity, it provides more accurate estimates of gestational age that prevent unnecessary inductions for post-term pregnancy. Screening detects multiple gestations, congenital anomalies, and IUGR, but direct health benefits from having this knowledge are unproved. Ultrasound has both positive and negative psychological effects on parents. The scans do not appear to harm childhood development. Even for the most established screening tests, the appropriateness of routine testing depends on subjective value judgments about the quality of supporting evidence and about the trade-offs between benefits and harms. Individuals, clinicians, policy makers, and governments must weigh the evidence in light of these values and the constraints imposed by available resources [115]. Serious placental insufficiency results in perinatal death or preterm birth from ischemic-thrombotic pathology, a process which has its origins in placental maldevelopment in the first trimester. A proportion of at-risk pregnancies may be identified from abnormalities in first- or second-trimester serum screening data, uterine artery Doppler wave-forms, or placental shape and texture at the time of the 18-20-week anatomical examination. In combination, these tests may be capable of recognizing a subset of at-risk pregnancies with 50% positive predictive value (PPV). Early recognition before fetal viability affords opportunities to direct women to regional perinatal care centers for enhanced maternal-fetal surveillance, corticosteroids to enhance fetal lung maturation, prophylactic measures to prevent preeclampsia, and optimal decision making around the time of delivery. The creation of regional screening programs to use screening data with a placental focus is likely to be cost-effective, because existing patterns of care are utilized. More importantly, this strategy can direct women to participate in clinical research programs designed to reduce morbidity and mortality from this common group of conditions [116]. Almost two-thirds of stillbirths that occur in the early preterm period (up to 32 weeks) can be predicted by uterine artery Doppler at 23 weeks. First-trimester screening studies have shown that an abnormal result increases the risk of subsequent fetal growth restriction, and such women are at particularly high risk when indices remain abnormal in the second trimester. Studies combining uterine artery Doppler with maternal serum markers have demonstrated that measurement of first-trimester maternal serum PAPP-A and free β-hCG improve sensitivities of second-trimester Doppler. As these are frequently measured in Down syndrome screening and they lend themselves in screening for preeclampsia, women with abnormal first- and second-trimester serum markers constitute a high-risk group. Maternal serum placental protein 13 (PP13) remains a promising method for early screening, although a recent study suggests lower sensitivities than initially reported. Uterine artery Doppler screening identifies women at high risk for developing adverse pregnancy outcomes. DR may be increased and FPR reduced by combination with maternal characteristics or serum markers [117]. One of the most important applications of Doppler ultrasonography in obstetrics is the detection of fetal anemia in pregnancies complicated by either red-cell alloimmunization or by other causes of fetal anemia. Doppler of the umbilical artery also has prognostic value in pregnancies affected by twin-to-twin transfusion syndrome (TTTS) undergoing in utero intervention. Another potential major application is the use of Doppler ultrasound in the management of IUGR fetuses. At the present time, there is no single test that appears superior to the other available tests for timing the delivery of the growth-restricted fetus. Therefore, the decision to deliver a fetus, especially at <32 weeks, remains mostly based on empirical management. Doppler may provide a more reliable and systematic basis for timing these deliveries (Figure 4) [118]. First-trimester risk assessment plays a major role in the contemporary pregnancy care. It has evolved significantly since its introduction in the 1990s when it essentially consisted of just the NT measurement. Today, it involves the measurement of several biophysical and biochemical markers and it is often combined with a cffDNA analysis as a secondary test. It can assess the risk for a wide array of major chromosomal and non-chromosomal defects as well as other pregnancy-related complications. The detailed ultrasound examination results in the detection of about half of major structural defects, determination of a very accurate gestational age, and identification of multiple pregnancies as well as their chorionicity. In addition, risk assessment for preeclampsia and early IUGR can be established at this stage. In case of an increased risk, the daily use of low-dose aspirin can be offered at a point in pregnancy when it still can have a positive impact. Additional screening tests for gestational diabetes and macrosomia are available. Contemporary first-trimester screening is essential to establish an individual risk profile and can be used to tailor the pregnancy care [119].

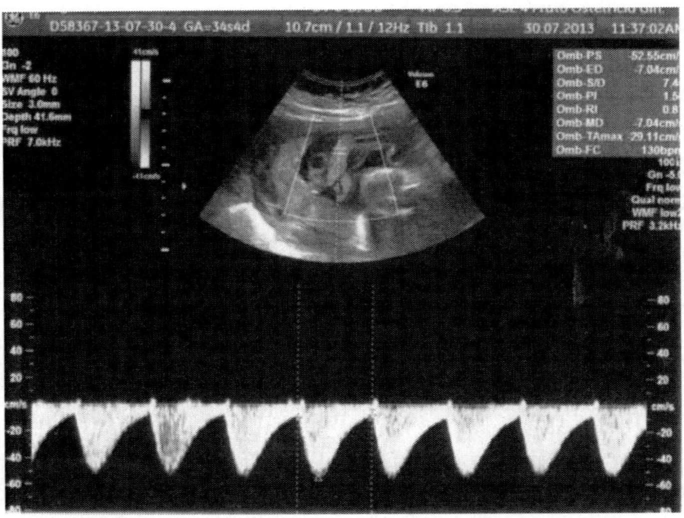

Figure 4. Doppler ultrasonography of the umbilical artery.

Over the past 25 years, the use of ultrasound in aneuploidy risk estimation has improved the way obstetrics is practiced. It allows patients to obtain more personalized risk assessment and has allowed many women a reasonable alternative to invasive testing. The addition of the so-called "soft markers" to the sonographic screening for aneuploidy has been extremely beneficial, especially when considered in combination with other ultrasound findings. The best estimate of risk seems to be achieved through the combined use of ultrasound, maternal serum screening, and maternal age. The literature supports the use of soft markers only when applied to the high-risk population, where the prevalence of aneuploidy is increased. If this information is applied to the low-risk populations, especially in isolation, the lower prevalence of aneuploidy makes the PPV too low to be of any value in counseling patients. As with many screening tests, it occasionally misses the diagnosis, and every patient needs to understand this potential shortcoming. It is a personal decision regarding their willingness to accept the risk of a missed diagnosis versus the risk of fetal loss from an invasive procedure. Although it is far from perfect, in the right hands and with appropriate counseling ultrasound is an excellent tool. This is such an important decision for women and their families, and it is worth the time it takes to explain the benefits and limitations of this test [120]. The importance of the clustering of sonographic markers forms the basis of the Genetic Sonogram Scoring Index (GSSI), such that individual markers are assigned point values based on their sensitivity and specificity in the detection of Down syndrome. The points acquired by each fetus are tabulated into a final "score" (Table 1) [121].

Table 1. The Genetic Sonogram Scoring Index (GSSI)

Finding	Score
Maternal age ≥40	2
Major anomaly	2
Nuchal fold ≥6 mm	2
Maternal age ≥35 and <40	1
Short femur (M:E ≤0.91)	1
Short humerus (M:E ≤0.90)	1
Renal pelvis dilation ≥4 mm	1
Hyperechoic bowel	1
Echogenic intracardiac focus	1
Maternal age <35	0

Adapted from [121].

Ultrasound screening at 16 to 20 weeks is one of the most common genetic screening and/or diagnostic tests used during pregnancy. The practical concern for ultrasound screening is false-positive and false-negative (missed or not present) results. The use and understanding of ultrasound soft markers and their screening relative risks (RR) is an important option in the care of pregnant women. Currently, the presence of a "significant" ultrasound marker adds risk to the likelihood of fetal pathology, but the absence of soft markers, except in controlled situations, should not be used to reduce fetal risk. The use of ultrasound in pregnancy has significant health and economic outcomes for families and the health care system, compared with no ultrasound use. The Society of Obstetricians and Gynecologists of Canada (SOGC) recommends a single "routine" ultrasound evaluation at 16 to 20 weeks in all pregnancies. Patients need to be counseled about the positive and negative findings that ultrasound may reveal so they are prepared for unexpected pregnancy knowledge and the possibility of further testing options being offered. The screening ultrasound at 16 to 20 weeks should evaluate eight markers, five of which (thickened nuchal fold, echogenic bowel, mild ventriculomegaly, echogenic focus in the heart, and choroid plexus cyst) are associated with an increased risk of fetal aneuploidy, and in some cases with non-chromosomal problems, while three (single umbilical artery, enlarged cisterna magna, and pyelectasis) are only associated with an increased risk of non-chromosomal abnormalities when seen in isolation. Identification of soft markers for fetal aneuploidy requires correlation with other risk factors, including history, maternal age, and maternal serum testing results. Soft markers identify a significant increase in fetal risk for genetic disease. Timely referral for confirmation, counseling, and investigation is required to maximize management options [122].

The evolving nature of screening for fetal aneuploidy has continued to feature strongly in recent literature. There is growing interest in early detailed ultrasound of fetal anatomy at the time of NT thickness assessment. Demonstration of tricuspid regurgitation and ductus venosus assessment have been shown to be beneficial additional second-line tests for aneuploidy screening in high-risk patients. Frontal-maxillary facial angle assessment has been explored as a new marker for aneuploidy. The limitations of first-trimester nasal bone measurement were reiterated while its measurement has been shown to be beneficial in the second trimester, especially when calculated with multiples of the median (MOM). As regards second-trimester screening, studies have explored the effectiveness of congenital heart defects (CHD) screening and the efficiency of the genetic sonogram for T21. The role of NT discordance in monochorionic twins has also been readdressed [123]. Improvements in the first-trimester screening and the recent implementation of NIPT for common aneuploidies have important impact on the prevalence of these conditions in the second-trimester ultrasound. Some studies suggest that soft markers in the second trimester of the fetus without structural anomalies have a minor or no role in Down syndrome detection in a prescreened population with reassuring results. However, NIPT could be offered as a next step in the management of such pregnancies if the calculated new composite risk for aneuploidy is increased. In the case of reassuring results, pregnancy follow-up for certain markers is advised. NIPT has emerged as a new method of prenatal testing and is feasible in the second trimester in women with increased new composite risk. However, apart from the Down syndrome screening, second-trimester ultrasound screening remains a powerful tool in screening for other fetal aneuploidies, structural anomalies, and pathological placental conditions and detection of specific soft markers that require pregnancy follow-up [124].

There is increasing evidence that about 50% of severe fetal anomalies can be diagnosed prior to 14 weeks of gestation. "Red flags" such as an increased nuchal or intracranial translucency, tricuspid valve regurgitation, a small bi-parietal diameter (BPD), a single umbilical artery, or an abnormal retro-nasal triangle should raise the sonographer's suspicion of a congenital defect and warrant a more thorough fetal assessment, which often includes trans-vaginal (TV) scanning. Care should, however, be taken not to over-interpret first-trimester findings as FPR of 3-4% have been reported. With more subtle findings, and especially if a heart defect is suspected, a sonographic reassessment after 15 weeks' gestation is indicated. Patients should be counseled that findings could worsen but also improve with time. Basic fetal anomaly screening should be recommended, piggybacked on the routine first-trimester (aneuploidy screening) ultrasound, both for low- and high-risk populations. First-trimester anatomy screening seems particularly useful in obese women, whose fetuses are difficult to screen at the mid-trimester ultrasound and in multiple gestation. NIPT using cffDNA can complement but should not replace first-trimester ultrasound [125]. The sonologist detects a soft marker during approximately 10% of routine second-trimester anatomy examinations and is often uncertain about what further management is appropriate. The era of ultrasound markers as a screen for fetal aneuploidy is coming to a close. The detection of these markers on an ultrasound examination should simply serve as a reminder to ensure that the patient was offered cffDNA screening or conventional analyte screening. cffDNA testing is revolutionizing screening. With normal results on a cffDNA test, many isolated soft markers, including choroid plexus cysts, echogenic intracardiac focus, mild rhizomelic limb shortening, and mild pyelectasis, are irrelevant from a genetic standpoint. However, further counseling and workup are indicated for ventriculomegaly, true fetal echogenic bowel, femur or humerus length measurement that is less than 2.5-percentile value, and pyelectasis to evaluate for the non-genetic associations with these findings [126].

Fetal NT can be measured in most pregnant women in the first and early second trimester. Following initial reports, recent studies of large populations of patients (>500 participants) at either high- or low-risk for fetal chromosomal abnormalities, demonstrate that nuchal thickness of >3 mm between 10- and 14-weeks' gestation by either TA or TV ultrasonography may serve as screening tool for fetal aneuploidy (Figure 5). Sensitivity and specificity rates improve when first-trimester maternal serum free β-hCG and PAPP-A levels are added to this ultrasonographic tool [127]. The size of translucency varies slightly with gestational age and crown-rump length (CRL) and is independent of maternal age. Most authors have used a nuchal thickness of ≥ 2.5 mm or ≥ 3 mm to define abnormal, although some have suggested that the normal variation with gestation requires that different thresholds be used at different gestational ages. The accuracy of NT measurement varies between examiners and between patients, likely in relation to examiner skill and image resolution. The small size of a NT, less than 3 mm in most cases, probably approximates the threshold of normal inter-examiner and intra-examiner variability. The presence of a thickened NT is associated with chromosomal abnormality and perhaps with structural abnormality even when the karyotype is normal. Because of the reported variations in the populations studied, the methods used, and the results of screening, it is inappropriate at this time to assign a numeric risk to any individual patient with this finding. However, in both high-risk and low-risk groups, the PPV appears to be high enough that patients with increased NT should be counseled by their obstetrician and prenatal diagnostic testing should be offered. Because early genetic diagnosis by CVS has a substantially higher procedure-associated loss rate than amniocentesis in the second trimester, many patients may elect to wait for chromosomal testing. If so, disappearance of nuchal thickening should not be taken as reassurance. As a screening test to be widely applied to a general or low-risk population, the utility of fetal NT measurement is uncertain. The reported sensitivity for identification of T21 has ranged from about 40% to 80%, and the sensitivity for identification of other aneuploidies may be lower than for Down syndrome. Currently, measurement of NT is not a substitute for the standard of obstetric care, which is to offer multiple-marker serum screening to every pregnant woman at 15 to 20 weeks. Similarly, it is inappropriate to substitute NT measurement for genetic counseling and CVS or amniocentesis in women above 35 years of age or those with a significant positive history. Finally, the data are not clear as to whether a normal NT decreases the likelihood of chromosomal abnormality in a high-risk population, and such women should not be discouraged from invasive testing because of a normal first-trimester ultrasound study. The data supporting the association between thickened NT and chromosomal abnormality are compelling. Combining first-trimester ultrasonography with early serum screening is currently being proving to be the most efficient means of screening for chromosomal anomaly [128].

The debate over the application of NT measurement in Down syndrome screening is still unresolved in some clinicians' minds. Although different authors report a range of sensitivities for Down syndrome, none question the validity of the association between increased NT and fetal aneuploidy The published literature reveals a lack of congruence over a standard, reproducible method for measuring NT. Only with the adoption of uniform methodology, and the establishment of international standards for NT measurement, is the true potential of this test likely to be realized. The increasing use of first-trimester ultrasound has focused attention on the value of this investigation in confirming fetal viability, estimation of gestational age, and screening for congenital abnormality [129]. First-trimester screening for Down syndrome has been proposed as a significant improvement with respect to second-trimester serum screening programs, because of apparently higher detection rates and an earlier gestational age at diagnosis. First-trimester NT on ultrasonography forms the basis of this new form of screening, although studies of its efficacy have yielded widely conflicting results, with DR ranging from 29% to 91%. Studies of first-trimester serum screening with measurements of PAPP-A and free β-hCG serum concentrations have been much more consistent, with Down syndrome DR of 55% to 63% at a 5% FPR. The combination of first-trimester ultrasonographic and serum screening has the potential to yield a Down syndrome detection rate of 80-90% at a 5% FPR, as we have seen before [130]. Because sonographic and biochemical markers appear to be largely independent, their combined risk results in improved detection rates compared with either method alone. The proposed "integrated" approach using a panel of first- and second-trimester markers suggests that further improvement in the screening performance is possible [131]. In fact, for a 5% FPR, the sensitivities are approximately 30% for maternal age alone, 60-70% for maternal age and second-trimester maternal serum biochemical testing, 75% for maternal age and first-trimester fetal NT scanning, and 90% for maternal age with fetal NT and maternal serum free β-hCG and PAPP-A at 11-14 weeks [132].

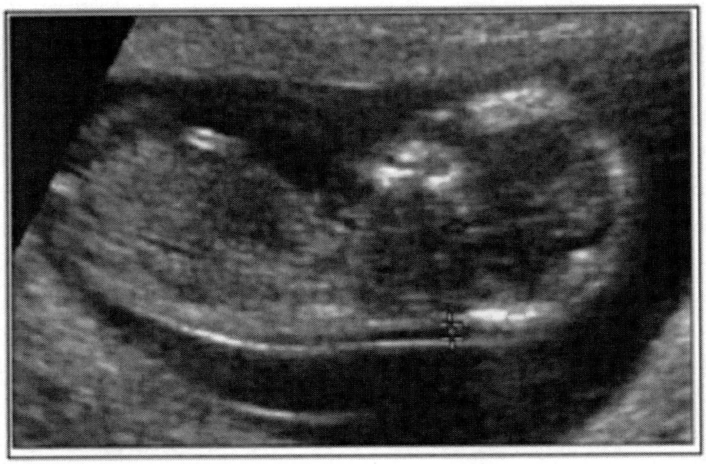

Figure 5. Ultrasonographic measurement of nuchal translucency (NT).

New first-trimester markers can substantially improve efficacy of screening. Recent reports on NT screening reiterate the importance of standardization of technique and quality control as proposed by the FMF in London. Effective quality control can be achieved through quantitative analysis of operator-specific data. 3D ultrasound does not provide substantially higher success rates in obtaining reliable NT measurements than two-dimensional (2D) ultrasound. New data confirm the previously reported association between increased NT and increased rate of spontaneous fetal loss, genetic syndromes, and a high prevalence (15%) of anomalies, among which cardiac defects are the commonest. Researchers agree that increased NT ought to be an indication for specialized echocardiography (Figure 6). Promising data have become available on new markers that can enhance first-trimester screening. It is estimated that when assessment of nasal bone and maternal serum analytes are taken into account, first-trimester screening can identify 97.5% of T21 pregnancies for a 5% FPR. It is stressed that parents need to be informed about the possible implications of screening before testing. Furthermore, the uptake of screening is likely to be relatively low among younger women [133]. There are evidences suggesting that 3D ultrasound allows to reduce the operator dependency in the visualization of standard diagnostic planes, thus reducing the examination time required for the obstetric ultrasound examination, with minimal impact on the visualization quality of the anatomic landmarks. Furthermore, operators with minimal experience may record cardiac or brain volumes that can be successfully analyzed off-line locally or sent by internet to experts for remote review. As a consequence, 3D ultrasonography promises to become the method of choice for diagnosis congenital structural defects [134]. For several years now, 3D and 4D ultrasound have been used as a complementary tool to 2D ultrasound for the evaluation of fetal morphology. This brings an improved morphological assessment of the fetus. Applications of the techniques are increasing, especially for the fetal face, heart, and extremities. The third field where fetal ultrasound is continuously providing important information is the knowledge of the natural history of diseases. This has brought significant improvement in the postnatal management of several diseases, especially urinary tract dilatation and broncho-pulmonary malformation [135]. The use of fetal MRI, in addition to prenatal genetic testing and sonography, has the potential to improve prenatal diagnosis of genetic disorders. MRI plays an important role in the evaluation of fetal abnormalities and malformations. Fetal MRI often enables a differential diagnosis, a determination of the extent of the disorder, the prognosis, and an improvement in therapeutic management. For counseling of parents, as well as to basically understand how genetic aberrations affect fetal development, it is of great importance to correlate different genotypes with fetal MRI data [136].

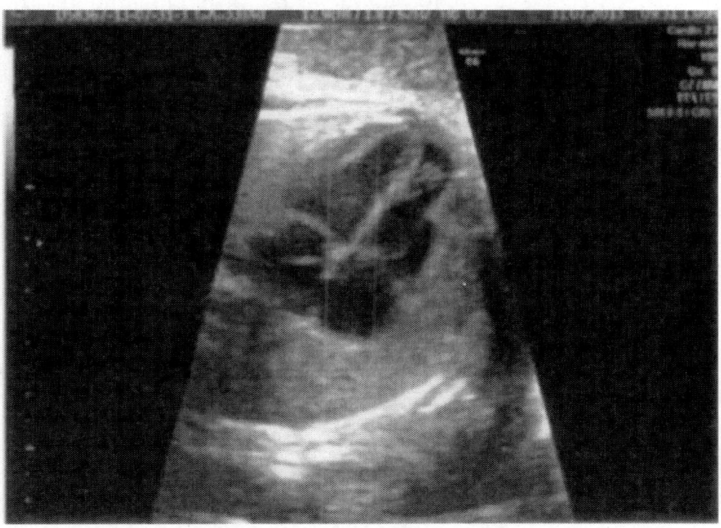

Figure 6. Fetal echocardiography.

DNA-Based Prenatal Diagnosis

Clinical molecular genetics has recently become recognized as a diagnostic discipline [137]. Rapid molecular biological methods for prenatal diagnosis of the most common aneuploidies, collectively known as rapid aneuploidy testing, are believed to be accurate and carry a low risk of misdiagnosis, but they differ in terms of labor-intensity and amenability to automation and high-throughput testing. These various techniques are so far not used as stand-alone tests, but some of them are routinely applied as a preliminary test that shortens the waiting time for classic cytogenetic karyotyping. In the future, mainly because of economic reasons, these methods may replace cytogenetics in the category of patients who make up the majority of those currently offered prenatal karyotyping: patients with moderately increased risk and no abnormalities detected by ultrasound [138].

Laboratory advances in molecular genetics have resulted in numerous clinical applications for DNA analysis [139]. The exponential increase in the discovery of human disease genes over the past 30 years has transformed DNA diagnostics from a minor research-based activity to a major professional operation. Mutation testing and linkage analysis are now used to provide prenatal or postnatal diagnosis for a wide range of monogenic disorders. The discovery of genes which confer susceptibility to common disorders has created demand for high-throughput testing for specific mutations or clinically relevant polymorphisms. Widespread genetic testing must be supported by adequate genetic counseling and by education of healthcare professionals in order to ensure the appropriate application of this information for the benefit of patients and their families [140]. In any pregnancy, there is an approximate 3% to 5% chance that a fetal complication will occur. The most familiar prenatal diagnostics cannot be performed until the fetus is well into gestation, and most involve invasive procedures along with their inherent risks. In light of these facts, many noninvasive prenatal screening (NIPS) and diagnostic tests have been developed, the newest using recombinant DNA technology in the examination of fetal cells. Through these procedures, genetic coding errors and chromosomal disruptions may be detected [141].

Molecular diagnosis is the detection of pathogenic mutations in DNA and RNA samples prepared from at-risk patients. Principles underlying DNA-based diagnosis originate from localization and identification of genes responsible for human disease and the characterization of pathogenic mutations; new diagnostic tests are in constant development. Indications for testing include diagnosis, carrier risk revision, prenatal diagnosis, presymptomatic diagnosis, and population screening. The majority of DNA diagnoses are performed in a reference laboratory in which the referring physician, rather that the patient, is the client of the laboratory. Thus, the role of the genetic counselor in a reference laboratory is quite different from traditional clinical practice. As with all clinical laboratory tests, molecular diagnostics are interpreted within the context of the patient's overall clinical presentation and are overlaid with regulatory programs of quality assurance, quality improvement, and quality control. The greatest challenges facing the clinical laboratory are genetic heterogeneity, cost control, regulatory and patent compliance, technology transfer, and the genetic education of the referring physician [142]. DNA-based testing has become possible for an increasing number of hereditary diseases as the responsible genes have been mapped to individual chromosomes and then isolated and characterized. The strategy for each test depends on the heterogeneity of mutations commonly causing the disease, the distribution of the mutations in the population, and the frequency of new mutations. In many cases, interpretation of the test result requires a comparison with relatives known to carry the abnormal gene. SCA is an example of a recessive mutation with a strong ethnic association and little genetic heterogeneity or new mutation. Cystic fibrosis also has a strong ethnic association and a low frequency of new mutation but greater heterogeneity. Fragile X affects all ethnic groups and often appears sporadic, but all cases have the same type of mutation, and a premutation can be found in all affected families [143].

The ability to diagnose human diseases at the DNA level has become possible because of a rapid development in DNA technology, particularly in the area of detection of single base substitutions. During the last decades, a new class of DNA markers, the restriction fragment length polymorphisms (RFLP), has been developed by molecular genetic techniques. Genetic linkage studies using RFLP have resulted in a large number of chromosome assignments of genes, making possible prenatal diagnosis and presymptomatic testing in many genetic disorders. Studies of the molecular basis of some of the mutant genes have brought to light a remarkable multiplicity and diversity of mutations that produce relatively few clinical phenotypes. Many genetic disorders including the thalassemias, familial hypercholesterolemia, Tay-Sachs disease, cystic fibrosis, and congenital adrenal hyperplasia (CAH), have been shown to be genetically heterogeneous. It is necessary, therefore, to know the precise mutation in order to make accurate diagnosis and restore proper enzyme or gene function [144]. Mutations in the genomic DNA of a particular gene may be inferred indirectly using linkage analysis and RFLP. However, direct detection of the mutation is the more favorable approach. The advent of the polymerase chain reaction (PCR) to amplify specific regions of genomic DNA or messenger RNA (mRNA) has enhanced the speed and sensitivity of many of the screening and diagnostic procedures. Screening methods have been developed that will detect close to 100% of all mutations. The methods include ribonuclease A cleavage, denaturing gradient gel electrophoresis, chemical cleavage of mismatch, and direct sequencing. Choice of method is based on a number of factors and will depend on the structure of the gene to be analyzed. Following identification of a mutation using one of the screening procedures, prenatal diagnosis and carrier testing can be offered. The overall aim is to develop a method that has the potential to determine the mutation present in an index case of a previously untested family in a few days, thus allowing any other relevant family member to be tested [145].

As we have said, current prenatal diagnosis has long relied on invasive methods such as amniocentesis and CVS. The invasive procedures amniocentesis and CVS are routinely applied in pregnancies at risk for fetal abnormalities and the results obtained are the gold standard for prenatal diagnosis. Because these methods of fetal cell procurement involve a 0.5-2% risk for fetal loss, they are recommended mainly in cases at high risk for fetal genetic or cytogenetic abnormalities. So, for over two decades, methods of first-trimester, noninvasive prenatal genetic diagnosis have been actively pursued by many investigators. As medical technology evolves, clinicians are increasingly choosing relatively painless noninvasive methods of patient diagnosis and treatment. There are two principles behind this: greater patient comfort and lower cost. Early during human development, the trophoblast lineage differentiates to commence placentation. Where the placenta contacts the uterine decidua, extravillous trophoblast (EVT) cells differentiate and invade maternal tissues. EVT cells, identified by expression of human leukocyte antigen G (HLA-G), invade into uterine blood vessels (endovascular EVT), as well as glands (endoglandular EVT), and open such luminal structures towards the intervillous space of the placenta. Endoglandular invasion diverts the contents of uterine glands to the intervillous space, while glands near the margin of the placenta that also contain endoglandular EVT cells open into the reproductive tract. Cells of the trophoblast lineage have thus been recovered from the uterine cavity and endocervical canal. An emerging noninvasive technology (trophoblast retrieval and isolation from the cervix [TRIC]) isolates and examines EVT cells residing in the cervix obtained during ongoing pregnancies (weeks 5-20) to explore their origin, biology, and relationship to pregnancy and fetal status. It has been hypothesized that endoglandular EVT cells at the margins of the expanding placenta enter the uterine cavity and are carried together with uterine secretion products to the cervix where they can be retrieved from a Pap smear. The literature describes a variety of invasive routes taken by EVT cells at the fetal-maternal interface that could displace them into the reproductive tract. Since the 1970s, investigators have attempted to recover trophoblast cells from the uterus or cervix for prenatal diagnostics. Trophoblast cells from Pap smears obtained at 5-20 weeks of gestation have been purified (>95% β-hCG positive) by immune-magnetic isolation with nanoparticles linked to anti-HLA-G (TRIC). The isolated cells contain the fetal genome, and have an EVT-like expression profile. Similar EVT-like cells appear in the lumen of uterine glands and can be observed entering the uterine cavity along the margins of the placenta, suggesting that they are the primary source of cervical trophoblast cells. Cells isolated by TRIC can be used to accurately genotype the embryo/fetus by targeted next generation sequencing (NGS). Biomarker protein expression quantified in cervical trophoblast cells after TRIC correlates with subsequent pregnancy loss, preeclampsia, and fetal growth restriction. A key remaining question is the degree to which EVT cells in the cervix might differ from those in the basal plate and placental bed. TRIC could one day provide a method of risk assessment for maternal and fetal disease, and reveal molecular pathways disrupted during the first trimester in EVT cells associated with placental maldevelopment. As perinatal interventions emerge for pregnancy disorders and inherited congenital disorders, TRIC could provide a key diagnostic tool for personalized precision medicine in obstetrics [146]. Isolation of fetal trophoblast from endocervical specimens remains an attractive approach, given the greater numbers of fetal cells than in maternal blood and the better potential for fetal cell identification based on markers specific for a single cell type (trophoblasts). Current studies demonstrate feasibility in identification and molecular analysis of fetal trophoblast cells for prenatal genetic testing. Sampling methods involving lavage, cytobrush, or aspiration of cervical specimens, however, have limitations in the recovery of trophoblasts. Clinical applications await further systematic studies to determine safety and accuracy in recovery [147].

Tears, hair, saliva, urine, and feces can also be used for diagnosis. The varied constituents in these biological materials can serve as biomarkers for the detection of both local and systemic diseases. Saliva, hair, tears, and other biological material, obtained via noninvasive methods, may serve as clinically informative biomarkers. These biomarkers may be used for: toxicology, psychological studies, disease detection, bio-monitoring, and drug abuse. The analysis of tears, hair, saliva, urine, and feces is a safe, noninvasive and useful diagnostic tool within groups of pregnant women, but further investigation is necessary to fully realize the promise of these novel diagnostic tools [148]. Isolating fetal cells and/or nucleic acids from maternal blood for genetic analysis is the least invasive method currently being investigated [149]. In fact, recent advances in cell separation technology and DNA analytic techniques leave little doubt as to the presence of fetal cells in the maternal circulation. The potential of using these cells for genetic analysis is compelling. The major hurdles that had to be traversed before this technology was universally adopted included the identification of appropriate sampling and separation methods yielding fetal cells amenable to genetic analysis by rapid DNA technologies, clinical studies of appropriate statistical power to validate and compare this approach to current genetic testing, and comparison of this approach to other noninvasive paradigms such as triple screening. Despite the tremendous value of noninvasive genetic screening, the rigorous course required to progress from description of scientific capability to validation of a clinical test must not be ignored or rushed for financial considerations [150].

Small amounts of DNA circulate in both healthy and diseased human plasma/serum, and increased concentrations of DNA are present in the plasma of cancer patients. Characteristics of tumor DNA have been found in genetic material extracted from the plasma of cancer patients. These features include decreased strand stability, the presence of specific oncogene or tumor-suppressor gene (TSG) mutations, micro-satellite alterations, immunoglobulin (Ig) rearrangements, and hypermethylation of several genes. The results obtained in many different cancers have opened a new research area indicating that plasma DNA might eventually be a suitable target for the development of noninvasive diagnostic, prognostic, and follow-up tests for cancer. Following the discovery of tumor-derived DNA in plasma or serum, cffDNA has also been found in maternal plasma and serum. This discovery provides an easily accessible source of fetal genetic material for prenatal diagnosis [151]. Thus, cell-free DNA refers to all noncapsulated DNA present in the blood stream which may originate from apoptotic cells as a part of the physiological cell turnover, or from cancer cells or fetal cells. Recent studies have highlighted the utility of cell-free DNA analysis for genetic profiling of cancer and NIPT besides many other clinical applications. For prenatal testing, cffDNA analysis provides an effective, noninvasive, and safer alternative to traditional amniocentesis and CVS tests. Also in cancer patients, cell-free DNA analysis is useful for genetic profiling and follow-up during treatment. However, standardization of methods of isolation and analysis has become crucial for the success of widespread use of cell-free DNA analysis [152]. During pregnancy, the fetal DNA increases to approximately 3-13% of the total circulating free DNA in maternal plasma. The very low amount of circulating cffDNA in maternal plasma is a crucial issue, and requires specific and optimized techniques for cffDNA purification from maternal plasma. In addition, highly sensitive detection approaches are required. In recent years, advanced cffDNA investigation approaches have allowed the application of NIPT to determine fetal sex, fetal RhD genotyping, aneuploidies, micro-deletions, and the detection of paternally inherited monogenic disorders. Finally, complex and innovative technologies such as digital PCR (dPCR) and NGS (exhibiting higher sensitivity and/or the capability to read the entire fetal genome from maternal plasma DNA) are expected to allow the detection, in the near future, of maternally inherited mutations that cause genetic diseases [153].

In contrast to the traditional teaching that the placenta forms an impermeable barrier, multiple studies show that both intact fetal cells and cell-free nucleic acids circulate freely in maternal blood. Complications of pregnancy, such as preeclampsia, or fetal cytogenetic abnormalities, such as T21, increase transfusion of both intact fetal cells and cell-free fetal nucleic acids into the maternal circulation. Abnormal fetal-maternal trafficking of nucleic acids is associated with fetal and placental pathology, and these observations lead to novel noninvasive diagnostic and screening tests. Real-time quantitative PCR amplification of deoxy-hypusine synthase 1 (DYS1) is used to measure the levels of male fetal DNA in case-control sets of serum or plasma taken from pregnant women. Women carrying fetuses with T21 or 13 (but not 18) have increased levels of fetal DNA in their fresh or archived serum and/or plasma samples. Women destined to develop preeclampsia have a characteristic biphasic elevation of cffDNA that precedes clinical symptoms. Data obtained from a variety of clinical scenarios suggest that the placenta is the predominant source of the circulating fetal nucleic acids, although apoptotic hematopoietic cells may contribute to the pool as well. cffDNA is elevated in a number of conditions associated with placental pathology. Fetal cell-free nucleic acids have potential for noninvasive monitoring of placental pathology [154]. Several new developments, which rely either on fluorescence in situ hybridization (FISH) or the combination of single-cell manipulation and subsequent PCR practices, which are common to the field of preimplantation genetics, have been tested. The research in the field yielded important observations regarding the traffic of cells between the fetus and the mother, which may provide a new insight into the development of disorders such as preeclampsia and the associated hemolysis, elevated liver enzymes, and low platelets (HELLP) syndrome [155]. As we have said before, it is well recognized that the levels of circulating cffDNA play a role in various complications of pregnancy. cffDNA is released due to apoptotic mechanisms occurring on trophoblastic cells, although recent in vivo studies support the existence of additional mechanisms. The increase in the levels of cffDNA can be used to predict pregnancy-related complications, such as preeclampsia, IUGR, preterm labor, placenta previa, and hyperemesis gravidarum, and has great value in the field of prenatal diagnosis and in common pregnancy-related complications, as it precedes the clinical symptoms of the disease. Gestational age is a factor that determines the elevation in cffDNA levels in response to pathological conditions. In conclusion, the detection of cffDNA levels has a number of valuable applications in prenatal screening. Thus, studies are focusing on unraveling the etiology of alterations in its levels under pathological conditions during pregnancy, in order to determine the potential predictive and diagnostic applications of this biomarker [156].

The development of a reproducible, reliable, noninvasive method based on retrieval of fetal cells from the maternal circulation will render testing feasible for the general population. A variety of cell separation methods recover fetal cells from maternal blood; these differ in cost-effectiveness and required expertise. Fetal cell types that are useful for prenatal diagnosis are terminally differentiated and are unlikely to persist postpartum since are rapidly cleared from the circulation following birth. Several cell types have been targeted to this end, mostly nucleated red blood cells (RBC), cluster D 34+ (CD34+) hematopoietic progenitors, and trophoblasts. Although these cell types have been unequivocally proven to be present in the maternal circulation, each bears a significant disadvantage: nucleated RBC cannot be expanded in culture, thereby ruling out metaphase chromosome analysis, an essential component of prenatal diagnosis. CD34+ cells do possess the potential for in vitro proliferation; however, they have been found to persist in the maternal circulation after delivery, thereby complicating diagnosis in consecutive pregnancies. Trophoblasts are not consistently detected in the maternal circulation [157]. So, many questions remain about the feasibility of using fetal cells from maternal blood for prenatal diagnosis. Although recently there has been more focus on clinically relevant methods, many studies have been performed using blood drawn after invasive procedures, and over a wide range of gestational ages. For methods to be applicable to clinical use, more work has been needed on isolating cells early in pregnancy, when termination is still an option for parents who are found to have an affected pregnancy. It is generally agreed that fetal nucleated erythrocytes are the most efficacious cell type for prenatal diagnosis, but it has not yet been shown definitively whether there is an ideal gestational age for sampling, whether AB0 incompatibility might limit availability of fetal cells, or whether the number of cells present might be different in normal versus abnormal pregnancies. Isolation of fetal erythroblasts from maternal blood should allow accurate NIPD of both aneuploidies and monogenic disorders. Expression of gamma-globin (γ-globin) in maternal erythroblasts and the inability to locate fetal erythroblasts reliably in all pregnancies have prevented its clinical application. In the absence of a highly specific fetal cell marker, enrichment, identification, and diagnosis, the three components of NIPD, have clearly defined objectives. Since fetal cells are rare in maternal blood, the sole purpose of enrichment is yield, to recover as many fetal cells as possible, even if purity is compromised at this stage. In contrast, the primary goal of identification is specificity; absolute certainty of fetal origin is required at this stage if the ultimate objective of diagnosis, accuracy, is to be achieved [158]. Advances in the understanding of cell surface and cytoplasmic protein expression have translated into better and more specific fetal cell identification. Fetal cells, once identified, are screened for the presence of aneuploidy using chromosome-specific probes on inter-phase nuclei. Significant progress in single-gene and single-cell analysis has expanded the diagnostic possibilities for noninvasive fetal testing. Although fetal cells are generally rare in maternal blood samples, they appear to be more common when the fetus has T21. This is beneficial for clinical diagnosis. Maternal-fetal cellular trafficking is the bidirectional passage of cells between mother and fetus during pregnancy. This results in the presence of fetal cells in the maternal circulation, known as fetal microchimerism, and maternal cells in the fetal circulation, known as maternal microchimerism. Furthermore, a large fetal-maternal transfusion occurs at the time of labor and delivery in all pregnant women. This may establish fetal cell microchimerism in the mother, which may be implicated in the subsequent development of diseases such as scleroderma that are more common in women. The biological role of this transplacental cellular trafficking during pregnancy is not known, although it has been implicated in development of the fetal immune system, tolerance mechanisms during pregnancy, tissue repair in autoimmune disease and cancer, and immune surveillance. Additionally, this trans-placental passage of cells has been implicated in the delicate balance between immunological priming and tolerance, which can influence the occurrence of autoimmune disease and transplantation outcomes. Ongoing studies are evaluating the utility of microchimerism in predicting the risk of graft rejection in transplantation [159]. The study of fetal cells in maternal blood, while technically challenging, provides a unique opportunity to explore the immune-biology of pregnancy [160].

The detection of certain fetal loci using cffDNA and conventional molecular analytic approaches is possible from 4-5 weeks gestation. To date, noninvasive first-trimester analysis for single-gene disorders has been limited by assay sensitivity and specificity, due to the background maternal DNA. cffDNA comprises only 3-6% of the total circulating cell-free DNA, therefore diagnoses are primarily limited to those caused by paternally inherited sequences as well as conditions that can be inferred by the unique gene expression patterns in the fetus and placenta. Broadly, the applications of this technology fall into two categories: first, high genetic risk families with inheritable monogenic diseases, including sex determination in cases at risk of X-linked diseases and detection of specific paternally inherited single-gene disorders; and second, routine antenatal care offered to all pregnant women, including prenatal screening/diagnosis for aneuploidy, particularly Down syndrome, and diagnosis of Rh factor status in RhD negative women. Already, sex determination and Rh factor diagnosis have been translated into clinical practice for high-risk individuals [161]. The anticipated ability to enrich the fetal component of cell-free DNA has increased the robustness of tests and permitted semi-quantitative analysis, broadening the scope of testing to include recessive disorders such as cystic fibrosis. Testing for large-scale mutations might remain limited by the fragmented nature of cffDNA and, when testing very early in gestation, careful ultrasound examination will be needed to determine the number of gestational sacs, because of the risk of discordant twin pregnancies, as we will say after [162]. Owing to many advantages, the adoption of NIPT in routine clinical practice was very rapid and global. As an example, NIPT has recently become a standard screening procedure for all pregnant women. On the other hand, invasive sampling procedures remain important, especially for their diagnostic value in the confirmation of NIPT positive findings and the detection of Mendelian disorders [163].

NIPT has been in clinical use for almost three decades; however, there is evidence that this technology will be more widely applied within the next few years. Guidance is therefore required to ensure that the procedure is offered in a way that is evidence-based and ethically and clinically acceptable. Four main themes emerged: perceived attributes of the test, regulation and ethical issues,

NIPT in practice, and economic considerations. However, there was a basic difference in the approach of actual or potential service users, who were very positive about the benefits of the technology, compared with other research participants, who were concerned with the potential moral and ethical outcomes of using this testing method [164]. NIPT has marked a revolution in aneuploidy screening because it allows a simple maternal blood test to detect Down syndrome in a fetus with a very high level of accuracy (at least 99.5% with a FPR of 0.2%). Results are available from 12 weeks gestation, giving a high level of reassurance for Down syndrome early in pregnancy. There are concerns, however, that the test is being offered without proper counseling and that women may not have a 12-week ultrasound to exclude significant structural abnormalities, therefore decreasing the early detection of severe abnormalities. In addition, the test is expensive and therefore prohibitive for many women and their families [165].

Prenatal aneuploidy screening has changed dramatically in recent years with increases in the types of chromosomal abnormalities reliably identified and in the proportion of aneuploid fetuses detected. Initially, screening was available only for T21 and T18 and was offered only to low-risk pregnancies. Improved detection with the quadruple- and first-trimester multiple marker screens led to the option of aneuploidy screening for women 35 years of age and older. cffDNA tests now screen for common autosomal trisomies and sex chromosome aneuploidies. cffDNA screening is particularly effective in older women because of higher PPV and lower FPR. Integrated first- and second-trimester multiple marker tests provide specific risks for T21, T18, and possibly T13, and may detect an even wider range of aneuploidies. Given current precision in risk assessment, based on maternal age and preferences for screening or diagnostic tests, counseling has become more complex [166, 167]. The introduction of cffDNA into clinical practice has changed the screening approach. Healthcare professionals and future parents tend to overestimate NIPT capabilities despite its relatively high cost and limited information. There are countries and regions that have already approved contingent screening test, while others are discussing the implementation of contingent screening versus universal use of NIPT. There are several recent meta-analyses debating whether to use NIPT for universal screening for trisomies and other fetal conditions. NIPT is a reasonable option as an advanced screening test for T21, 18, and 13 only. Introducing screening by NIPT instead of a first-trimester screening will cause the loss of other valuable information including accurate dating of pregnancy and diagnosing major structural fetal abnormalities and multiple pregnancies at an early gestational age. Additionally, the opportunity to screen for early preeclampsia will be lost. Currently, the price for NIPT is still high adding extra strain on publicly funded health systems [168].

Fetal nucleic acids in maternal plasma have opened up new possibilities for NIPD of chromosomal aneuploidies. The predominance of admixed maternal genetic material in circulation demands innovative means for identification and analysis of cffDNA and RNA. One approach is based on the measurement of the allelic ratio of single-nucleotide polymorphisms (SNP) in the coding region of placental mRNA. Another approach is through the analysis of DNA fragments with different patterns of DNA methylation between fetal and maternal DNA. One other alternative is to enrich the fractional concentration of fetal DNA in maternal plasma using physical or chemical methods. Finally, the development of more precise dPCR-based methods for fetal nucleic acid analysis has further catalyzed the developments in this area [169]. dPCR approaches have been developed for the detection of nucleic acids of low abundance, such as cffDNA, and represent an attractive and sensitive alternative to conventional methods, particularly in the field of NIPD from current and emerging uses, such as fetal gender determination, RhD genotyping, or monogenic disorders prenatal testing, to future applications, such as the diagnosis and monitoring of pregnancy-related disorders [170]. DNA methylation in the human genome is largely programmed and shaped by transcription factor binding and interaction between DNA methyltransferases and histone marks during gamete and embryo development. Normal methylation profiles can be modified at single or multiple loci, more frequently as consequences of genetic variants acting in cis or in trans, or in some cases stochastically or through interaction with environmental factors. For many developmental disorders, specific methylation patterns or signatures can be detected in blood DNA. The recent use of high-throughput assays investigating the whole genome has largely increased the number of diseases for which DNA methylation analysis provides information for their diagnosis [171].

Over the past 20 years, NIPT, which uses massive parallel sequencing (MPS) to align and count DNA fragments floating in the plasma of pregnant women, has become integrated into prenatal care. Professional societies currently recommend offering NIPT as an advanced screen to pregnant women at high risk for fetal aneuploidy, reserving invasive diagnostic procedures for those at the very highest risk. Clinical performance in Clinical Laboratory Improvement Amendments (CLIA)-certified, College of American Pathologists (CAP)-accredited laboratories appears to be equivalent to prior clinical validation studies, with high sensitivities and specificities and very high negative predictive values (NPV). The main impact on clinical care has been a reduction in invasive procedures. Test accuracy is affected by the fetal fraction, the percentage of fetal DNA in the total amount of circulating cffDNA. Fetal fraction is in turn affected by maternal body mass index (BMI), gestational age, type of aneuploidy, singleton vs multiples, and mosaicism. Three studies comparing NIPT to serum or combined screening for autosomal aneuploidy all show that NIPT has significantly lower FPR (approximately 0.1%), even in all-risk populations. A significant number of the discordant positive cases have underlying biological reasons, including CPM, maternal mosaicism, cot-win demise, or maternal malignancy. NIPT performs well as an advanced screen for whole chromosome aneuploidy [172]. In fact, cffDNA-based NIPT using maternal blood is highly sensitive for detecting fetal trisomies. However, false-positive and false-negative results can occur, which prevents NIPT from being a diagnostic test. Fetal-placental mosaicism is one of the main reasons for discordant test results. It is therefore important to understand this phenomenon to enable more comprehensive and appropriate genetic counseling. Publications are emerging demonstrating that genome-wide approaches to analyzing cffDNA can detect chromosomal aneuploidy other than the common trisomies. Despite the high accuracy of current cffDNA-based NIPT, a substantial number of false-positive and false-negative test results remain. Biological causes, such as fetal or CPM have been identified using advanced bio-informatics algorithms. Fetal-placental mosaicism can occur as part of normal pregnancy development, hence clinical practice standards recommend confirmation of positive NIPT results with a diagnostic karyotype or micro-array study. cffDNA-based NIPT for fetal chromosomal aneuploidies is not diagnostic because of false-positive and false-negative test results. Recently, novel algorithms have been described that identify pregnancies with an increased risk of fetal-placental mosaicism. Reporting the presence of fetal-placental mosaicism during pregnancy can influence risk estimation and improve genetic counseling [173].

Molecular laboratory techniques are increasingly important in the evaluation of fetuses at risk for a single-gene disorder or chromosomal abnormality and for the detection of genetic or other conditions that can lead to an adverse fetal or maternal outcome. The localization and identification of novel disease genes allows for mutation analysis or linkage studies on fetuses at risk for these disorders. Since publication of the PCR technique in 1985 [174], there has been an explosion of reports on its use in medicine and science, both as a diagnostic technique and as a research tool, in the characterization of genetic defects, prenatal diagnosis, carrier testing, HLA typing, detecting microorganisms, identifying activated oncogenes and in the characterization of leukemias and lymphomas, and in biomedical research [175]. PCR is a rapid method for generating a 10^6- to 10^7-fold increase in the number of copies of a discrete DNA or RNA sequence. The ability to amplify DNA by the PCR technique has revolutionized our ability to test for genetic mutations. The technique is being used for rapid prenatal diagnosis and carrier testing of several inherited disorders. Many different assay systems are available for analyzing the amplified DNA and RNA. These techniques can be performed easily on material from adults, children, fetuses, and even single cells from blastomeres and polar bodies. The DR of the screening test, as well as the frequency of the mutation in the study population and the technical limitations of the procedure, will determine the usefulness of a positive or negative result. PGD provides a paradigm for the ease of use of PCR-based testing, yet also underscores the problems encountered with genetic screening because of the multitude of possible mutations and the possible misinterpretation of results [176]. PCR has been shown to be a powerful tool in allowing amplification and identification of very small amounts of fetal DNA. However, this is limited to cases in which a specific and unique gene from the father is sought. This means that there is the potential to diagnose many paternally inherited autosomal dominant diseases and some autosomal recessive diseases, in which the parents have different and identifiable mutations. However, when parents are both carriers of the same autosomal recessive mutations, or when the disease is X-linked, PCR will not aid in prenatal diagnosis. Cytogenetic analysis of fetal cells by FISH after cell sorting is another useful method of prenatal diagnosis, but requires relatively pure samples of fetal cells or an independent marker that allows easy microscopic identification. The latter might be accomplished by identifying fetal cells through their expression of embryonic hemoglobin or because they contain HLA-G mRNA. Methods such as immunophenotyping that allow the selective identification of fetal cells by microscopy, and can be used in conjunction with FISH, may be extremely valuable because they may allow the genetic analysis of only the few fetal cells within a background preponderance of maternal cells [177].

An understanding of biological parameters governing this phenomenon, such as the concentration and molecular size of circulating fetal DNA, has guided PCR diagnostic applications. Early efforts focused on the detection of paternally inherited sequences, which were absent in the maternal genome, in maternal plasma. Recent developments in precise measurement technologies such as dPCR have allowed the detection of minute allelic imbalances in plasma and have catalyzed analysis of single-gene disorders such as the hemoglobinopathies and hemophilia. The advent of MPS has enabled the robust detection of fetal trisomies in maternal plasma. Recent proof-of-concept studies have detected a chromosomal translocation and a micro-deletion and have deduced a genome-wide genetic map of a fetus from maternal plasma. Techniques using PCR, mass spectrometry, and sequencing have been developed for the purposes of detecting fetal-specific sequences, such as paternally inherited or de novo mutations, or determining allelic balance or chromosome dosage. Clinical applications of these methods include fetal sex determination and blood group typing, which are currently available commercially. Other uses of cffDNA and RNA are the detection of single-gene disorders, chromosomal abnormalities, and inheritance of parental polymorphisms across the whole fetal genome. The concentration of cffDNA may also provide predictive capabilities for pregnancy-associated complications [178]. After PCR, mutations producing single-gene disorders can be detected by several different methods, including endonuclease digestion and gel electrophoresis (applicable when a mutation affects an endonuclease recognition site), gel electrophoresis (used for detection of deletions), and hybridization to an oligonucleotide probe specific for a mutation. Less often, gene sequencing of a PCR product is used to rapidly identify a mutation. In addition, the PCR technique can be applied to polymorphism analysis to provide diagnosis by linkage analysis. In other areas, PCR is being used to detect and characterize microbial pathogens and to characterize mutations associated with carcinogenesis. The PCR method is useful in situations in which the amount of DNA sample is limited, such as in forensics and prenatal testing, or in which the quality of the DNA sample is poor [179]. New assays or techniques for mutation detection in single-gene disorders such as amplification refractory mutation system PCR, fluorescent PCR, hetero-duplex analysis, and the protein truncation test are now applied in prenatal diagnosis. Recent advances in molecular cytogenetics, such as comparative genomic hybridization (CGH), the primed in situ labeling technique, the development of new telomeric probes, and spectral karyotyping have been evaluated for their role in prenatal diagnosis of chromosomal abnormalities. These methods have greatly improved the accuracy and applicability of PGD or diagnosis on fetal cells isolated from maternal blood [180].

Several studies have been performed to assess the diagnostic value of using small tandem repeat (STR) markers and quantitative fluorescent PCR

(QF-PCR) assays for the rapid detection of aneuploidies involving chromosomes 21, 18, and 13 [181-184]. The results of these investigations have documented the diagnostic advantages of this approach to perform prenatal tests using amniotic and chorionic samples, or fetal nucleated cells retrieved from peripheral maternal blood or endocervical samples. The use of two or more STR markers for each autosome facilitates the diagnosis of aneuploidies, while avoiding the need to employ internal non-polymorphic markers. Multiplex quantitative fluorescent analyses can be performed in about six hours from the collection of the samples and, although targeted to specific abnormalities, they can exclude the presence of the most frequent chromosomal disorders. QF-PCR can be exploited to analyze DNA present in single or clumps of cells and thus to perform prenatal diagnosis on maternal peripheral blood or TC cell samples and on preimplantation embryos [185]. Microscopic karyotype analysis of cultured cells has been regarded as the gold standard for prenatal diagnosis for over 45 years. Since the first application of this technique to prenatal testing in the early 1970's, this procedure has proved to be highly reliable for identifying chromosome copy number abnormalities (aneuploidy) and large structural rearrangements in fetal cells obtained invasively by either amniocentesis or CVS. Recognizing the need for more rapid testing methods which do not require cell culture, molecular techniques have been developed for prenatal diagnosis of the most common chromosome disorders (T21, 13, 18, and sex chromosome aneuploidies) where results are available within a day or two. This involves FISH and microscopy analysis of fetal cells or QF-PCR on fetal DNA. Both methods are reliable, and the risk for misdiagnosis is low, although slightly higher for FISH. FISH is also more labor intensive than QF-PCR, the latter lending itself more easily to automation. These tests have been used as a preamble to full chromosome analysis by microscopy. However, there is a trend to apply the tests as "stand-alone" tests for women who are at relatively low risk of having a baby with a chromosome disorder, in particular that associated with advanced age or results of maternal serum screening programs. These women comprise the majority of those currently offered prenatal diagnosis with respect to fetal chromosome disorders and if introduced on a larger scale, the use of FISH and QF-PCR would lead to substantial economic savings. The implication, on the other hand, is that around 1 in 500 to 1 in 1000 cases with a mentally and/or physically disabling chromosome disorder would remain undiagnosed [186]. In the prenatal DNA diagnostic setting, fetal DNA is usually tested for a specific single-gene disorder for which the fetal risk is 25% or more. In contrast, cytogenetic testing is often used to detect fetal chromosomal abnormalities in cases that involve a wider range of indications. Classic cytogenetic and DNA-based testing methods provide a range of aberrations detected with different levels of genomic resolution. FISH and QF-PCR have been introduced to this field in order to answer specific diagnostic questions. However, both FISH and QF-PCR suffer the disadvantage in that they are difficult to scale to a comprehensive, genome-wide screen. More recently developed molecular cytogenetic methods provide powerful tools to bridge the technical divide between these related areas. One such hybrid method is micro-array-based CGH. CMA has been applied to clinical testing for unbalanced gains or losses of genomic regions associated with genetic disorders. This technology is poised to have a substantial impact on clinical genetics, including prenatal genetic testing [187].

Array-CGH is a comprehensive, genome-wide screening strategy for detecting DNA copy number imbalances which can be rapid, less labor-intensive than karyotype banding analysis, and is highly amenable to automation. Array-CGH can be used for prenatal diagnosis and may address many of the limitations of both conventional microscopic cytogenetic analyses and the more recently employed rapid-screening strategies [188]. Array-CGH is transforming clinical cytogenetics with its ability to interrogate the human genome at increasingly high resolution. Array-CGH testing in the prenatal population provides diagnostic information over conventional karyotyping. Array-CGH is used on prenatal samples or on postnatal samples following termination of pregnancy for structural abnormalities that were detected on an ultrasound scan. There appears to be an increased detection rate of chromosomal imbalances, compared with conventional karyotyping, when array-CGH techniques are employed in the prenatal population. However, some are copy number imbalances that are not clinically significant. This carries implications for prenatal counseling and maternal anxiety [189]. For these reasons, routine chromosome analysis, which has been the gold standard for prenatal cytogenetic diagnosis, may be replaced by micro-array technology with increased diagnostic capability for smaller, submicroscopic genetic alterations associated with postnatal morbidity. Micro-array technology has been shown to increase our ability to make a diagnosis of known or new chromosomal deletion syndromes in pediatric populations with developmental delay [190]. In fact, the ability of CMA to detect submicroscopic genetic abnormalities has revolutionized the clinical diagnostic approach to individuals with intellectual disability, neurobehavioral phenotypes, and congenital malformations. The recognition of the underlying copy number variants (CNV) in respective individuals may allow not only for better counseling and anticipatory guidance but also for more specific therapeutic interventions in some cases. The use of CMA technology in prenatal diagnosis is emerging and promises higher sensitivity for several highly penetrant, clinically severe micro-deletion and micro-duplication syndromes. Genetic counseling complements the diagnostic testing with CMA, given the presence of CNV of uncertain clinical significance, incomplete penetrance, and variable expressivity in some cases. While oligonucleotide arrays with high-density exonic coverage remain the gold standard for the detection of CNV, SNP arrays allow for detection of consanguinity and most cases of UPD and provide a higher sensitivity to detect low-level mosaic aneuploidies [191].

Cytogenetic studies have demonstrated that duplications or deletions of entire chromosomes or microscopically visible aberrations are associated with specific congenital disorders. The subsequent development and application of micro-array-based assays have established the importance of CNV as a substantial source of genetic diversity in the human genome. Pathogenic CNV are associated not only with birth defects and cancers, but also with neurodevelopmental disorders at birth or neurodegenerative diseases in adulthood, such as intellectual disability and autism. Unfortunately, the limited knowledge of the phenotypic effects of most CNV has led to the classification of many CNV as genomic imbalances of unknown clinical significance. This has caused many clinicians to resist the introduction of micro-array technologies in detecting CNV in a genome-wide manner for prenatal applications [192]. Evaluation of CNV by CMA has significant advantages over standard metaphase karyotyping and is quickly becoming the primary means of postnatal genetic evaluation for neonates and infants with dysmorphic features or cognitive difficulties. Use in certain prenatal situations such as the fetus with structural anomalies or those who are stillborn appears to add important, clinically relevant information. There are a broad range of array designs available and recent research has focused on the appropriate design for prenatal testing. Patient counseling may occasionally be difficult because of the uncertain phenotype associated with some array findings [193].

A high rate of concordance between conventional methods of detecting chromosomal abnormalities (e.g., FISH and karyotyping) and CMA was reported in the prenatal setting with CMA providing more comprehensive and detailed results as it investigates the whole genome at higher resolution. In preimplantation genetic screening (PGS), CMA is replacing FISH and the selection of embryos based on CMA has already resulted in live births. For ongoing pregnancies and miscarriages, CMA eliminates tissue culture failures and artifacts and allows a quick turnaround time. The detection of submicroscopic imbalances (or CNV) is beneficial when the imbalance has a clear clinical consequence but is challenging for previously undescribed imbalances, particularly for ongoing pregnancies. Recurrent CNV have been documented in patients with reproductive disorders; CMA enhances reproductive medicine as it facilitates better understanding of the genetic aspects of human development and reproduction and more informed patient management [194]. CMA technology represents the technical convergence of molecular genetics and cytogenetics, and is rapidly revolutionizing modern cytogenetics. Expected genomic aberrations are accurately identified and provide readily interpretable results that are suitable for clinical risk stratification and therapeutic strategies. The application of array technology in prenatal genetic diagnosis provides distinct advantages over conventional cytogenetic analysis in detecting both the majority of microscopic and submicroscopic chromosomal abnormalities. In the last few years, the validity of array technology has become obvious to medical and laboratory communities involved in prenatal diagnostic testing [195], so that prenatal array-CGH testing has by and large replaced routine karyotyping in many healthcare settings. While this will lead to more diagnoses, uncertain, unexpected, or unhelpful findings are also likely to increase. This is the case for array-CGH in any setting [196]. To assist clinical laboratories in validation of micro-array methodologies for constitutional applications, the ACMG has produced revised professional standards and guidelines [197]. However, CMA comes with an increased need and role for genetic counseling, because the potential genomic information available is exponentially increased. CMA also can be performed on a small number of preimplantation embryonic cells for assessment of the embryo's reproductive potential. Implementation of these new genomic techniques in an IVF setting has already demonstrated significant improvements in reproductive outcome [198].

As we have said, CMA assesses chromosomal copy number alterations and affords higher resolution when compared with standard karyotype. There is high-quality evidence for the added detection of clinically significant copy number alterations with CMA in prenatal diagnosis when the traditional karyotype is normal. Other potential advantages of CMA include a quicker turnaround time and utilization in clinical situations with a high probability of non-dividing cells (i.e., intrauterine fetal demise, spontaneous miscarriage, and third-trimester amniocentesis). CMA may be beneficial when prenatally detected structural anomalies are associated with specific micro-deletions and micro-duplications or to assess for CNV when a de novo balanced rearrangement or marker chromosome is diagnosed. Use of CMA includes the detection of CNV of uncertain significance [199]. In the prenatal diagnosis test, compared with karyotyping, micro-array technology could identify the extra-cell genetic information with clinical significance, aneuploids, and nonparallel translocations. CMA is able to detect changes as small as 5-10 kb in size, a resolution up to 1000 times higher than that of conventional karyotyping [200]. However, its disadvantage is that it could not identify parallel translocations and triploids [201].

Karyotyping, the gold standard used for diagnosis of chromosomal abnormalities, is being progressively replaced by rapid aneuploidy testing (RAT) techniques such as QF-PCR, FISH, and multiplex ligation-dependent probe amplification for diagnosing the common aneuploidies, or CMA for comprehensive genome-wide testing. However, due to technical limitations, current RAT is confined to the detection of common aneuploidies 13, 18, 21, and sex chromosomes. To overcome the limitations of RAT, a bacterial artificial chromosomes (BAC)-on-beads (BoBs™) assay technology has been introduced for the detection of the common aneuploidies as well as specific micro-deletion syndromes. The BoBs assay is a bead-based multiplex assay using polystyrene beads impregnated with two spectrally distinct infrared fluorochromes to create a liquid array of up to 100 unique spectral signatures that supports the analysis of that scale of simultaneous hybridization assays on a minute DNA sample [202]. Genome-wide methods have been, or can be, successfully applied on total DNA (DNA-seq), methylated DNA immune-precipitation (with tiling array), micro-RNA (Megaplex), and total RNA (RNA-seq). Chromosome- or gene-specific assays have been successively applied on placenta RNA (allele ratio) or DNA multiplex ligation-dependent probe amplification (MLPA). The technical advances for noninvasive aneuploidy tests based on cffDNA and placental mRNA in maternal plasma have been enormous. Multi-marker assays including genome-wide approaches with the option of qualitative information on variation (polymorphism or mutation) besides quantitative information are the preferred methods of choice [203].

Different methodologies of development of NIPT for tracking aneuploidies, including sex chromosomes, have been made available for clinical use, for some micro-deletions and triploids, and for exclusion of paternity. These exams make use of three methodological tools: massively parallel shotgun sequencing (MPSS), targeted massively parallel sequencing (TMPS), and SNP. Genetic tests, despite the high cost, cover a broader range of clinical applications, have the advantage that can be performed early, with high accuracy and low FPR. NIPT stand out for being applied earlier during the pregnancy with high accuracy and low FPR, including a broad spectrum of clinical applications. The TMPS is a recent technique used to evaluate aneuploidy that shows greater accuracy and lower cost than the MPSS, but that is limited to being applied only to the most common aneuploidies. The SNP technique can search for more genetic conditions, besides presenting better accuracy [204]. MPSS and TMPS perform similarly in terms of clinical sensitivity and specificity for the detection of fetal T31, T18, T13, and sex chromosome aneuploidy. However, no study compared the two approaches head-to-head in the same cohort of patients. The accuracy of NIPT as a prenatal screening test has been mainly evaluated as a second-tier screening test to identify pregnancies at very low risk of fetal aneuploidies (T21, T18, and T13), thus avoiding invasive procedures. Genomics-based NIPT methods appear to be sensitive and highly specific for detection of fetal T21, T18, and T13 in high-risk populations. There is paucity of data on the accuracy of NIPT as a first-tier aneuploidy screening test in a population of unselected pregnant women. With respect to the replacement of invasive tests, the performance of NIPT observed is not sufficient to replace current invasive diagnostic tests. Given the current data on the performance of NIPT, invasive fetal karyotyping is still the required diagnostic approach to confirm the presence of a chromosomal abnormality prior to making irreversible decisions relative to the pregnancy outcome. However, most of the NIPT studies were prone to bias, especially in terms of the selection of participants [205]. Nevertheless, methods using MPS are now being implemented almost worldwide. Substantial progress has been made from initially testing for aneuploidies of chromosomes 13, 18, and 21, to testing for sex chromosome aneuploidies, additional autosomal aneuploidies, as well as partial deletions and duplications genome-wide. Although NIPT is associated with significantly reduced risks for the fetus in comparison to existing invasive prenatal diagnostic methods, it presents several implementation challenges [206]. The advent of new digital counting technologies, including dPCR and MPS, has provided the opportunity to quantify the cffDNA molecules in maternal plasma in an unprecedentedly precise manner [207]. So, it was the introduction of MPS that allowed NIPT to become a widely used clinical test [208].

The ability to gain genetic information from the fetus in the mother's blood during pregnancy has been a long-desired goal of research in prenatal medicine. The detection of fetal DNA in maternal blood, coupled with the development of the powerful techniques of NGS finally transferred this analysis into clinical practice. Following the commercial introduction of NIPT for aneuploidies, there has been a very strong demand, which has fostered an extremely rapid development and improvement of technology. Publications in this field are so numerous so that it is challenging to keep up with the latest state-of-the-art [209]. NIPS has emerged as a highly accurate method of screening for fetal Down syndrome, with a DR and specificity approaching 100%. Challenging the widespread use of this technology are cost and the paradigm shift in counseling that accompanies any emerging technology. The expense of the test is expected to decrease with increased utilization, and well beyond the current NIPS technology, its components (fetal genome measurements, sequencing technology, and bio-informatics) will be utilized alone or in combinations to interrogate the fetal genome. The end goal is simple: to offer patients information early in pregnancy about fetal genomes without incurring procedural risks. This will allow patients an opportunity to make informed reproductive and pregnancy management decisions based on precise fetal genomic information [210]. Rapidly developing NGS technologies produce a large amount of data across the whole human genome and allow a large number of DNA samples to be analyzed simultaneously. Screening cffDNA obtained from maternal blood using NGS technologies has provided new opportunities for NIPD of fetal aneuploidies. One of the major challenges to the analysis of fetal abnormalities is the development of accurate and reliable algorithms capable of analyzing large numbers of short sequence reads. Several such algorithms have recently been developed. The main considerations for clinical development for NIPD and screening tests using DNA sequencing are: accuracy, intellectual property, cost, and the ability to screen for a wide range of chromosomal abnormalities and genetic defects. The cost of the diagnostic test depends on the sequencing method, diagnostic algorithm, and volume of the tests. If the cost of sequencing equipment and reagents remains at or around current levels, targeted approaches for sequencing-based aneuploidy testing and SNP-based methods are preferred [211]. However, obstetric care providers must become familiar with the advantages and disadvantages of the utilization of this approach as analysis of cffDNA moves into clinical practice. Once informed, clinicians can provide efficient pretest and post-test counseling with the goal of avoiding patient harm. It is in the public's best interest that test results contain key elements and that laboratories adhere to established quality control and proficiency testing standards. The analysis of cffDNA in maternal circulation for fetal aneuploidy screening is likely the first of major steps toward the eventual application of fetal WGS/WES [212].

As newborn screening success stories gained general confirmation during the past 50 years, scientists quickly discovered diagnostic tests for a host of genetic disorders that could be treated at birth. Outstanding progress in sequencing technologies over the last two decades has made it possible to comprehensively profile newborn screening and identify clinically relevant genomic alterations. With the rapid developments in WGS and WES recently, we can detect newborns at the genomic level and be able to direct the appropriate diagnosis to the different individuals at the appropriate time, which is also encompassed in the concept of precision medicine. Besides, we can develop novel interventions directed at the molecular characteristics of genetic diseases in newborns. The implementation of genomics in newborn screening programs would provide an effective premise for the identification of the majority of genetic aberrations and primarily help in accurate guidance in treatment and better prediction. However, there are some debates correlated with the widespread application of genome sequencing in newborn screening due to some major concerns such as clinical analysis, result interpretation, storage of sequencing data, and communication of clinically relevant mutations to pediatricians and parents, along with the ethical, legal, and social implications (ELSI). If WGS or WES is to be incorporated into newborn screening practice, considerations about these challenges should be carefully regarded and tackled properly to adapt the requirement of genome sequencing in the era of precision medicine [213]. Exome sequencing may provide an even higher detection rate of genetic anomalies and may be more commonly applied in the future. Exome sequencing may be a useful prenatal genetic diagnostic tool in cases with ultrasound anomalies with previously normal chromosomal micro-array and/or karyotype. As more data become available, technology improves, and costs fall [214], WES is increasingly being used in the prenatal setting. The emerging data support the clinical utility of prenatal WES based on its diagnostic yield, which can be as high as 80% for certain ultrasound findings. However, detailed practice and laboratory guidelines, addressing the indications for prenatal WES and the surrounding technical, interpretation, ethical, and counseling issues, are still lacking [215]. Prenatal exome sequencing is beneficial, but more research is needed to better understand the clinical utility, circumstances for ideal use, feasibility, and costs of offering rapid exome sequencing as a routine option for prenatal genetic testing [216].

A variety of approaches for NIPT using NGS have been developed, which have been rapidly transforming clinical practices nowadays. In such approaches, the fetal DNA fraction is a pivotal parameter governing the overall performance and guaranteeing the proper clinical interpretation of testing results [217]. Recently, the introduction of a new tool called WIthin SamplE COpy Number aberration DetectOR (WISECONDOR) marked a new era in prenatal screening using NGS of fetal DNA in maternal blood. WISECONDOR detects copy number aberrations at a resolution that is almost comparable to classic karyotyping and requires only shallow sequencing, making NIPS cost-effective. This emphasizes the role of NGS in the daily clinical practice of prenatal diagnosis and will require reorganization of clinical genetics laboratories to accommodate NGS. For prenatal diagnostics, WISECONDOR introduces an exciting development that will substantially improve the information provided to pregnant couples regarding their fetus's well-being [218]. Optical genome mapping (OGM) is a novel method that fills this void by being able to detect all classes of structural variations, including CNV. OGM is being adopted by laboratories as a tool for both postnatal constitutional genetic disorders and hematological malignancies. OGM has the potential to become a standard of care in prenatal genetic testing based on its capability to comprehensively identify large balanced and unbalanced structural variations (currently the strength of karyotyping and metaphase FISH), CNV (by CMA), repeat contraction disorders (by Southern blotting), and multiple repeat expansion disorders (by PCR-based methods or Southern blotting). NGS methods are excellent at detecting sequence variants, but they are unable to accurately resolve repeat regions of the genome, which limits their ability to detect all classes of structural variations. Notably, multiple molecular methods are used to identify repeat expansion and contraction disorders in routine clinical laboratories around the world. With NIPT becoming the standard of care screening assay for all global pregnancies, OGM can provide a high-resolution, cytogenomic assay to be employed following a positive NIPT screen or for high-risk pregnancies with an abnormal ultrasound. Accurate detection of all types of genetic disorders by OGM, such as live-born aneuploidies, sex chromosome anomalies, micro-deletion/micro-duplication syndromes, repeat expansion/contraction disorders is key to reducing the global burden of genetic disorders [219].

NIPD for single gene disorders has lagged behind due to complexities of technology development, lack of investment, and the need for validation samples for rare disorders. Publications are emerging demonstrating a variety of technical approaches and feasibility of clinical application. Techniques for analysis of cffDNA including dPCR, NGS, and relative haplotype dosage have been used most often for assay development. Analysis of circulating fetal cells in the maternal blood is still being investigated as a viable alternative and, more recently, TC trophoblast cells. Studies exploring ethical and social issues are generally positive but raise concerns around the routinization of prenatal testing. Further work is necessary to make testing available to all patients with a pregnancy at risk of a single-gene disorder, and it remains to be seen if the development of more powerful technologies such as isolation and analysis of single cells will shift the emphasis of NIPD. As testing becomes possible for a wider range of conditions, more ethical questions will become relevant [220]. Emerging genomic technologies, largely based around NGS, have expanded the analyses to the sub-chromosomal aneuploidies. However, further clinical validation studies are needed to better characterize this technology. These tests bring advantage through providing a higher diagnostic yield, without risks of miscarriage than previously available diagnostic test, but also raise the question of harms related to an increase in uncertain and unknown results. In view of the revolution brought about by the NIPT, numerous scientific societies have published recommendations regarding the appropriate application of cffDNA screening in pregnancy [221]. ACMG Clinical Laboratory Practice Resources are developed primarily as an educational tool for clinical laboratory geneticists to help them provide quality clinical laboratory genetic services. Adherence to these practice resources is voluntary and does not necessarily assure a successful medical outcome. This Clinical Laboratory Practice Resource should not be considered inclusive of all proper procedures and tests or exclusive of other procedures and tests that are reasonably directed to obtaining the same results. In determining the propriety of any specific procedure or test, the clinical laboratory geneticist should apply his or her own professional judgment to the specific circumstances presented by the individual patient or specimen. Clinical laboratory geneticists are encouraged to document in the patient's record the rationale for the use of a particular procedure or test, whether or not it is in conformance with this Clinical Laboratory Practice Resource. They also are advised to take notice of the date any particular guideline was adopted, and to consider other relevant medical and scientific information that becomes available after that date. It also would be prudent to consider whether intellectual property interests may restrict the performance of certain tests and other procedures. Since NIPS is a screening test, diagnostic testing is recommended to confirm all cases of screen-positive NIPS results. For cytogenetics laboratories performing confirmatory testing on prenatal diagnostic samples, a standardized testing algorithm is needed to ensure that the appropriate testing takes place. This algorithm includes diagnostic testing by either CVS or amniocentesis samples and encompasses chromosome analysis, FISH, and CMA [222].

Congenital malformations are permanent changes produced by abnormality of development in a body structure during prenatal life.

Population-based studies place the incidence of major malformations at about 2-3% of all live births. The etiology is mostly due multi-factorial inheritance or unknown (50-80%). Congenital anomalies cause ~7% of all neonatal deaths, many of which have no identified pathophysiological cause. Because accurate and robust laboratory tests are unavailable for most birth defects, physicians rely on imaging such as ultrasound and MRI. Biomarkers from human body fluids are considered a powerful diagnostic tool to assess human disease and health as it mirrors an individual's condition. Minimally invasive "liquid biopsies" from blood samples are highly valuable for diagnosis, prognosis, risk assessment, and treatment of many conditions. Recent large-scale analysis ("'omics") have enabled researchers to identify novel biomarkers in different areas. To accurately facilitate the early detection of congenital anomalies, the identification of biomarkers from maternal plasma should be promoted. This approach will uncover new opportunities in prenatal diagnosing and likely lead to a better understanding of the pathogenesis of congenital anomalies [223]. The continuum and gradual shift from genetics to genomics will offer new possibilities for diagnosis, treatment, prediction, and prevention of congenital malformations. Prenatal genetics has evolved over the last decade to include application of new 'omics technologies to improve perinatal care [224].

Central to translational medicine trend is the ability to sequence, annotate, and interpret the genomic variants in a given patient to guide precision diagnosis and personalized treatment. This new section intends to promote the translation of emerging genomic technologies into clinical applications. The coverage extends to basic, translational, and clinical studies related to human genomics and genetics [225]. Genomics has many tools including pathogenomics, pharmacogenomics, nutrigenomics, and bio-informatics. Pathogenomics will help to discover new genes or susceptibility genes and genetic variants with a role in the pathogenesis of congenital malformations. Pharmacogenomics will identify genetic variants affecting the response to drugs and it should be applied to study drug-induced birth defects. Nutrigenomics will determine the impact of diet on genome stability and how genotype determines nutritional requirements. Bio-informatics then will collect and store obtained data, which will facilitate analysis of systems biology questions involving relationships between genes, their variants, and biological functions. This knowledge should be translated into more sensitive and specific genetic tests [226].

Post-genomics technologies that explore the proteins (proteomics) and transcripts (transcriptomics) released by the placenta into the maternal circulation offer new opportunities to identify genes and their protein products that are key diagnostic markers of disease (in particular Down syndrome), and might replace the current screening markers in use for prediction of risk of Down syndrome. In the ideal situation, these markers are sufficiently diagnostic not to require invasive sampling of fetal genetic material. Post-genomics techniques might also offer better opportunities for defining fetal cell-specific markers that might enhance their isolation from maternal blood samples [227]. In addition to specific fetal genetic disorders, the whole fetal genome, transcriptome, and methylome have been revealed by deep sequencing of maternal plasma. The analysis of the fetal transcriptome and methylome may yield valuable information on fetal and maternal health [228]. Sequencing of fetal exomes offers broad diagnostic capability for pregnancies with unexpected fetal anomalies, improving the yield and accuracy of diagnoses and allowing better counseling for parents. The challenge now is to translate these approaches into mainstream use in the clinic. As technology continues to advance, future developments may be toward noninvasive fetal WES or WGS and a universal method for NIPD without the need to sequence both parents or an affected proband. Expansion of cffDNA analysis to include the transcriptome and the methylome is likely to yield clinical benefits for monitoring other pregnancy-related pathologies such as preeclampsia and IUGR [229]. Metabolomics opens up new avenues for biomarker discovery in different branches of medicine, including perinatology. Chromosomal aberration, preterm delivery, CHD, spina bifida, chorioamnionitis, and low birth weight (LBW) are the main perinatal pathologies. Investigations using untargeted metabolomics have found the candidate metabolites for diagnostic biomarkers. Untargeted metabolomics is a powerful tool which can shed a new light on prenatal diagnostics. It helps to discover affected metabolic pathways that may help to reveal disease pathogenesis and propose potential biomarkers. Among others, glycerol and 2- and 3-hydroxybutyrate (HB) were proposed as markers of chromosomal aberration. Serum metabolic signature of preterm delivery was characterized by increased lipids and decreased levels of hypoxanthine, tryptophane, and pyroglutamic acid. Lower-level lipids and vitamin D3 metabolites together with increased bilirubin level in maternal serum were associated with macrosomia. However, to give a real value to those assays and allow their clinical application multi-center, large cohort validation studies are necessary [230].

Although some have wondered whether the sequencing of the human genome has led to major advances in medicine, in fact there are multiple examples where genomics has been integrated into medical practice. In the area of prevention, genomic approaches are now used for NIPT of fetal DNA in the maternal circulation, for expanded preconceptional screening for carrier status, for autosomal recessive disorders, and for assessment of risk of common disease. NIPT is the vanguard of genomic medicine. In only ten years, this screening test has revolutionized prenatal care globally and opened up new prospects for personalized medicine for the fetus. There are widespread implications for increasing the scope of human genetic variation that can be detected before birth, and for discovering more about fetal-maternal and placental biology. These include an urgent need to develop pretest education for all pregnant women and consistent post-test management recommendations for those with discordant test results. The reduction in invasive testing has had downstream effects on specialist training and caused many countries to re-examine their national approaches to prenatal screening. In the area of diagnosis, major advances have been made in cytogenomics and in use of WES or WGS. In therapeutics, pharmacogenetic testing is now feasible, tumor genome sequencing is being used to guide cancer therapy, and genomic discoveries are enabling development of new targeted therapies. Ultimately, it is possible that genome sequencing may be done for all individuals on a routine basis, though there remain significant technical, ethical, and medical systems challenges to be overcome [231]. In fact, the accumulating datasets of genomic information on pregnant women and their fetuses raise ethical issues regarding consent for future data mining and intellectual property. It is likely that integration of genomics into medical practice will occur gradually over a long period of time, but the process is now well underway [232].

The US HGP is a federally funded effort to produce a detailed genetic and physical map of all human chromosomes. Because of their central role in reproduction and care-giving, women are likely to be affected differently, and more significantly, by the information the HGP generates. It is important to identify inequities that may emerge from gender differences and to consider ways in which they may be avoided, reduced, or overcome. Although this type of analysis is one of the goals of the ELSI Program of the National Center for Human Genome Research (NCHGR), now *National Human Genome Research Institute* (NHGRI), few studies have focused explicitly on the impact of the HGP on women. Identification of gender differences as they affect both research and clinical practice and the psycho-social, legal, and ethical implications of the HGP should evoke and inform public discussion and policies that may be generated by these issues [233]. The technologies developed for the HGP, the recent surge of available DNA sequences resulting from it and the increasing pace of gene discoveries and characterization have all contributed to new technical platforms that have enhanced the spectrum of disorders that can be diagnosed prenatally. The importance of determining the disease-causing mutation or the informativeness of linked genetic markers before embarking upon a DNA-based prenatal diagnosis is, however, still emphasized. Different FISH technologies provide increased resolution for the elucidation of structural chromosome abnormalities that cannot be resolved by more conventional cytogenetic analyses, including micro-deletion syndromes, cryptic or subtle duplications and translocations, complex rearrangements involving many chromosomes, and marker chromosomes. Inter-phase FISH and the QF-PCR are efficient tools for the rapid prenatal diagnosis of selected aneuploidies, the latter being considered to be most cost-effective if analyses are performed on a large scale. There is some debate surrounding whether this approach should be employed as an adjunct to karyotyping or whether it should be used as a stand-alone test in selected groups of women [234].

After the mapping and sequencing of the human genome, medical professionals from essentially all specialties turned their attention to investigating the role genes play in health and disease. Until recently, medical genetics was considered a specialty of minor practical relevance. This view has changed with the development of new diagnostic and therapeutic possibilities. It is now realized that genetic disease represents an important part of medical practice. Achievements in cancer genetics, in the field of prenatal diagnostics (including carrier testing for common recessive disorders), and in newborn screening for treatable metabolic disorders reinforce the rapidly expanding role of genetics in medicine. Diagnosing a genetic disorder not only allows for disease-specific management options but also has implications for the affected individual's entire family. A working understanding of the underlying concepts of genetic disease with regard to chromosome, single gene, mitochondrial, and multi-factorial disorders is necessary for today's practicing physician. Routine clinical practice in virtually all medical specialties will soon require integration of these fundamental concepts for use in accurate diagnosis and ensuring appropriate referrals for patients with genetic disease and their families [235]. Therefore, the sequencing of the human genome should be regarded as a milestone in a road that stretches years into the future. Researchers will benefit from the catalog of human genes in studies of the genetics of disease susceptibility and the cell biology of gene interactions. Clinicians will increasingly offer genetic or biochemical testing to identify those at highest risk for a number of diseases. Drug discovery will eventually follow newly possible studies of gene expression and protein function. However, the HGP eventually shapes medicine, it is certain that physicians, particularly obstetricians and gynecologists, will need to be well versed in the scientific and ethical issues involved, inasmuch as we will likely be at the center of the most heated debates [236]. The rapid development in molecular biological technologies makes it possible to screen and to diagnosis thousands of genetic conditions, mutations, and also predispositions to chronic diseases or traits, either prenatally or after birth. The arrival of the molecular genetic era also leads to many new ethical, social, and medical-legal problems and dilemmas that obstetricians will have to face in the near future. There is an urgent need for the development of a new model for provision of genetic screening and diagnosis [237].

In summary, screening for fetal aneuploidy in pregnant women using cffDNA has increased dramatically since the technology became commercially available in 2011. Since that time, numerous trials have demonstrated high sensitivity and specificity to screen for common aneuploidies in high-risk populations. Studies assessing the performance of these tests in low-risk populations have also demonstrated improved DR compared with traditional, serum-based screening strategies. Concurrent with the increased use of this technology has been a decrease in invasive procedures (amniocentesis and CVS). As the technology becomes more widely understood, available, and utilized, challenges regarding its clinical implementation have become apparent. Some of these challenges include test failures, false-positive and false-negative results, limitations in PPV in low-prevalence populations, and potential maternal health implications of abnormal results. In addition, commercial laboratories are expanding screening beyond common aneuploidies to include micro-deletion screening and WGS [238]. With the ability to decipher the entire fetal genome from maternal plasma DNA, we foresee that an increasing of NIPT will be available for detecting many single-gene disorders in the near future [239]. The roles that cell-free fetal nucleic acid testing assume in the existing framework of prenatal screening and invasive diagnostic testing will depend on factors such as costs, clinical validity and utility, and perceived benefit-risk ratios for different applications. As cffDNA and RNA testing continues to be developed and translated, significant ethical, legal, and social questions will arise that will need to be addressed by those with a stake in the use of this technology. Understanding the ethical, legal, and social aspects in light of such rapid developments is thus a priority for future research [240]. In fact, the goal of prenatal cytogenetic testing is to provide reassurance to the couple seeking testing for their pregnancy, identify chromosome abnormalities in the fetus, if present, and provide treatments and medical management for affected babies. Cytogenetic analysis of banded chromosomes has been the standard for identifying chromosome abnormalities in the fetus for over 40 years. With chromosome analysis, whole chromosome aneuploidies and large structural rearrangements can be identified. The sequencing of the human genome has provided the resources to develop molecular tools that allow higher resolution observations of human chromosomes. The future holds the promise of sequencing that may identify chromosomal imbalances and deleterious single nucleotide variants [241].

Prenatal Diagnosis in Multiple Gestations

The incidence of twins, triplets, and high-order multiples has increased dramatically in the last two decades secondary to greater reliance on fertility treatments and to delayed childbearing. Offspring of a multiple gestation are at increased risk for both chromosomal and structural abnormalities. Prenatal diagnosis in these patients is challenging. Options for screening tests are limited. Invasive diagnostic procedures are complex. Likewise, physicians and patients may be faced with the dilemma of deciding how to manage discordant results [242]. Multiple gestations account for 1-2% of all pregnancies but contribute disproportionately to the incidence of both perinatal loss and fetal structural abnormalities. Ultrasound examination provides essential information about screening for, and the management of, such defects, including accurate determination of chorionicity, assessment of risk, invasive testing, and selective termination if appropriate [243]. Screening for aneuploidy in twins and higher-order multiples present complex practical and ethical issues that limit its provision to women [244]. Chromosomal anomalies and Mendelian diseases are more frequent in multiple gestations than in singletons. Prenatal diagnosis is recommended in multiple pregnancies whenever indicated. Invasive testing using amniocentesis or CVS can be performed safely. CVS has a significant advantage over amniocentesis because it offers rapid karyotyping and biochemical and DNA studies at an early stage of pregnancy. Only experienced centers should perform these procedures because of the technical aspects and the expertise needed in handling discordant results [245]. Accurate determination of chorionicity is vital and an inability to determine this should trigger consideration for referral to a specialist. The choice of screening method for detection of chromosomal abnormality is limited, and existing data demonstrates the advantages of NT screening. The possibility of obtaining discordant results and options for management should be discussed in advance. Invasive tests are technically more difficult and associated with a higher risk of procedure-related pregnancy loss than less invasive methods. Repeat invasive testing is required more often in multiple pregnancies than in singleton pregnancies. Selective termination is technically feasible in both mono- and dichorionic pregnancies, although the risks are higher with the former. It is likely to be more acceptable than high-order multi-fetal reduction performed in the absence of fetal abnormality [246].

Summary Guidelines

Prenatal diagnostic and screening tests are routinely offered to all women in pregnancy. Advances in technology have led to an expansion in available testing. As technology improves, women are facing increasingly complex decisions regarding the quantity and quality of information they wish to have regarding their fetus. The rapid development of prenatal genetic testing and screening tools and choices constantly challenges clinicians to stay up-to-date on current best practice. Recently published (2016-2017) national guidelines and updates on prenatal genetic screening and testing including ACOG committee opinions and practice bulletins, Society for Maternal-Fetal Medicine (SMFM) consult series publications, and an ACMG position statement on carrier screening, cffDNA screening, CMA, NGS, and prenatal diagnostic testing, contain many updates and changes to previous screening and testing strategies, most of which are consistent between professional societies. Although many new technologies have been integrated into prenatal diagnosis, some newer technologies are not yet routinely recommended for widespread use, often because of lack of clinical trials and validation studies. Prenatal screening and testing options are rapidly expanding. To provide best-practice prenatal care, obstetric care providers should educate themselves about the most up-to-date recommendations and be prepared to interpret and apply these guidelines to their patients. Society guidelines are largely in agreement [247]. Prenatal testing for chromosomal abnormalities is designed to provide an accurate assessment of a patient's risk of carrying a fetus with a chromosomal disorder. A wide variety of prenatal screening and diagnostic tests are available; each offers varying levels of information and performance, and each has relative advantages and limitations. When considering screening test characteristics, no one test is superior in all circumstances, which results in the need for nuanced, patient-centered counseling from the obstetric care professional and complex decision making by the patient. Each patient should be counseled in each pregnancy about options for testing for fetal chromosomal abnormalities. It is important that obstetric care professionals be prepared to discuss not only the risk of fetal chromosomal abnormalities but also the relative benefits and limitations of the available screening and diagnostic tests. Testing for chromosomal abnormalities should be an informed patient choice based on provision of adequate and accurate information, the patient's clinical context, accessible health care resources, values, interests, and goals. All patients should be offered both screening and diagnostic tests, and all patients have the right to accept or decline testing after counseling [248].

Pregnancy screening for fetal aneuploidy (T13, T18, and T21) started in the mid-1960s, using maternal age as the screening test. New developments in maternal serum and ultrasound screening have made it possible to offer all pregnant patients a noninvasive screening test to assess their risk of having a fetus with aneuploidy to determine whether invasive prenatal diagnostic testing is necessary. Invasive prenatal diagnosis would be offered to women who screen above a set risk cut-off level on noninvasive screening or to pregnant women whose personal, obstetric, or family history places them at increased risk. Currently available noninvasive screening options include maternal age combined with one of the following:

1. first-trimester screening (NT, maternal age, and maternal serum biochemical markers);
2. second-trimester serum screening (maternal age and maternal serum biochemical markers); or
3. two-step integrated screening, which includes first- and second-trimester serum screening with or without NT (integrated prenatal screen and serum integrated prenatal screening, contingent and sequential).

Reducing the number of prenatal invasive procedures done when maternal age is the only indication will have the benefit of reducing the numbers of normal pregnancies lost because of complications of invasive procedures. Any screening test has an inherent FPR, which may result in undue anxiety. It is not possible at this time to undertake a detailed cost-benefit analysis of the implementation of this guideline, since this would require health surveillance and research and health resources not presently available; however, these factors need to be evaluated in a prospective approach by provincial and territorial initiatives. All pregnant women, regardless of age, should be offered, through an informed counseling process, the option of a prenatal screening test for the most common clinically significant fetal aneuploidies in addition to a second-trimester ultrasound for dating, assessment of fetal anatomy, and detection of multiples. Counseling must be non-directive and must respect a woman's right to accept or decline any or all of the testing or options offered at any point in the process. Maternal age alone is a poor minimum standard for prenatal screening for aneuploidy, and it should not be used a basis for recommending invasive testing when NIPS for aneuploidy is available. Invasive prenatal diagnosis for cytogenetic analysis should not be performed without multiple marker screening results except for women who are at increased risk of fetal aneuploidy:

1. because of ultrasound findings;
2. because the pregnancy was conceived by IVF with intracytoplasmic sperm injection (ICSI); or
3. because the woman or her partner has a history of a previous child or fetus with a chromosomal abnormality or is a carrier of a chromosome rearrangement that increases the risk of having a fetus with a chromosomal abnormality.

At minimum, any prenatal screen offered to women who present for care in the first trimester should have a DR of 75% with no more than a 3% FPR. The performance of the screen should be substantiated by annual audit. The minimum standard for women presenting in the second trimester should be a screen that has a DR of 75% with no more than a 5% FPR. The performance of the screen should be substantiated by annual audit. First-trimester NT should be interpreted for risk assessment only when measured by sonographers or sonologists trained and accredited for this service and when there is ongoing quality assurance, and it should not be offered as a screen without biochemical markers in singleton pregnancies. Evaluation of the fetal nasal bone in the first trimester should not be incorporated as a screen unless it is performed by sonographers or sonologists trained and accredited for this service and there is ongoing quality assurance. For women who undertake first-trimester screening, second-trimester serum α-FP screening and/or ultrasound examination is recommended to screen for open NTD. Timely referral and access are critical for women and should be facilitated to ensure women are able to undergo the type of screening test they have chosen as first-trimester screening. The first steps of integrated screening (with or without NT), contingent or sequential screening are performed in an early and relatively narrow time window. Ultrasound dating should be performed if menstrual or conception dating is unreliable. For any abnormal serum screen calculated on the basis of menstrual dating, an ultrasound should be done to confirm gestational age. The presence or absence of soft markers or anomalies in the 18- to 20-week ultrasound can be used to modify the a priori risk of aneuploidy established by age or prior screening. Information such as gestational dating, maternal weight, ethnicity, insulin-dependent diabetes mellitus (IDDM), and use of assisted reproduction technologies (ART) should be provided to the laboratory to improve accuracy of testing. Health care providers should be aware of the screening modalities available in their province or territory. A reliable system needs to be in place ensuring timely reporting of results. Screening programs should be implemented with resources that support audited screening and diagnostic laboratory services, ultrasound, genetic counseling services, patient and health care provider education, and high-quality diagnostic testing, as well as resources for administration, annual clinical audit, and data management. In addition, there must be the flexibility and funding to adjust the program to new technology and protocols [249, 250].

Findings of isolated or multiple fetal anomalies on prenatal ultrasound examination always lead to stressful times for women and families. Although a proportion of such anomalies can be explained by chromosomal abnormalities (aneuploidy, unbalanced translocation, deletions, or duplications), others may represent recognizable syndromes with another genetic basis (micro-deletion or autosomal dominant, recessive, or X-linked inheritance). Providing accurate information and relevant reproductive genetic counseling to these women and families will allow them to make informed decisions. This is not easily accomplished because of the limited information available prenatally. When a fetal structural anomaly is identified, the pregnant woman should be offered a timely consultation with a trained genetic counselor and with a maternal-fetal medicine specialist and/or a medical geneticist. The counseling should be unbiased and respectful of the patient's choice, culture, religion, and beliefs. Patients should be informed that prenatal ultrasound at 18 to 20 weeks can detect major structural anomalies in approximately 60% of such cases. When a fetal structural anomaly is suspected or identified, a referral to a tertiary ultrasound unit should be made as soon as possible to optimize therapeutic options. In ongoing pregnancies with fetal structural anomalies, ultrasound examination should be repeated (at a frequency depending on the anomaly) to assess the evolution of the anomaly and attempt to detect other anomalies not previously identified, as this may influence the counseling as well as the obstetric or perinatal management. Once a fetal structural anomaly is identified by 2D ultrasound, other imaging techniques such as fetal echocardiography, 3D obstetric ultrasound, ultra-fast fetal MRI, and, occasionally, fetal X-ray and fetal computerized tomography (CT) scan (using a low-dose protocol) may be helpful in specific cases. Parental imaging should be considered in specific cases, depending on the fetal anomaly identified (e.g., potential dominant inheritance). Parental blood testing and invasive prenatal testing may also be required to clarify the diagnosis for a fetus with isolated or multiple structural anomalies. Women should receive information regarding the abnormal ultrasound findings in a clear, sympathetic, and timely fashion, and in a supportive environment that ensures privacy. Referral to the appropriate pediatric or surgical sub-specialists should be considered to provide the most accurate information possible concerning the anomaly or anomalies and the associated prognosis. Parents should be informed that major or minor fetal structural anomalies, whether isolated or multiple, may be part of a genetic syndrome, sequence, or association, despite a normal fetal karyotype. If early or urgent postnatal management may be required, delivery at a center that can provide the appropriate neonatal care should be considered. When any congenital structural anomaly has been identified prenatally, a comprehensive newborn assessment is essential for diagnosis and counseling on the etiology, prognosis, and recurrence risk for future pregnancies, especially when the etiology has not been clearly identified prenatally. In cases of termination of pregnancy, stillbirth, or neonatal death, the health professional should encourage the performance of a complete autopsy by a perinatal or pediatric pathologist to provide maximum information on the diagnosis and etiology of the structural fetal anomaly or anomalies. When a complete autopsy is refused, the health professional should encourage the performance of at least a partial or external autopsy (including X-rays and photographs) [251]. The Biochemistry, *Ultrasound*, Nuchal Translucency (BUN) and First and Second Trimester Evaluation of Risks (FASTER) studies, two prospective multicenter trials in the US, validated the accuracy and DR of first- and second-trimester screening previously reported abroad. These studies, coupled with the 2007 release of the ACOG Practice Bulletin that endorsed first-trimester screening as an alternative to traditional second-trimester multiple marker screening, led to an explosion of screening options available to pregnant women. ACOG also recommended that invasive diagnostic testing for chromosome aneuploidy be made available to all women regardless of maternal age. More recently, another option known as NIPT became available to screen for chromosome aneuploidy. While screening and testing options may be limited due to a variety of factors, healthcare providers need to be aware of the options in their area in order to provide their patients with accurate and reliable information. If not presented clearly, patients may feel overwhelmed at the number of choices available [252].

NIPS that uses cffDNA from the plasma of pregnant women offers tremendous potential as a screening method for fetal aneuploidy. A number of laboratories have validated different techniques for the use of cffDNA as a screening test for fetal aneuploidy. All tests have a high sensitivity and specificity for T18 and T21, regardless of which molecular technique is used. Women whose results are not reported, indeterminate, or uninterpretable (a "no call" test result) from cffDNA screening should receive further genetic counseling and be offered comprehensive ultrasound evaluation and diagnostic testing because of an increased risk of aneuploidy. Patients should be counseled that cffDNA screening does not replace the precision obtained with diagnostic tests, such as CVS or amniocentesis and, therefore, is limited in its ability to identify all chromosome abnormalities. cffDNA screening does not assess risk of fetal anomalies such as NTD or ventral wall defects. Patients who are undergoing cffDNA screening should be offered maternal serum α-FP screening or ultrasound evaluation for risk assessment. The cffDNA screening test should not be considered in isolation from other clinical findings and test results. Management decisions, including termination of the pregnancy, should not be based on the results of the cffDNA screening alone. Patients should be counseled that a negative cffDNA test result does not ensure an unaffected pregnancy. Given the performance of conventional screening methods, the limitations of cffDNA screening performance, and the limited data on cost-effectiveness in the low-risk obstetric population, conventional screening methods remain the most appropriate choice for first-line screening for most women in the general obstetric population [253, 254]. It is now possible to choose standard chromosome analysis or QF-PCR for the prenatal diagnosis of chromosomal abnormalities, or to perform both tests, depending on the clinical indication for testing. The use of a rapid aneuploidy DNA test for women at increased risk of having a pregnancy affected by a common aneuploidy will have the benefit of providing rapid and accurate results to women at increased risk of fetal Down syndrome, T13, T18, and sex chromosome aneuploidy or triploidy. It will also promote better use of laboratory resources and reduce the cost of prenatal diagnosis. However, a small percentage of pregnancies with a potentially clinically significant chromosomal abnormality will remain undetected by QF-PCR but detectable by conventional cytogenetics. QF-PCR is a reliable method to detect trisomies and should replace conventional cytogenetic analysis whenever prenatal testing is performed solely because of an increased risk of aneuploidy in chromosomes 13, 18, 21, X, or Y. As with all tests, pretest counseling should include a discussion of the benefits and limitations of the test. In the initial period of use, education for health care providers will be required. Both conventional cytogenetics and QF-PCR should be performed in all cases of prenatal diagnosis referred for a fetal ultrasound abnormality (including an increased NT measurement >3.5 mm) or a familial chromosomal rearrangement. Cytogenetic follow-up of QF-PCR findings of T13 and 21 is recommended to rule out inherited Robertsonian translocations. However, the decision to set up a back-up culture for all cases that would allow for traditional cytogenetic testing if indicated by additional clinical or laboratory information should be made by each center offering the testing according to the local clinical and laboratory experience and resources. Other technologies for the rapid detection of aneuploidy may replace QF-PCR if they offer a similar or improved performance for the detection of T13, 18, 21, and sex chromosome aneuploidy [255].

Professional guidelines support the use of CMA as a first-tier test in place of standard karyotype for the evaluation of fetal chromosomes when one or more anomaly is detected by ultrasound. These same guidelines indicate that either CMA or standard karyotype can be offered for prenatal diagnosis with a phenotypically normal fetus. Additionally, recent work continues to validate the use of NIPT for the detection of aneuploidy in the high-risk population. This testing utilizes cffDNA in the maternal circulation to predict fetal karyotype with greater sensitivity and specificity than maternal serum screening or first-trimester screening. Data continue to accumulate supporting NIPT use in an all-risk or low-risk population. Additionally, NIPT is clinically available to screen for a selected number of micro-deletion syndromes, broadening the scope of population-based screening to include conditions not previously evaluated, although there are limited data available regarding this application. As prenatal diagnosis becomes increasingly complex, there is a need for the education of both patients and providers regarding the benefits and limitations of the testing strategies available to them [256]. Array-CGH is not recommended in pregnancies at low risk for a structural chromosomal abnormality; for example, advanced maternal age, positive maternal serum screen, previous trisomy, or the presence of soft markers on fetal ultrasound.

Array-CGH may be an appropriate diagnostic test in cases with fetal structural abnormalities detected on ultrasound or fetal MRI; it could be done in lieu of a karyotype if rapid aneuploidy screening is negative and an appropriate turnaround time for results is assured. Any pregnant woman who qualifies for micro-array-CGH testing should be seen in consultation by a medical geneticist before testing so that the benefits, limitations, and possible outcomes of the analysis can be discussed in detail. The difficulties of interpreting some CNV should also be discussed. This will allow couples to make an informed decision about whether or not they wish to pursue such prenatal testing [257]. cffDNA testing should be an informed patient choice after pretest counseling and should not be part of routine prenatal laboratory assessment. cffDNA testing should not be offered to low-risk women or women with multiple gestations because it has not been sufficiently evaluated in these groups. A negative cffDNA test result does not ensure an unaffected pregnancy. A patient with a positive test result should be referred for genetic counseling and should be offered invasive prenatal diagnosis for confirmation of test results [258].

There is a need for specific guidelines for prenatal screening and diagnosis in twins. These guidelines should assist health care providers in the approach to this aspect of prenatal care of women with twin pregnancies. Fetal NT combined with maternal age is an acceptable first-trimester screening test for aneuploidies (e.g., Down syndrome and T18) in twin pregnancies. First-trimester serum screening combined with NT may be considered in twin pregnancies. It provides some improvement over the performance of screening by NT and maternal age by decreasing the FPR. Integrated screening with NT plus first- and second-trimester serum screening is an option in twin pregnancies. Further prospective studies are required in this area, since it has not been validated in prospective studies in twins. Non-directive counseling is essential when invasive testing is offered. When CVS is performed in nonmonochorionic multiple pregnancies, a combination of TA and TC approaches or a TA only approach appears to provide the best results to minimize the likelihood of sampling errors. All pregnant women, regardless of age, should be offered, through an informed counseling process, the option of a prenatal screening test for the most common clinically significant fetal aneuploidies. In addition, they should be offered a second-trimester ultrasound for dating, assessment of fetal anatomy, and detection of multiples. Counseling must be non-directive and must respect a woman's right to accept or decline any or all of the testing or options offered at any point in the process. When NIPS for aneuploidy is available, maternal age alone should not be an indication for invasive prenatal diagnosis in a twin pregnancy. If NIPS is not available, invasive prenatal diagnosis in twins should be offered to women aged 35 and over. Chorionicity has a major impact on the prenatal screening process and should be determined by ultrasound in the first trimester of all twin pregnancies. When screening is done by NT and maternal age, a pregnancy-specific risk should be calculated in monochorionic twins. In dichorionic twins, a fetus-specific risk should be calculated. During amniocentesis, both amniotic sacs should be sampled in monochorionic twin pregnancies, unless monochorionicity is confirmed before 14 weeks and the fetuses appear concordant for growth and anatomy. Prior to invasive testing or in the context of twins discordant for an abnormality, selective reduction should be discussed and made available to those requesting the procedure after appropriate counseling. Monitoring for disseminated intravascular coagulopathy (DIC) is not indicated in dichorionic twin pregnancies undergoing selective reduction [259].

Conclusion

Rapid advances in the field of human genetics have led to an increase in the availability of genetic diagnostic tests [260]. There has been an explosion of new information in molecular biology that will change the ways in which we practice medicine in the future. These laboratory advances in disease detection at the DNA level are quickly finding clinical application in prenatal diagnosis. An understanding of some basic concepts of DNA laboratory techniques and their applications is increasingly important in obstetrics and gynecology today [261]. The recent explosion of scientific and technical knowledge in the field of molecular biology has allowed us to make important advances in our understanding of the molecular basis of many human diseases. This technology has now entered the clinical laboratory where identification of specific genetic sequences can aid in the precise diagnosis of hematological and other malignancies, inherited diseases, specific infectious agents, and inherited predisposition to disease. In addition, it can be applied to prenatal diagnosis, paternity testing, identification of minimal residual disease following treatment, and assessment of drug sensitivity or resistance. In many cases in diagnostic pathology, the need for molecular analysis often is not realized until after a critical tissue specimen has been fixed, embedded, and examined microscopically [262].

The study of human genetics and developments therein have truly made great strides in recent years. The tendency to immediately introduce new technology into medical practice, however, suggests the urgent need to consider the ethics of our recently developed and developing technological prowess, as well as the long- and short-term impacts of these changes. In response to the increasing number of prospective parents who want to have a prenatal assessment of normal fetal well-being, voluntary ultrasound screening programs have developed. New available techniques make the diagnosis of fetal maldevelopments more frequent and more precise. The procedures seems safe within the limits of current practice. As for the isolation of fetal cells from maternal circulation for prenatal diagnosis, large clinical pilot trials have been needed to especially determine the method's sensitivity and specificity for use in either screening or diagnosis. This approach should be under tight control to avoid potential misuse [263]. The enormous progress witnessed in the field of prenatal diagnosis during the past five decades is likely to continue into the future. Improved imaging techniques are likely to enhance the resolution of noninvasively obtained fetal images considerably over their current excellent quality. Although this undoubtedly will be true for ultrasonography, the increased speed of MRI equipment may offer a new realm of imaging possibilities. Computerized image processing, analysis, and 3D reconstructions all should make interpretation of fetal images easier and more understandable to the non-specialist. Advances in molecular genetics will continue to accelerate, greatly expanding the range and accuracy of prenatal diagnosis. The alert pediatrician who is sensitive to genetic issues may, by early detection of pediatric disorders and careful family history assessment, be in a position to identify families at risk for serious genetic conditions and provide the opportunity to make informed decisions on reproductive options that avert a major tragedy. The pediatrician, working with obstetric colleagues, should be part of a team effort to support families going through prenatal testing. Familiarity with these rapidly changing technologies will make it far easier to support the family needing additional explanation about prenatal diagnosis issues [264].

Reproductive genetic technology provides unprecedented opportunities for pregnant women and their families to obtain direct information about the genetic makeup of their developing fetus. Ultrasonography, maternal serum markers, amniocentesis, CVS, and per-cutaneous umbilical blood sampling already offer opportunities for prenatal diagnosis in early pregnancy. New techniques, such as preimplantation, prenatal diagnosis, and fetal cell sorting offer opportunities in even earlier stages of pregnancy [265]. These methods have the advantage of providing earlier diagnosis in addition to being noninvasive and of less psychological traumas. PGD is another new growing field offering the genetic diagnosis prior to implantation [266]. Molecular genetic technology is diffusing from the research laboratory to the clinical laboratory, where it has already begun to influence prenatal diagnosis and counseling. In the very near future, this technology will be applied more generally, using population-based screening strategies. Pilot programs have evaluated the technical feasibility and efficacy of recombinant DNA techniques for newborn screening follow-up. DNA-based population screening has been considered for heterozygous carriers of an autosomal recessive disorder such as cystic fibrosis in order to identify carrier couples at risk of having an affected child. Implementation of these new technologies requires two key factors: machines and people. Machines are required to automate molecular genetic procedures, which are currently personnel-intensive, so that the expense can be reduced and the procedures made more cost-effective. The people who are required are health professionals knowledgeable in the clinical aspects of the target disorders, as well as in the DNA laboratory testing. These professionals will be able to facilitate sample acquisition and information exchange among the laboratory, the primary health care provider, and the families requesting consultation [267].

Fetal aneuploidies are among the most common causes of miscarriages, perinatal mortality, and neurodevelopmental impairment. During the last 70 years, many efforts have been made in order to improve prenatal diagnosis and prenatal screening of these conditions [268]. The most common referral indication is a raised risk of Down syndrome, and diagnosis has, until recently, been carried out by culture of cells from invasive prenatal sampling, followed by full karyotype analysis, with a waiting time of around two weeks for results. First-trimester screening is presently offered to all pregnant women as a means of prenatal screening for Down syndrome, T18, and T13. NT measurement is a fundamental component of the screening protocol. A woman whose fetus' NT is greater than the 95th percentile is also at increased risk for a multiplicity of other adverse pregnancy and pediatric outcomes, and as a consequence, counseling of patients about their testing options and range of pregnancy outcomes has become complex and difficult. The increased risk for chromosome abnormalities, CHD, and pregnancy loss in the presence of an increased NT is well documented. What has not been clearly defined is the incidence of other genetic syndromes, congenital defects, and adverse pregnancy and pediatric outcomes in the presence of increased NT. Currently, Noonan syndrome is the only molecular genetic condition that has been shown to have a clear association with the finding of increased NT in the first trimester [269].

Newborn screening has been a mainstay of genetic testing for several decades. Recent advances in newborn screening and molecular genetics are transforming our understanding of the genetic basis of diseases that affect individuals of all ages. It is essential for clinicians to understand the methods and goals of newborn screening, the principles of genetics, and the methods of molecular analysis including Southern blots, PCR amplification, DNA sequence analysis, Reverse Transcriptase PCR (RT-PCR), MLPA, FISH, CGH, as well as fetal ultrasonography. This understanding and applications of these tools can lead to genetic diagnoses by identifying risks from newborn screening results or family histories, selecting appropriate tests, and understanding the implications of test results to the patient and their families [270]. Molecular biological techniques, pervasive in genetics and in medicine, are shifting the focus of such testing from enzymology to molecular diagnosis. Concomitant developments in the isolation of fetal cells from maternal blood enable molecular analysis to be performed not just postnatally, but in fact as early as the late first trimester. Potential advantages of first-trimester prenatal diagnosis of those disorders currently performed postnatally include more reproductive options for couples, and, in selected cases, the fact that certain genetic disorders can be treated much earlier in development, thereby potentially ameliorating the outcome of these disorders. Thus, the future of newborn screening will belong as much to the obstetrician as to the pediatrician, if not more so [271]. PCR has undergone rapid improvement since its initial development, such that the technique currently permits rapid, accurate, and predictive tests to be made in the field of prenatal diagnosis and has greatly aided forensic medicine. PCR has also facilitated advances in other fields, in particular PGD, virology, bacteriology, and cancer therapy [272]. More recent developments in FISH and QF-PCR techniques have led to rapid one-two days reporting for Down syndrome, opening the way to the possibility of targeted testing based on referral indication, thus reducing the incidence of difficult counseling issues and potentially unnecessary pregnancy terminations following the unexpected discovery of anomalies such as balanced chromosome rearrangements [273].

The future of prenatal diagnosis must lie in the noninvasive diagnosis of Down syndrome using fetal cells from maternal circulation. The discovery of cffDNA in maternal blood enabled the development of DNA-based NIPT. NIPT for chromosomal aneuploidy detection was first applied for clinical use a few years ago, resulting in a paradigm shift in prenatal testing. Apart from the use of cell-free fetal nucleic acids for the detection of fetal genetic or chromosomal diseases, the analysis of cell-free placental RNA and DNA methylation signatures allows the noninvasive monitoring of placental function. These developments have allowed the screening and identification of a range of pregnancy-associated diseases, providing a holistic approach to prenatal management. Recently, genome-wide fetal transcriptome and methylome can be obtained from maternal plasma, which allow the identification of novel biomarkers and the elucidation of the pathogenesis of maternal and fetal diseases. In fact, some studies demonstrated the feasibility of applying the RNA and DNA methylation analysis techniques for prenatal disease assessment [274]. NIPT utilizes cffDNA present in maternal peripheral blood to detect chromosomal abnormalities. The detection of T21, T18, and T13 in the fetus has become a common screening method during pregnancy and has been widely applied in routine clinical testing because of its analytical and clinical validity. Currently, NIPT involving CNV and other frequent single-gene disorders is being widely studied, and it plays an important and indispensable role in prenatal detection. The multiple approaches that have been reported and validated by various laboratories have different merits and limitations. Their clinical validity, utility, and application vary with different diseases. Before implementation of NIPT into clinical practice, a list of criteria that the application must meet is crucial. Essential parameters such as clinical sensitivity, clinical specificity, PPV, and NPV are required to properly evaluate the clinical validity and utility of NIPT [275].

NGS and other genomic technologies are transforming prenatal and reproductive screening and testing for fetal genetic disorders at an unprecedented pace. Original approaches of screening and testing for fetal genetic and genomic disorders were focused on a few more prevalent conditions that were easily diagnosable with pregenomic era diagnostic tools. First, CMA analysis and then NGS brought technology capable of more detailed genomic evaluation to prenatal genetic screening and diagnosis. This has facilitated parallel introduction of a variety of new tests on maternal blood samples, including expanded carrier screening and cffDNA-based noninvasive screening for fetal aneuploidy, selected CNV, and single-gene disorders. Genomic tests on fetal DNA samples, obtained primarily through amniocentesis or CVS, include CMA analysis and gene panel and exome sequencing. All these form the diagnostic pillar of the emerging field of fetal precision medicine, but their implementation is associated with ethical, counseling, and healthcare resource utilization challenges [276]. Two recent studies [277, 278] demonstrate the potential of applying the latest genome-sequencing technologies to preconception carrier testing and NIPD. These studies shine new light on old ethical, legal, and social concerns associated with genetic technology and deserve careful discussion [279]. Since the completion of the human genome map, genomics, proteomics, and pharmacogenomics have become popular headings. Collaborative approaches of clinicians, geneticists, pathologists, biochemists, and molecular biologists have contributed significantly to the prenatal diagnosis, genetic counseling, and prevention of single-gene disorders, and in some instances to successful treatment. DNA technology widens the range to predictive risk testing for multi-factorial disorders manifesting in adulthood. This offers new perspectives for potential patients and their close relatives, but also poses new psycho-social and ethical problems. Despite high expectations of new technologies in the development of new medicines for multi-factorial disorders, examples of previous studies on the molecular etiology and pathogenesis of monogenic diseases indicate that a long way is ahead of us. Also, the treatment of rare disorders and equal access to cure and care in the Third World need great attention [280].

The field of prenatal screening and diagnosis has undergone enormous progress over the past four decades. Most of this period has been characterized by gradual improvements in the technical and public health aspects of prenatal screening for Down syndrome. Compared to the direct analysis of fetal cells from amniocentesis or CVS, noninvasive approaches using maternal blood or ultrasound have the great advantage of posing no risk of miscarriage to the pregnancy. Recent advances in molecular genetics and DNA sequencing have revolutionized both the accuracy and the range of noninvasive testing for genetic abnormalities using cffDNA in maternal plasma. Many of these advances have already been incorporated into clinical care, including diagnosis of fetal blood group and aneuploidy screening. The accelerated pace of these recent developments is creating not just technical and logistical challenges, but is also magnifying the ethical and public policy issues traditionally associated with this field [281]. Multidisciplinary clinics are the most efficient means of providing antenatal genetic diagnosis. Advances in techniques such as ultrasonography and molecular genetics will extend the services available, and the impact of this will be felt by the community. Education of the medical profession and the public in this area is necessary so that informed decision-making can take place [282].

References

[1] Thorlacius, L. S., Blakney, G., Krahn, J., Bamforth, F. and Higgins, T. N. (2006). Biochemistry testing associated with pregnancy and the newborn period – A lot has changed since you were a baby! *Clin Biochem*, 519-541.

[2] Longo, L. D. Fundamental and clinical research and patient care: a triad for progress in reproductive medicine. (1988). *Am J Obstet Gynecol*, 6-12.

[3] Johnson, C. A. (1988). Prenatal screening. *Am Fam Physician*, 175-183.

[4] Rappaport, V. J. (2008). Prenatal diagnosis and genetic screening – Integration into prenatal care. *Obstet Gynecol Clin North Am*, 435-458.

[5] Smith, J. F. Jr. (2008). Fetal health assessment using prenatal diagnostic techniques. *Curr Opin Obstet Gynecol*, 152-156.

[6] Driscoll, D. A., Wenstrom, K. D. and Williams, J. 3rd; ACOG Committee on Genetics. (2002). ACOG Technology Assessment in Obstetrics and Gynecology. Number 1, July 2002. Genetics and molecular diagnostic testing. *Obstet Gynecol*, 193-211.

[7] Whittaker, L. (1996). Clinical applications of genetic testing: implications for the family physician. *Am Fam Physician*, 2077-2084.

[8] Control of hereditary diseases. Report of a WHO Scientific Group. (1996). *World Health Organ Tech Rep Ser*, 1-84.

[9] LeGrys, V. A., Leinbach, S. S. and Silverman, L. M. (1987). Clinical applications of DNA probes in the diagnosis of genetic diseases. *Crit Rev Clin Lab Sci*, 255-274.

[10] Bamforth, F. J. (1994). Laboratory screening for genetic disorders and birth defects. *Clin Biochem*, 333-342.

[11] Wieacker, P. and Steinhard, J. (2010). The prenatal diagnosis of genetic diseases. *Dtsch Arztebl Int*, 857-862.

[12] Ferguson-Smith, M. A. (2008). Cytogenetics and the evolution of medical genetics. *Genet Med*, 553-559.

[13] Cowan, R. S. (1993). Aspects of the history of prenatal diagnosis. *Fetal Diagn Ther*, 10-17.

[14] Bedei, I., Wolter, A., Weber, A., Signore, F. and Axt-Fliedner, R. (2021). Chances and Challenges of New Genetic Screening Technologies (NIPT) in Prenatal Medicine from a Clinical Perspective: A Narrative Review. *Genes (Basel)*, 501.

[15] Mărginean, C., Brînzaniuc, K., Mühlfay, G., Horvath, K. and Mărginean, O. (2010). The three-dimensional ultrasonography of the fetal face – History and progress. *Rev Med Chir Soc Med Nat Iasi*, 1058-1063.

[16] Aucamp, J., Bronkhorst, A. J., Badenhorst, C. P. and Pretorius, P. J. (2016). A historical and evolutionary perspective on the biological significance of circulating DNA and extracellular vesicles. *Cell Mol Life Sci*, 4355-4381.

[17] Chiu, R. W. and Lo, Y. M. (2013). Clinical applications of maternal plasma fetal DNA analysis: translating the fruits of 15 years of research. *Clin Chem Lab Med*, 197-204.

[18] Mennuti, M. T. (2008). Genetic screening in reproductive health care. *Clin Obstet Gynecol*, 3-23.

[19] Bittles, A. H. (2013). Genetics and global healthcare. *J R Coll Physicians Edinb*, 7-10.

[20] Burke, W., Tarini, B., Press, N. A. and Evans, J. P. (2011). Genetic screening. *Epidemiol Rev*, 148-164.

[21] Ram, K. T. and Klugman, S. D. (2010). Best practices: antenatal screening for common genetic conditions other than aneuploidy. *Curr Opin Obstet Gynecol*, 139-145.

[22] Cunniff, C. and Hudgins, L. (2010). Prenatal genetic screening and diagnosis for pediatricians. *Curr Opin Pediatr*, 809-813.

[23] Wojcik, M. H., Reimers, R., Poorvu, T. and Agrawal, P. B. (2020). Genetic diagnosis in the fetus. *J Perinatol*, 997-1006.

[24] Yagel, S. and Anteby, E. (1998). A rational approach to prenatal screening and intervention. *Hum Reprod*, 1126-1128.

[25] McCabe, L. L. and McCabe, E. R. (2004). Genetic screening: carriers and affected individuals. *Annu Rev Genomics Hum Genet*, 57-69.

[26] Cunniff, C.; American Academy of Pediatrics Committee on Genetics. (2004). Prenatal screening and diagnosis for pediatricians. *Pediatrics*, 889-894.

[27] Dolan, S. M. and Moore, C. (2007). Linking family history in obstetric and pediatric care: assessing risk for genetic disease and birth defects. *Pediatrics*, S66-70.

[28] Walter, J. H. (2009). Genes, patients, families, doctors – Mutation analysis in clinical practice. *J Inherit Metab Dis*, 441-446.

[29] Hsairi, M., Mehdi, F., Bellaaj, R. and Kassis, M. (2018). Health screening strategies in Maghreb countries: Situation Analysis and perspectives. *Tunis Med*, 688-695.

[30] Vallance, H. and Ford, J. (2003). Carrier testing for autosomal-recessive disorders. *Crit Rev Clin Lab Sci*, 473-497.

[31] Simpson, J. L. (1991). Screening for fetal and genetic abnormalities. *Baillieres Clin Obstet Gynaecol*, 675-696.

[32] Zinberg, R. E., Kornreich, R., Edelmann, L. and Desnick, R. J. (2001). Prenatal genetic screening in the Ashkenazi Jewish population. *Clin Perinatol*, 367-382.

[33] Eng, C. M. and Desnick, R. J. (2001). Experiences in molecular-based prenatal screening for Ashkenazi Jewish genetic diseases. *Adv Genet*, 275-296.

[34] Tunçbilek, E. and Ozgüç, M. (2007). Application of medical genetics in Turkey. *Turk J Pediatr*, 353-359.

[35] Jaber, L. and Halpern, G. J. (2006). Consanguinity among the Arab and Jewish populations in Israel. *Pediatr Endocrinol Rev*, 437-446.

[36] Rosner, G., Rosner, S. and Orr-Urtreger, A. (2009). Genetic testing in Israel: an overview. *Annu Rev Genomics Hum Genet*, 175-192.

[37] (2016). Practice Bulletin No. 162 Summary: Prenatal Diagnostic Testing for Genetic Disorders. *Obstet Gynecol*, 976-978.

[38] (2016). Practice Bulletin No. 162: Prenatal Diagnostic Testing for Genetic Disorders. *Obstet Gynecol*, e108-e122.

[39] Chitty, L. (1998). Prenatal screening for chromosome abnormalities. *Br Med Bull*, 839-856.

[40] (2016). Practice Bulletin No. 163 Summary: Screening for Fetal Aneuploidy. *Obstet Gynecol*, 979-981.

[41] (2016). Practice Bulletin No. 163: Screening for Fetal Aneuploidy. *Obstet Gynecol*, e123-e137.

[42] Kuppermann, M., Goldberg, J. D., Nease, R. F. Jr. and Washington, A. E. (1999). Who should be offered prenatal diagnosis? The 35-year-old question. *Am J Public Health*, 160-163.

[43] Hawk, A. F. and Saller, D. N. (2012). Screening for fetal aneuploidy: is maternal age relevant? *Clin Obstet Gynecol*, 217-225.

[44] Chitty, L. S. (1998). Antenatal screening for aneuploidy. *Curr Opin Obstet Gynecol*, 91-96.

[45] Evans, M. I., O'Brien, J. E., Dvorin, E. and Johnson, M. P. (1994). Biochemical screening. *Curr Opin Obstet Gynecol*, 453-458.

[46] Kilshaw, D. (1989). Screening for fetal abnormalities during pregnancy. *Med Lab Sci*, 244-249.

[47] Chitty, L. S. and Bobrow, M. (1994). Techniques in current use in prenatal diagnosis. *Int J Technol Assess Health Care*, 604-627.

[48] South, S. T., Chen, Z. and Brothman, A. R. (2008). Genomic medicine in prenatal diagnosis. *Clin Obstet Gynecol*, 62-73.

[49] Lowther, G. W. and Whittle, M. J. (1997). Prenatal diagnosis in the United Kingdom – An overview. *Eur J Hum Genet*, 84-89.

[50] Kabra, M. (2003). Prenatal diagnosis. *Indian J Pediatr*, 81-85.

[51] American College of Obstetricians and Gynecologists. (2007). ACOG Practice Bulletin No. 88, December 2007. Invasive prenatal testing for aneuploidy. *Obstet Gynecol*, 1459-1467.

[52] Papp, C. and Papp, Z. (2003). Chorionic villus sampling and amniocentesis: what are the risks in current practice? *Curr Opin Obstet Gynecol*, 159-165.

[53] Van Opstal, D. and Srebniak, M. I. (2016). Cytogenetic confirmation of a positive NIPT result: evidence-based choice between chorionic villus sampling and amniocentesis depending on chromosome aberration. *Expert Rev Mol Diagn*, 513-520.

[54] Wilson, R. D., Gagnon, A., Audibert, F., Campagnolo, C. and Carroll, J.; Genetics Committee. (2015). Prenatal Diagnosis Procedures and Techniques to Obtain a Diagnostic Fetal Specimen or Tissue: Maternal and Fetal Risks and Benefits. *J Obstet Gynaecol Can*, 656-668.

[55] (1995). Chorionic villus sampling and amniocentesis: recommendations for prenatal counseling. Centers for Disease Control and Prevention. *MMWR Recomm Rep*, 1-12.

[56] Eisenberg, B. and Wapner, R. J. (2002). Clinical procedures in prenatal diagnosis. *Best Pract Res Clin Obstet Gynaecol*, 611-627.

[57] Monni, G., Pagani, G., Stagnati, V., Iuculano, A. and Ibba, R. M. (2016). How to perform transabdominal chorionic villus sampling: a practical guideline. *J Matern Fetal Neonatal Med*, 1499-1505.

[58] Alfirevic, Z., Navaratnam, K. and Mujezinovic, F. (2017). Amniocentesis and chorionic villus sampling for prenatal diagnosis. *Cochrane Database Syst Rev*, CD003252.

[59] Reece, E. A. (1997). Early and midtrimester genetic amniocenteses. Safety and outcomes. *Obstet Gynecol Clin North Am*, 71-81.

[60] Seeds, J. W. (2004). Diagnostic mid trimester amniocentesis: how safe? *Am J Obstet Gynecol*, 607-615.

[61] Doran, T. A. (1990). Chorionic villus sampling as the primary diagnostic tool in prenatal diagnosis. Should it replace genetic amniocentesis? *J Reprod Med*, 935-940.

[62] Jenkins, T. M. and Wapner, R. J. (1999). First trimester prenatal diagnosis: chorionic villus sampling. *Semin Perinatol*, 403-413.

[63] Wapner, R. J. (1997). Chorionic villus sampling. *Obstet Gynecol Clin North Am*, 83-110.

[64] Kalousek, D.K. and Vekemans, M. (1996). Confined placental mosaicism. *J Med Genet*, 529-533.

[65] Schreck, R. R., Falik-Borenstein, Z. and Hirata, G. (1990). Chromosomal mosaicism in chorionic villus sampling. *Clin Perinatol*, 867-888.

[66] Wilkins-Haug, L. (1993). The emerging genetic theories of unstable DNA, uniparental disomy, and imprinting. *Curr Opin Obstet Gynecol,* 179-185.

[67] Tantravahi, U. and Wheeler, P. (2003). Molecular genetic testing for prenatal diagnosis. *Clin Lab Med*, 481-502.

[68] Eggermann, T. (2020). Prenatal Detection of Uniparental Disomies (UPD): Intended and Incidental Finding in the Era of Next Generation Genomics. *Genes (Basel)*, 1454.

[69] Wax, J. R. and Blakemore, K. J. (1992). What can be learned from cordocentesis? *Clin Lab Med*, 503-522.

[70] Hare, J. Y. and Ludomirsky, A. (1994). Cordocentesis: direct access to the fetal circulation for evaluating fetal wellbeing and thyroid function. *Curr Opin Obstet Gynecol*, 440-444.

[71] Wax, J. R. and Blakemore, K. J. (1993). Fetal blood sampling. *Obstet Gynecol Clin North Am*, 533-562.

[72] Ralston, S. J. and Craigo, S. D. (2004). Ultrasound-guided procedures for prenatal diagnosis and therapy. *Obstet Gynecol Clin North Am*, 101-123.

[73] Geaghan, S. M. (2012). Fetal laboratory medicine: on the frontier of maternal-fetal medicine. *Clin Chem*, 337-352.

[74] Cadrin, C. and Golbus, M. S. (1993). Fetal tissue sampling – Indications, techniques, complications, and experience with sampling of fetal skin, liver, and muscle. *West J Med*, 269-272.

[75] Reece, E. A. (1997). Embryoscopy and early prenatal diagnosis. *Obstet Gynecol Clin North Am*, 111-121.

[76] Antonucci, I., Provenzano, M., Rodrigues, M., Pantalone, A., Salini, V., Ballerini, P., Borlongan, C. V. and Stuppia, L. (2016). Amniotic Fluid Stem Cells: A Novel Source for Modeling of Human Genetic Diseases. *Int J Mol Sci*, 607.

[77] Prusa, A. R. and Hengstschlager, M. (2002). Amniotic fluid cells and human stem cell research: a new connection. *Med Sci Monit*, RA253-257.

[78] Geifman-Holtzman, O. and Ober Berman, J. (2008). Prenatal diagnosis: update on invasive versus noninvasive fetal diagnostic testing from maternal blood. *Expert Rev Mol Diagn*, 727-751.

[79] Mujezinovic, F. and Alfirevic, Z. (2012). Technique modifications for reducing the risks from amniocentesis or chorionic villus sampling. *Cochrane Database Syst Rev*, CD008678.

[80] Rose, N. C. and Eller, A. G. (2014). The impact of noninvasive fetal evaluation: its effect on education, training, and the maintenance of clinical competence in prenatal diagnosis. *Curr Opin Obstet Gynecol*, 117-123.

[81] Bubb, J. A. and Matthews, A. L. (2004). What's new in prenatal screening and diagnosis? *Prim Care*, 561-582.

[82] Wilson, R. D. (2000). Amniocentesis and chorionic villus sampling. *Curr Opin Obstet Gynecol*, 81-86.

[83] Shulman, L. P. and Elias, S. (1993). Amniocentesis and chorionic villus sampling. *West J Med*, 260-268.

[84] Ball, R. H. (2004). Invasive fetal testing. *Curr Opin Obstet Gynecol*, 159-162.

[85] Green, P. and Alfirevic, Z. (2005). The evidence base for fetal medicine. *Best Pract Res Clin Obstet Gynaecol*, 75-83.

[86] Nicolini, U. (1993). Prenatal diagnosis and fetal therapy. *Curr Opin Obstet Gynecol*, 50-55.

[87] Stojilkovic-Mikic, T. and Rodeck, C. H. (2003). Screening for chromosomal anomalies: first or second trimester, biochemical or ultrasound? *Ann Acad Med Singap*, 583-588.

[88] ACOG Committee on Practice Bulletins. (2007). ACOG Practice Bulletin No. 77: screening for fetal chromosomal abnormalities. *Obstet Gynecol*, 217-227.

[89] Vaiopoulos, A. G., Athanasoula, K. C., Papantoniou, N. and Kolialexi, A. (2013). Review: advances in non-invasive prenatal diagnosis. *In Vivo*, 165-170.

[90] Simpson, J. L. (1995). Noninvasive screening for prenatal genetic diagnosis. *Bull World Health Organ*, 799-804.

[91] Snow, T. M. and Coble, M. (2018). Maternal Prenatal Screening and Serologies. *Adv Neonatal Care,* 431-437.

[92] Bock, J. L. (1992). Current issues in maternal serum alpha-fetoprotein screening. *Am J Clin Pathol*, 541-554.

[93] Drugan, A., Dvorin, E., Obrien, J. E., Johnson, M. P. and Evans, M. I. (1991). Alpha-fetoprotein. *Curr Opin Obstet Gynecol*, 230-234.

[94] Ashwood, E. R. (1992). Evaluating health and maturation of the unborn: the role of the clinical laboratory. *Clin Chem*, 1523-1529.

[95] Ross, H. L. and Elias, S. (1997). Maternal serum screening for fetal genetic disorders. *Obstet Gynecol Clin North Am*, 33-47.

[96] Evans, M. I., O'Brien, J. E., Dvorin, E., Harrison, H. and Bui, T. H. (2001). Second-trimester biochemical screening. *Clin Perinatol*, 289-301.

[97] Budorick, N. E. and O'Boyle, M. K. (2003). Prenatal diagnosis for detection of aneuploidy: the options. *Radiol Clin North Am*, 695-708.

[98] Driscoll, D. A. and Gross, S. J.; Professional Practice and Guidelines Committee. (2008). First trimester diagnosis and screening for fetal aneuploidy. *Genet Med*, 73-75.

[99] Nicolaides, K. H. (2005). First-trimester screening for chromosomal abnormalities. *Semin Perinatol*, 190-194.

[100] Nicolaides, K. H. (2004). Nuchal translucency and other first-trimester sonographic markers of chromosomal abnormalities. *Am J Obstet Gynecol*, 45-67.

[101] Sherer, D. M., Bombard, A. T., Kellner, L. H. and Divon, M. Y. (1997). Noninvasive first-trimester screening for fetal aneuploidy. *Obstet Gynecol Surv*, 123-129.

[102] Kagan, K. O., Sonek, J., Wagner, P. and Hoopmann, M. (2017). Principles of first trimester screening in the age of non-invasive prenatal diagnosis: screening for chromosomal abnormalities. *Arch Gynecol Obstet*, 645-651.

[103] Breathnach, F. M. and Malone, F. D. (2007). Screening for aneuploidy in first and second trimesters: is there an optimal paradigm? *Curr Opin Obstet Gynecol*, 176-182.

[104] Reddy, U. M. and Wapner, R. J. (2007). Comparison of first and second trimester aneuploidy risk assessment. *Clin Obstet Gynecol*, 442-453.

[105] Martin, J. N. Jr. and Cowan, B. D. (1990). Biochemical assessment and prediction of gestational well-being. *Obstet Gynecol Clin North Am*, 81-93.

[106] Hecher, K., Snijders, R. and Nicolaides, K. (1993). Screening for fetal chromosomal abnormalities by maternal serum biochemistry and ultrasound examination of fetal morphology. *Curr Opin Obstet Gynecol*, 170-178.

[107] Wagner, R. K. and Calhoun, B. C. (1998). The routine obstetric ultrasound examination. *Obstet Gynecol Clin North Am*, 451-463.

[108] Pathak, S. and Lees, C. (2009). Ultrasound structural fetal anomaly screening: an update. *Arch Dis Child Fetal Neonatal Ed*, F384-F390.

[109] Carlson, D. E. and Platt, L. D. (1992). Ultrasound detection of genetic anomalies. *J Reprod Med*, 419-426.

[110] Sanders, R. C. (1991). Prenatal diagnosis of structural abnormalities. *Curr Opin Obstet Gynecol*, 259-265.

[111] Hyett, J., Mogra, R. and Sonek, J. (2014). First trimester ultrasound assessment for fetal aneuploidy. *Clin Obstet Gynecol*, 142-158.

[112] Evans, M. I., O'Brien, J. E. and Critchfield, G. (1998). Detection of anomalies: alternatives to ultrasound. *Ann N Y Acad Sci*, 191-199.

[113] Levi, S. (1998). Routine ultrasound screening of congenital anomalies. An overview of the European experience. *Ann N Y Acad Sci*, 86-98.

[114] Papp, Z. and Fekete, T. (2003). The evolving role of ultrasound in obstetrics/gynecology practice. *Int J Gynaecol Obstet*, 339-346.

[115] Woolf, S. H. (2001). The accuracy and effectiveness of routine population screening with mammography, prostate-specific antigen, and prenatal ultrasound: a review of published scientific evidence. *Int J Technol Assess Health Care*, 275-304.

[116] Whittle, W., Chaddha, V., Wyatt, P., Huppertz, B. and Kingdom, J. (2006). Ultrasound detection of placental insufficiency in women with

"unexplained" abnormal maternal serum screening results. *Clin Genet*, 97-104.

[117] Papageorghiou, A. T. and Leslie, K. (2007). Uterine artery Doppler in the prediction of adverse pregnancy outcome. *Curr Opin Obstet Gynecol*, 103-109.

[118] Mari, G. and Hanif, F. (2008). Fetal Doppler: umbilical artery, middle cerebral artery, and venous system. *Semin Perinatol*, 253-257.

[119] Kagan, K. O., Sonek, J., Wagner, P. and Hoopmann, M. (2017). Principles of first trimester screening in the age of non-invasive prenatal diagnosis: screening for other major defects and pregnancy complications. *Arch Gynecol Obstet*, 635-643.

[120] Stewart, T. L. (2004). Screening for aneuploidy: the genetic sonogram. *Obstet Gynecol Clin North Am*, 21-33.

[121] Bromley, B. and Benacerraf, B. R. (2003). The Genetic Sonogram Scoring Index. *Semin Perinatol*, 124-129.

[122] Van den Hof, M. C. and Wilson, R. D; Diagnostic Imaging Committee, Society of Obstetricians and Gynaecologists of Canada; Genetics Committee, Society of Obstetricians and Gynaecologists of Canada. (2005). Fetal soft markers in obstetric ultrasound. *J Obstet Gynaecol Can*, 592-636.

[123] Flood, K. and Malone, F. D. (2008). Screening for fetal abnormalities with ultrasound. *Curr Opin Obstet Gynecol*, 139-145.

[124] Stefanovic, V. (2015). Soft markers for aneuploidy following reassuring first trimester screening: what should be done? *Curr Opin Obstet Gynecol*, 151-158.

[125] Van Mieghem, T., Hindryckx, A. and Van Calsteren, K. (2015). Early fetal anatomy screening: who, what, when and why? *Curr Opin Obstet Gynecol*, 143-150.

[126] Winter, T. C. and Rose, N. C. (2018). How to Integrate Cell-Free DNA Screening With Sonographic Markers for Aneuploidy: An Update. *AJR Am J Roentgenol*, 906-912.

[127] Sherer, D. M. and Manning, F. A. (1999). First-trimester nuchal translucency screening for fetal aneuploidy. *Am J Perinatol*, 103-120.

[128] Jackson, M. and Rose, N. C. (1998). Diagnosis and management of fetal nuchal translucency. *Semin Roentgenol*, 333-338.

[129] Hyett, J. and Thilaganathan, B. (1999). First trimester screening for fetal abnormalities. *Curr Opin Obstet Gynecol*, 563-569.

[130] Malone, F. D., Berkowitz, R. L., Canick, J.A. and D'Alton, M. E. (2000). First-trimester screening for aneuploidy: research or standard of care? *Am J Obstet Gynecol*, 490-496.

[131] Souter, V. L. and Nyberg, D. A. (2001). Sonographic screening for fetal aneuploidy: first trimester. *J Ultrasound Med*, 775-790.

[132] Nicolaides, K. H., Bindra, R., Heath, V. and Cicero, S. (2002). One-stop clinic for assessment of risk of chromosomal defects at 12 weeks of gestation. *J Matern Fetal Neonatal Med*, 9-18.

[133] Snijders, R. and Smith, E. (2002). The role of fetal nuchal translucency in prenatal screening. *Curr Opin Obstet Gynecol*, 577-585.

[134] Rizzo, G., Pietrolucci, M., Aiello, E., Mammarella, S., Bosi, C. and Arduini, D. (2011). The role of three-dimensional ultrasound in the diagnosis of fetal congenital anomalies: a review. *Minerva Ginecol*, 401-410.

[135] Avni, F. E., Cos, T., Cassart, M., Massez, A., Donner, C., Ismaili, K. and Hall, M. (2007). Evolution of fetal ultrasonography. *Eur Radiol*, 419-431.

[136] Hengstschläger, M. (2006). Fetal magnetic resonance imaging and human genetics. *Eur J Radiol*, 312-315.

[137] Elles, R. (1997). An overview of clinical molecular genetics. *Mol Biotechnol*, 95-104.

[138] Dudarewicz, L., Holzgreve, W., Jeziorowska, A., Jakubowski, L. and Zimmermann, B. (2005). Molecular methods for rapid detection of aneuploidy. *J Appl Genet*, 207-215.

[139] Gupta, G. K. and Bianchi, D. W. (1997). DNA diagnosis for the practicing obstetrician. *Obstet Gynecol Clin North Am*, 123-142.

[140] Mathew, C. G. (1999). DNA diagnostics: goals and challenges. *Br Med Bull*, 325-339.

[141] Bozzette, M. (2002). Recent advances in prenatal screening and diagnosis of genetic disorders. *AACN Clin Issues*, 501-510.

[142] Amos, J. and Gold, B. (1998). Testing environment for single-gene disorders in U.S. reference laboratories. *Hum Mutat*, 293-300.

[143] Maddalena, A., Bick, D. P. and Schulman, J. D. (1992). Molecular diagnosis of genetic disease. *J Reprod Med*, 437-444.

[144] Myrianthopoulos, N. C. (1987). Molecular approaches in the prenatal diagnosis and therapy of genetic disorders. *Fetal Ther*, 160-168.

[145] Forrest, S. and Cotton, R. G. (1990). Methods of detection of single base substitutions in clinical genetic practice. *Mol Biol Med*, 451-459.

[146] Moser, G., Drewlo, S., Huppertz, B. and Armant, D. R. (2018). Trophoblast retrieval and isolation from the cervix: origins of cervical trophoblasts and their potential value for risk assessment of ongoing pregnancies. *Hum Reprod Update*, 484-496.

[147] Bischoff, F. Z. and Simpson, J. L. (2006). Endocervical fetal trophoblast for prenatal genetic diagnosis. *Curr Opin Obstet Gynecol*, 216-220.

[148] Zygula, A., Kosinski, P. and Wielgos, M. (2019). Saliva, hair, tears, and other biological materials obtained non-invasively for diagnosis in pregnancy: a literature review. *Ginekol Pol*, 475-481.

[149] Lamvu, G. and Kuller, J. A. (1997). Prenatal diagnosis using fetal cells from the maternal circulation. *Obstet Gynecol Surv*, 433-437.

[150] Senyei, A. E. and Wassman, E. R. (1993). Fetal cells in the maternal circulation. Technical considerations for practical application to prenatal diagnosis. *Obstet Gynecol Clin North Am*, 583-598.

[151] Anker, P. and Stroun, M. (2000). Circulating DNA in plasma or serum. *Medicina (B Aires)*, 699-702.

[152] Nandi, K., Verma, R., Dawar, R. and Goswami, B. (2020). Cell free DNA: revolution in molecular diagnostics – The journey so far. *Horm Mol Biol Clin Investig*, /j/hmbci.2020.41.issue-1/hmbci-2019-0012/hmbci-2019-0012.xml.

[153] Breveglieri, G., D'Aversa, E., Finotti, A. and Borgatti, M. (2019). Non-invasive Prenatal Testing Using Fetal DNA. *Mol Diagn Ther*, 291-299.

[154] Bianchi, D. W. (2004). Circulating fetal DNA: its origin and diagnostic potential – A review. *Placenta*, S93-S101.

[155] Holzgreve, W., Di Naro, E., Garvin, A. M., Troeger, C. and Hahn, S. (1998). Prenatal diagnosis using fetal cells enriched from maternal blood. *Croat Med J*, 115-120.

[156] Sifakis, S., Koukou, Z. and Spandidos, D. A. (2015). Cell-free fetal DNA and pregnancy-related complications (review). *Mol Med Rep*, 2367-2372.

[157] Guetta, E., Simchen, M. J., Mammon-Daviko, K., Gordon, D., Aviram-Goldring, A., Rauchbach, N. and Barkai, G. (2004). Analysis of fetal blood cells in the maternal circulation: challenges, ongoing efforts, and potential solutions. *Stem Cells Dev*, 93-99.

[158] Ho, S. S., O'Donoghue, K. and Choolani, M. (2003). Fetal cells in maternal blood: state of the art for non-invasive prenatal diagnosis. *Ann Acad Med Singap*, 597-603.

[159] Jeanty, C., Derderian, S. C. and Mackenzie, T. C. (2014). Maternal-fetal cellular trafficking: clinical implications and consequences. *Curr Opin Pediatr*, 377-382.

[160] Bianchi, D. W. (1998). Current knowledge about fetal blood cells in the maternal circulation. *J Perinat Med*, 175-185.

[161] Wright, C. F. and Burton, H. (2009). The use of cell-free fetal nucleic acids in maternal blood for non-invasive prenatal diagnosis. *Hum Reprod Update,* 139-51. doi: 10.1093/humupd/dmn047. Epub 2008 Oct 22.

[162] Norbury, G. and Norbury, C. J. (2008). Non-invasive prenatal diagnosis of single gene disorders: how close are we? *Semin Fetal Neonatal Med*, 76-83.

[163] Pös, O., Budiš, J. and Szemes, T. (2019). Recent trends in prenatal genetic screening and testing. *F1000Res*, F1000 Faculty Rev-764.

[164] Skirton, H. and Patch, C. (2013). Factors affecting the clinical use of non-invasive prenatal testing: a mixed methods systematic review. *Prenat Diagn*, 532-541.

[165] Woolcock, J. and Grivell, R. (2014). Noninvasive prenatal testing. *Aust Fam Physician*, 432-434.

[166] Dashe, J. S. (2016). Aneuploidy Screening in Pregnancy. *Obstet Gynecol*, 181-194.

[167] Robinson, C., van den Boom, D. and Bombard, A. T. (2014). Noninvasive prenatal detection of aneuploidy. *Clin Obstet Gynecol*, 210-225.

[168] Suciu, I., Galeva, S., Abdel Azim, S., Pop, L. and Toader, O. (2021). First-trimester screening-biomarkers and cell-free DNA. *J Matern Fetal Neonatal Med*, 3983-3989.

[169] Lo, Y. M. (2009). Noninvasive prenatal detection of fetal chromosomal aneuploidies by maternal plasma nucleic acid analysis: a review of the current state of the art. *BJOG*, 152-157.

[170] Nectoux, J. (2018). Current, Emerging, and Future Applications of Digital PCR in Non-Invasive Prenatal Diagnosis. *Mol Diagn Ther*, 139-148.

[171] Cerrato, F., Sparago, A., Ariani, F., Brugnoletti, F., Calzari, L., Coppedè, F., De Luca, A., Gervasini, C., Giardina, E., Gurrieri, F., Lo Nigro, C., Merla, G., Miozzo, M., Russo, S., Sangiorgi, E., Sirchia, S. M., Squeo, G. M., Tabano, S., Tabolacci, E., Torrente, I., Genuardi, M., Neri, G. and Riccio, A. (2020). DNA Methylation in the Diagnosis of Monogenic Diseases. *Genes (Basel)*, 355.

[172] Bianchi, D. W. and Wilkins-Haug, L. (2014). Integration of noninvasive DNA testing for aneuploidy into prenatal care: what has happened since the rubber met the road? *Clin Chem*, 78-87.

[173] Neofytou, M. (2020). Predicting fetoplacental mosaicism during cfDNA-based NIPT. *Curr Opin Obstet Gynecol*, 152-158.

[174] Saiki, R. K., Scharf, S., Faloona, F., Mullis, K. B., Horn, G. T., Erlich, H. A. and Arnheim, N. (1985). Enzymatic amplification of beta-globin genomic sequences and restriction site analysis for diagnosis of sickle cell anemia. *Science*, 1350-1354.

[175] Wright, P. A. and Wynford-Thomas, D. (1990). The polymerase chain reaction: miracle or mirage? A critical review of its uses and limitations in diagnosis and research. *J Pathol*, 99-117.

[176] Ben-Ezra, J. M. (1995). Amplification methods in the molecular diagnosis of genetic diseases. *Clin Lab Med*, 795-815.

[177] Steele, C. D., Wapner, R. J., Smith, J. B., Haynes, M. K. and Jackson, L. G. (1996). Prenatal diagnosis using fetal cells isolated from maternal peripheral blood: a review. *Clin Obstet Gynecol*, 801-813.

[178] Sayres, L. C. and Cho, M. K. (2011). Cell-free fetal nucleic acid testing: a review of the technology and its applications. *Obstet Gynecol Surv*, 431-442.

[179] Boehm, C. D. (1989). Use of polymerase chain reaction for diagnosis of inherited disorders. *Clin Chem*, 1843-1848.

[180] Van den Veyver, I. B. and Roa, B. B. (1998). Applied molecular genetic techniques for prenatal diagnosis. *Curr Opin Obstet Gynecol*, 97-103.

[181] Mansfield, E. S. (1993). Diagnosis of Down syndrome and other aneuploidies using quantitative polymerase chain reaction and small tandem repeat polymorphisms. *Hum Mol Genet*, 43-50.

[182] Pertl, B., Yau, S. C., Sherlock, J., Davies, A. F., Mathew, C. G. and Adinolfi, M. (1994). Rapid molecular method for prenatal detection of Down's syndrome. *Lancet*, 1197-1198.

[183] Pertl, B., Weitgasser, U., Kopp, S., Kroisel, P. M., Sherlock,, J. and Adinolfi, M. (1996). Rapid detection of trisomies 21 and 18 and sexing by quantitative fluorescent multiplex PCR. *Hum Genet*, 55–59.

[184] Adinolfi, M., Sherlock, J. and Pertl, B. (1995). Rapid detection of selected aneuploidies by quantitative fluorescent PCR. *Bioessays*, 661–664.

[185] Adinolfi, M., Pertl, B. and Sherlock, J. (1997). Rapid detection of aneuploidies by microsatellite and the quantitative fluorescent polymerase chain reaction. *Prenat Diagn*, 1299-1311.

[186] Hultén, M. A., Dhanjal, S. and Pertl, B. (2003). Rapid and simple prenatal diagnosis of common chromosome disorders: advantages and disadvantages of the molecular methods FISH and QF-PCR. *Reproduction*, 279-297.

[187] Roa, B. B., Pulliam, J., Eng, C. M. and Cheung, S. W. (2005). Evolution of prenatal genetics: from point mutation testing to chromosomal microarray analysis. *Expert Rev Mol Diagn*, 883-892.

[188] Rickman, L., Fiegler, H., Carter, N. P. and Bobrow, M. (2005). Prenatal diagnosis by array-CGH. *Eur J Med Genet*, 232-240.

[189] Hillman, S. C., Pretlove, S., Coomarasamy, A., McMullan, D. J., Davison, E. V., Maher, E. R. and Kilby, M. D. (2011). Additional information from array comparative genomic hybridization technology over conventional karyotyping in prenatal diagnosis: a systematic review and meta-analysis. *Ultrasound Obstet Gynecol*, 6-14.

[190] Wilson, R. D., Blight, C. and Langlois, S. (2009). Diagnosing chromosomal abnormalities from "big" to "small" with molecular cytogenetic technology. *J Obstet Gynaecol Can*, 414-421.

[191] Schaaf, C. P., Wiszniewska, J. and Beaudet, A. L. (2011). Copy number and SNP arrays in clinical diagnostics. *Annu Rev Genomics Hum Genet*, 25-51.

[192] Choy, K. W., Setlur, S. R., Lee, C. and Lau, T. K. (2010). The impact of human copy number variation on a new era of genetic testing. *BJOG*, 391-398.

[193] Savage, M. S., Mourad, M. J. and Wapner, R. J. (2011). Evolving applications of microarray analysis in prenatal diagnosis. *Curr Opin Obstet Gynecol*, 103-108.

[194] Rajcan-Separovic, E. (2012). Chromosome microarrays in human reproduction. *Hum Reprod Update*, 555-567.

[195] Kang, J. U. and Koo, S. H. (2012). Clinical implementation of chromosomal microarray technology in prenatal diagnosis. (Review). *Mol Med Rep*, 1219-1222.

[196] Wellesley, D. G. and Lucassen, A. (2014). Prenatal diagnosis of chromosomal imbalances. *Arch Dis Child Fetal Neonatal Ed*, F338-F341.

[197] South, S. T., Lee, C., Lamb, A. N., Higgins, A. W. and Kearney, H. M.; Working Group for the American College of Medical Genetics and Genomics Laboratory Quality Assurance Committee. (2013). ACMG Standards and Guidelines for constitutional cytogenomic microarray analysis, including postnatal and prenatal applications: revision 2013. *Genet Med*, 901-909.

[198] Wapner, R. J. and Levy, B. (2014). The impact of new genomic technologies in reproductive medicine. *Discov Med*, 313-318.

[199] Lo, J. O., Shaffer, B. L., Feist, C. D. and Caughey, A. B. (2014). Chromosomal microarray analysis and prenatal diagnosis. *Obstet Gynecol Surv*, 613-621.

[200] Batzir, N. A., Shohat, M. and Maya, I. (2015). Chromosomal Microarray Analysis (CMA) a Clinical Diagnostic Tool in the Prenatal and Postnatal Settings. *Pediatr Endocrinol Rev*, 448-454.

[201] Xu, H. B., Yang, H., Liu, G. and Chen, H. (2014). Systematic review of accuracy of prenatal diagnosis for abnormal chromosome diseases by microarray technology. *Genet Mol Res*, 9115-9121.

[202] Choy, R. K., Chen, Y., Sun, X. F., Kwok, Y. K. and Leung, T. Y. (2014). BACs-on-beads: a new robust and rapid detection method for prenatal diagnosis. *Expert Rev Mol Diagn*, 273-280.

[203] Go, A. T., van Vugt, J. M. and Oudejans, C. B. (2011). Non-invasive aneuploidy detection using free fetal DNA and RNA in maternal plasma: recent progress and future possibilities. *Hum Reprod Update*, 372-382.

[204] Andari, M. V. C., Bussamra, S. L. C., Tedesco, T. G. D., Peixoto, P. A. B., Pares, P. D. B. S., Braga, A., Araujo Júnior, E. and Aoki, T. (2020).

Noninvasive prenatal testing: benefits and limitations of the available tests. *Ceska Gynekol*, 41-48.

[205] Badeau, M., Lindsay, C., Blais, J., Nshimyumukiza, L., Takwoingi, Y., Langlois, S., Légaré, F., Giguère, Y., Turgeon, A. F., Witteman, W. and Rousseau, F. (2017). Genomics-based non-invasive prenatal testing for detection of fetal chromosomal aneuploidy in pregnant women. *Cochrane Database Syst Rev*, CD011767.

[206] Thung, D. T., Beulen, L., Hehir-Kwa, J. and Faas, B. H. (2015). Implementation of whole genome massively parallel sequencing for noninvasive prenatal testing in laboratories. *Expert Rev Mol Diagn*, 111-124.

[207] Sun, K., Jiang, P. and Chan, K. C. (2015). The impact of digital DNA counting technologies on noninvasive prenatal testing. *Expert Rev Mol Diagn*, 1261-1268.

[208] Guseh, S. H. (2020). Noninvasive prenatal testing: from aneuploidy to single genes. *Hum Genet*, 1141-1148.

[209] Manegold-Brauer, G., Hahn, S. and Lapaire, O. (2014). What does next-generation sequencing mean for prenatal diagnosis? *Biomark Med*, 499-508.

[210] Gregg, A. R., Van den Veyver, I. B., Gross, S. J., Madankumar, R., Rink, B. D. and Norton, M. E. (2014). Noninvasive prenatal screening by next-generation sequencing. *Annu Rev Genomics Hum Genet*, 327-347.

[211] Nepomnyashchaya, Y. N., Artemov, A. V., Roumiantsev, S. A., Roumyantsev, A. G. and Zhavoronkov, A. (2013). Non-invasive prenatal diagnostics of aneuploidy using next-generation DNA sequencing technologies, and clinical considerations. *Clin Chem Lab Med*, 1141-1154.

[212] Gregg, A. R., Gross, S. J., Best, R. G., Monaghan, K. G., Bajaj, K., Skotko, B. G., Thompson, B. H. and Watson, M. S. (2013). ACMG statement on noninvasive prenatal screening for fetal aneuploidy. *Genet Med*, 395-398.

[213] Yang, L., Chen, J. and Shen, B. (2017). Newborn Screening in the Era of Precision Medicine. *Adv Exp Med Biol*, 47-61.

[214] Hopkins, M. K., Dugoff, L. and Kuller, J. A. (2020). Exome Sequencing and Its Emerging Role in Prenatal Genetic Diagnosis. *Obstet Gynecol Surv*, 317-320.

[215] Abou Tayoun, A. and Mason-Suares, H. (2020). Considerations for whole exome sequencing unique to prenatal care. *Hum Genet*, 1149-1159.

[216] Pratt, M., Garritty, C., Thuku, M., Esmaeilisaraji, L., Hamel, C., Hartley, T., Millar, K., Skidmore, B., Dougan, S. and Armour, C. M. (2020). Application of exome sequencing for prenatal diagnosis: a rapid scoping review. *Genet Med*, 1925-1934.

[217] Peng, X. L. and Jiang, P. (2017). Bioinformatics Approaches for Fetal DNA Fraction Estimation in Noninvasive Prenatal Testing. *Int J Mol Sci*, 453.

[218] Straver, R., Sistermans, E. A. and Reinders, M. J. (2014). Introducing WISECONDOR for noninvasive prenatal diagnostics. *Expert Rev Mol Diagn*, 513-515.

[219] Sahajpal, N. S., Barseghyan, H., Kolhe, R., Hastie, A. and Chaubey, A. (2021). Optical Genome Mapping as a Next-Generation Cytogenomic Tool for Detection of Structural and Copy Number Variations for Prenatal Genomic Analyses. *Genes (Basel)*, 398.

[220] Allen, S., Young, E. and Bowns, B. (2017). Noninvasive prenatal diagnosis for single gene disorders. *Curr Opin Obstet Gynecol*, 73-79.

[221] D'ambrosio, V., Squarcella, A., Vena, F., Di Mascio, D., Corno, S., Pajno, C., Piccioni, M. G., Brunelli, R., Pizzuti, A., Benedetti Panici, P. and Giancotti, A. (2019). Update in non-invasive prenatal testing. *Minerva Ginecol*, 44-53.

[222] Cherry, A. M., Akkari, Y. M., Barr, K. M., Kearney, H. M., Rose, N. C., South, S. T., Tepperberg, J. H. and Meck, J. M. (2017). Diagnostic cytogenetic testing following positive noninvasive prenatal screening results: a clinical laboratory practice resource of the American College of Medical Genetics and Genomics (ACMG). *Genet Med*, 845-850.

[223] Wagner, R., Tse, W. H., Gosemann, J. H., Lacher, M. and Keijzer, R. (2019). Prenatal maternal biomarkers for the early diagnosis of congenital malformations: A review. *Pediatr Res*, 560-566.

[224] Vora, N. L. and Hui, L. (2018). Next-generation sequencing and prenatal 'omics: advanced diagnostics and new insights into human development. *Genet Med*, 791-799.

[225] Liu, W. (2019). Journal of Translational Medicine advances in Translational Genomics and Genetics Era. *J Transl Med*, 134.

[226] Shawky, R. M. and Sadik, D. I. (2011). The role of genomics in prevention or reducing the impact of congenital malformations. *Genet Couns*, 135-141.

[227] Avent, N. D., Plummer, Z. E., Madgett, T. E., Maddocks, D. G. and Soothill, P. W. (2008). Post-genomics studies and their application to non-invasive prenatal diagnosis. *Semin Fetal Neonatal Med*, 91-98.

[228] Wong, F. C. and Lo, Y. M. (2016). Prenatal Diagnosis Innovation: Genome Sequencing of Maternal Plasma. *Annu Rev Med*, 419-432.

[229] Mellis, R., Chandler, N. and Chitty, L. S. (2018). Next-generation sequencing and the impact on prenatal diagnosis. *Expert Rev Mol Diagn*, 689-699.

[230] Parfieniuk, E., Zbucka-Kretowska, M., Ciborowski, M., Kretowski, A. and Barbas, C. (2018). Untargeted metabolomics: an overview of its usefulness and future potential in prenatal diagnosis. *Expert Rev Proteomics*, 809-816.

[231] Korf, B. R. (2013). Integration of genomics into medical practice. *Discov Med*, 241-248.

[232] Hui, L. and Bianchi, D. W. (2017). Noninvasive Prenatal DNA Testing: The Vanguard of Genomic Medicine. *Annu Rev Med*, 459-472.

[233] Mahowald, M. B., Levinson, D. and Cassel, C. (1996). The new genetics and women. *Milbank Q*, 239-283.

[234] Bui, T. H., Blennow, E. and Nordenskjöld, M. (2002). Prenatal diagnosis: molecular genetics and cytogenetics. *Best Pract Res Clin Obstet Gynaecol*, 629-643.

[235] Ensenauer, R. E., Reinke, S. S., Ackerman, M. J., Tester, D. J., Whiteman, D.A. and Tefferi, A. (2003). Primer on medical genomics. Part VIII: Essentials of medical genetics for the practicing physician. *Mayo Clin Proc*, 846-857.

[236] Schimpf, M. O. and Domino, S. E. (2001). Implications of the Human Genome Project for obstetrics and gynecology. *Obstet Gynecol Surv*, 437-443.

[237] Lau, T. K. and Leung, T. N. (2005). Genetic screening and diagnosis. *Curr Opin Obstet Gynecol*, 163-169.

[238] Grace, M. R., Hardisty, E., Dotters-Katz, S. K., Vora, N. L. and Kuller, J. A. (2016). Cell-Free DNA Screening: Complexities and Challenges of Clinical Implementation. *Obstet Gynecol Surv*, 477-487.

[239] Liao, G. J., Gronowski, A. M. and Zhao, Z. (2014). Non-invasive prenatal testing using cell-free fetal DNA in maternal circulation. *Clin Chim Acta*, 44-50.

[240] Lo, Y. M. and Chiu, R. W. (2012). Genomic analysis of fetal nucleic acids in maternal blood. *Annu Rev Genomics Hum Genet*, 285-306.

[241] Shaffer, L. G. and Rosenfeld, J. A. (2013). Microarray-based prenatal diagnosis for the identification of fetal chromosome abnormalities. *Expert Rev Mol Diagn*, 601-611.

[242] Cleary-Goldman, J., D'Alton, M. E. and Berkowitz, R. L. (2005). Prenatal diagnosis and multiple pregnancy. *Semin Perinatol*, 312-320.

[243] Sebire, N. J. and Nicolaides, K. H. (1998). Screening for fetal abnormalities in multiple pregnancies. *Baillieres Clin Obstet Gynaecol*, 19-36.

[244] Odibo, A. O., Lawrence-Cleary, K. and Macones, G. A. (2003). Screening for aneuploidy in twins and higher-order multiples: is first-trimester nuchal translucency the solution? *Obstet Gynecol Surv*, 609-614.

[245] Appelman, Z. and Furman, B. (2005). Invasive genetic diagnosis in multiple pregnancies. *Obstet Gynecol Clin North Am*, 97-103.

[246] Bhide, A. and Thilaganathan, B. (2004). What prenatal diagnosis should be offered in multiple pregnancy? *Best Pract Res Clin Obstet Gynaecol*, 531-542.

[247] Post, A. L., Mottola, A. T. and Kuller, J. A. (2017). What's New in Prenatal Genetics? A Review of Current Recommendations and Guidelines. *Obstet Gynecol Surv*, 610-617.

[248] American College of Obstetricians and Gynecologists' Committee on Practice Bulletins – Obstetrics; Committee on Genetics; Society for Maternal-Fetal Medicine. (2020). Screening for Fetal Chromosomal Abnormalities: ACOG Practice Bulletin, Number 226. *Obstet Gynecol*, e48-e69.

[249] Summers, A. M., Langlois, S., Wyatt, P. and Douglas Wilson, R.; Members of the SOGC Genetics Committee; Members of the CCMG Committee on Prenatal Diagnosis; Members of the SOGC Diagnostic Imaging Committee. (2007). Prenatal screening for fetal aneuploidy. *J Obstet Gynaecol Can*, 146-161.

[250] Chitayat, D., Langlois, S. and Douglas Wilson, R.; SOGC Genetics Committee; CCMG Prenatal Diagnosis Committee. (2011). Prenatal screening for fetal aneuploidy in singleton pregnancies. *J Obstet Gynaecol Can*, 736-750.

[251] Gagnon, A; Genetics Committee. (2009). Evaluation of prenatally diagnosed structural congenital anomalies. *J Obstet Gynaecol Can*, 875-881.

[252] Wilson, K. L., Czerwinski, J. L., Hoskovec, J. M., Noblin, S. J., Sullivan, C. M., Harbison, A., Campion, M. W., Devary, K., Devers, P. and Singletary, C. N. (2013). NSGC practice guideline: prenatal screening and diagnostic testing options for chromosome aneuploidy. *J Genet Couns*, 4-15.

[253] (2015). Committee Opinion Summary No. 640: Cell-Free DNA Screening For Fetal Aneuploidy. *Obstet Gynecol*, 691-692.

[254] (2015). Committee Opinion No. 640: Cell-Free DNA Screening For Fetal Aneuploidy. *Obstet Gynecol*, e31-e37.

[255] Langlois, S. and Duncan, A.; SOGC Genetics Committee; CCMG Prenatal Diagnosis Committee. (2011). Use of a DNA method, QF-PCR, in the prenatal diagnosis of fetal aneuploidies. *J Obstet Gynaecol Can*, 955-960.

[256] Hardisty, E. E. and Vora, N. L. (2014). Advances in genetic prenatal diagnosis and screening. *Curr Opin Pediatr*, 634-638.

[257] Duncan, A. and Langlois, S.; SOGC Genetics Committee; CCMG Prenatal Diagnosis Committee. (2011). Use of array genomic hybridization

technology in prenatal diagnosis in Canada. *J Obstet Gynaecol Can*, 1256-1259.

[258] American College of Obstetricians and Gynecologists Committee on Genetics. (2012). Committee Opinion No. 545: Noninvasive prenatal testing for fetal aneuploidy. *Obstet Gynecol*, 1532-1534.

[259] Audibert, F. and Gagnon, A.; Genetics Committee of the Society of Obstetricians and Gynaecologists of Canada; Prenatal Diagnosis Committee of the Canadian College of Medical Geneticists. (2011). Prenatal screening for and diagnosis of aneuploidy in twin pregnancies. *J Obstet Gynaecol Can*, 754-767.

[260] Jackson-Cook, C. and Pandya, A. (1995). Strategies and logistical requirements for efficient testing in genetic disease. *Clin Lab Med*, 839-857.

[261] Isada, N. B. and Blakemore, K. J. (1993). Basic concepts in molecular (DNA) diagnosis. *Obstet Gynecol Clin North Am*, 413-420.

[262] Crisan, D. and Mattson, J. C. (1993). Retrospective DNA analysis using fixed tissue specimens. *DNA Cell Biol*, 455-464.

[263] Holzgreve, W., Nippert, I., Gänshirt-Ahlert, D., Schloo, R. and Miny, P. (1993). Immediate and long-term applications of technology. *Clin Obstet Gynecol*, 476-484.

[264] DiLiberti, J. H., Greenstein, M. A. and Rosengren, S. S. (1992). Prenatal diagnosis. *Pediatr Rev*, 334-342.

[265] Davis, J. G. (1993). Reproductive technologies for prenatal diagnosis. *Fetal Diagn Ther*, 28-38.

[266] Addar, M. H. (2000). New trends in prenatal screening for chromosomal abnormalities. *Saudi Med J*, 429-432.

[267] McCabe, E. R. (1991). Genetic screening for the next decade: application of present and new technologies. *Yale J Biol Med*, 9-14.

[268] Carbone, L., Cariati, F., Sarno, L., Conforti, A., Bagnulo, F., Strina, I., Pastore, L., Maruotti, G. M. and Alviggi, C. (2020). Non-Invasive Prenatal Testing: Current Perspectives and Future Challenges. *Genes (Basel)*, 15.

[269] Alamillo, C. M., Fiddler, M. and Pergament, E. (2012). Increased nuchal translucency in the presence of normal chromosomes: what's next? *Curr Opin Obstet Gynecol*, 102-108.

[270] Cogan, J. D. and Phillips, J. A. 3rd. (2006). New methods in genetic diagnosis including prenatal diagnosis. *Pediatr Endocrinol Rev*, 424-433.

[271] Evans, M. I. and Levy, H. L. (1999). The future of newborn screening belongs to obstetricians. *Acta Paediatr Suppl*, 55-57.

[272] Lynch, J. R. and Brown, J. M. (1990). The polymerase chain reaction: current and future clinical applications. *J Med Genet*, 2-7.

[273] Ogilvie, C. M. (2003). Prenatal diagnosis for chromosome abnormalities: past, present and future. *Pathol Biol (Paris)*, 156-160.

[274] Hui, W. W. and Chiu, R. W. (2016). Noninvasive prenatal testing beyond genomic analysis: what the future holds. *Curr Opin Obstet Gynecol*, 105-110.

[275] Shi, J., Zhang, R., Li, J. and Zhang, R. (2019). Novel perspectives in fetal biomarker implementation for the noninvasive prenatal testing. *Crit Rev Clin Lab Sci*, 374-392.

[276] Sabbagh, R. and Van den Veyver, I. B. (2020). The current and future impact of genome-wide sequencing on fetal precision medicine. *Hum Genet*, 1121-1130.

[277] Lo, Y. M., Chan, K. C., Sun, H., Chen, E. Z., Jiang, P., Lun, F. M., Zheng, Y. W., Leung, T. Y., Lau, T. K., Cantor, C. R. and Chiu, R. W. (2010). Maternal plasma DNA sequencing reveals the genome-wide genetic and mutational profile of the fetus. *Sci Transl Med*, 61ra91.

[278] Bell, C. J., Dinwiddie, D. L., Miller, N. A., Hateley, S. L., Ganusova, E. E., Mudge, J., Langley, R. J., Zhang, L., Lee, C. C., Schilkey, F. D., Sheth, V., Woodward, J. E., Peckham, H. E., Schroth, G. P., Kim, R. W. and Kingsmore, S. F. Carrier testing for severe childhood recessive diseases by next-generation sequencing. *Sci Transl Med*, 65ra4.

[279] Jackson, L. and Pyeritz, R. E. (2011). Molecular technologies open new clinical genetic vistas. *Sci Transl Med*, 65ps2.

[280] Galjaard, H. (2002). New names for old disciplines. *J Inherit Metab Dis*, 139-156.

[281] Hui, L. (2019). Noninvasive Approaches to Prenatal Diagnosis: Historical Perspective and Future Directions. *Methods Mol Biol*, 45-58.

[282] Benzie, R. J. (1979). Antenatal genetic diagnosis: current status and future prospects. *Can Med Assoc J*, 685-692.

Chapter 2

Tubal Ectopic Pregnancy: Treatment Update

Cristina de Miguel López[1,*], MD,
Enrique Achiaga Sánchez[1], MD,
María Teresa Gómez García[2,3], PhD,
Gema Serrano García[1], MD, Lidia Gómez Muñoz[1]
and Antonio Nicolás Amezcua Recover[2,3], PhD

[1]Obstetrics and Gynecology Department,
University and Hospital Complex of Albacete, Spain
[2]Obstetrics and Gynecology Department of the University and Hospital Complex of Albacete, Spain
[3]Medical Science Department, School of Medicine of Albacete,
Universidad de Castilla-La Mancha, Spain

Abstract

Ectopic pregnancy is defined as a pregnancy implanted at a place other than the endometrial line of the uterine body, mostly the fallopian tube (96%). In these days, EP remains the leading cause of early pregnancy related death. Diagnosis of this condition is usually made via transvaginal ultrasound. Serial serum beta-human chorionic gonadotrophin (β-hCG) measurement may help to differentiate normal from abnormal pregnancies and rise suspicion of an ectopic pregnancy.

Choosing between expectant, medical or surgical treatment is based on clinical characteristics, medical conditions, radiologic and laboratory findings as well as patient-informed choice based on discussion of each

---

* Corresponding Author's E-mail: cdmiguel@sescam.jccm.es.

In: A Closer Look at Pregnancy and Childbirth
Editor: Louise J. Salgado
ISBN: 978-1-68507-658-0

approach. In this chapter, our aim is to collect the latest evidence on treatment for tubal ectopic pregnancy, as well as to highlight the impact that drugs and surgical techniques used for this purpose may have.

Expectant management is restricted to a limited number of patients who must be asymptomatic, be aware of the clinical implications and have a serum β-hCG concentration below 1500 mIU/mL

Although surgical approach is the prop of treatment, medical therapy has shown similar success rates in selected patients. The main pharmacologic agent used for ectopic pregnancy treatment is metothrexate (MTX), a drug which inhibits dihydrofolate reductase, leading to the inhibition of DNA synthesis, repair, and cellular replication. MTX is usually administered intramuscularly at a single dose of 50mg/m2. The candidates to this line of treatment are those patients who are hemodynamically stable, have serum β-hCG concentration below 5000 mIU/mL, do not present fetal cardiac activity on the ultrasound scan and do not have any contraindications for the use of this drug. Some other drugs have been proposed to be used in combination with MTX-based therapy such as mifepristone - a progesterone antagonist - and gefitinib, a selective inhibitor of the tyrosine kinase domain of epidermal growth factor receptor. However, none of these drugs have managed to oust MTX as treatment of choice.

Patients who meet the inclusion criteria to receive medical treatment are generally candidates to surgery. Emergency surgical treatment is indicated for patients with hemodynamic instability or evidence of an ongoing ruptured ectopic mass. In stable or asymptomatic women, surgery is necessary in heterotopic pregnancies, if medical treatment is contraindicated or follow-up cannot be achieved or if the patient has a concurrent abnormality that may be solved in the same procedure. Laparoscopic approach is preferable. Salpingectomy should be performed in women with severe tubal damage, significant bleeding and in cases of desired fertility with a healthy contralateral tube. Salpingostomy is technically more difficult and needs serial β-hCG measurements but it should be performed in cases of previous contralateral salpingectomy or tubal damage and reproductive wish.

Keywords: tubal ectopic pregnancy, methrotexate, laparoscopy, salpingectomy, salpingostomy

Introduction

Ectopic pregnancy is defined as gestational sac implantation outside the uterine cavity and is estimated to account for 1.5% to 2% of all pregnancies

(Chang et al. 2003). Tubal ectopic pregnancy is the most common of all blastocyst implantation disorders: at least 90% of all ectopic pregnancies occur in the fallopian tube, and 80% implant in the ampullary portion of the fallopian tube (Wong and Clark 1968). The condition has become more common in recent decades, mainly due to assisted-reproduction techniques (ART), although this rise has fortunately not been accompanied by higher rates of mortality or severe morbidity. Early diagnosis before fallopian tube rupture and greater treatment efficacy have lowered mortality (Chang et al. 2003), although tubal ectopic pregnancy still accounts for 4% of maternal deaths in the U.S. in the early 21st century ("Ectopic Pregnancy Mortality - Florida, 2009-2010." 2012).

The current therapeutic armamentarium includes expectant management of tubal ectopic pregnancy, medical treatment with methotrexate (MTX) at different doses and via different routes of administration, conservative surgery (salpingostomy), radical surgery (salpingectomy), and new medical strategies (mifepristone, gefitinib).

We review the indications for each of the different therapeutic options and present the success rates, economic costs, risk of failure, prognosis of fertility, risk of another ectopic pregnancy, and follow-up time to full cure.

Expectant Management

The first author to report his experience in this field was Lund (LUND 1955) in 1955. Among all the articles published by 2004, only two well-designed studies compared expectant management with medical treatment. One was a double-blind clinical trial conducted by Korhonen et al. to compare expectant management with low-dose MTX (Korhonen, Stenman, and Ylöstalo 1996). This study included 60 patients diagnosed with ectopic pregnancy by vaginal ultrasound and serum β-hCG levels. The inclusion criteria were as follows: a) mild symptoms, b) β-hCG increase < 50% in 48 hours, c) ectopic pregnancy diameter < 40 mm, d) no ultrasound signs of intra-abdominal bleeding, and e) no other reason for laparoscopy. Patients were randomized to oral MTX 2.5 mg for 5 days or oral placebo for 5 days. Patients were then monitored by serial tests every 48 hours (complete blood count, chemistry, β-hCG levels) and vaginal ultrasound at 5 and 12 days. Surgical laparoscopy was performed in cases of abdominal pain and/or intra-abdominal hemorrhaging diagnosed by ultrasound. Laparoscopy was not required for cure in 77% of patients in each group. There were no differences in recovery time between the groups.

Mean serum β-hCG levels were low at 211 IU/L (range, 20-1343) in the group managed expectantly and 395 IU/L (range, 61-4279) in the MTX group. These authors concluded that low-dose oral MTX seems to be no more effective than placebo in women with ectopic pregnancy selected for expectant management.

The other study was a small clinical trial that compared prostaglandin therapy (local and systemic) with expectant management. A total of 23 patients with unruptured ectopic pregnancy and β-hCG levels < 2500 IU/L were included. The results showed that expectant management should only be recommended in a few selected cases, as it was significantly less successful than prostaglandin therapy (odds ratio [OR], 0.08; 95% confidence interval [CI], 0.02-0.39) (Egarter, Kiss, and Husslein 1991).

All these data are also included in the 2007 Cochrane Database System Review (Hajenius et al. 2007). Sadly, few conclusions can be drawn from this review since the treatment arm in both clinical trials included drugs (oral MTX and prostaglandins) that are no longer used in the clinical practice.

The METEX study (van Mello et al. 2013) is a multicenter, randomized clinical trial conducted in the Netherlands between April 2007 and January 2012. This study included 73 patients older than age 18 who were hemodynamically stable, had been diagnosed by ultrasound with ectopic pregnancy (ectopic ring or ectopic mass and/or fluid in the pouch of Douglas), and plateaued serum β-hCG levels < 1500 IU/L. Patients with signs of shock or fallopian tube rupture, an embryo with a positive heartbeat, or any contraindication for MTX were excluded. Patients who signed the informed consent were randomized to the expectant management group (32 patients) or a single intramuscular MTX injection of 1 mg/kg body weight (41 women) within 24 hours after randomization. The results showed no significant differences in cure rate between the two groups; 76% of patients treated with MTX (31/41) achieved negative β-hCG levels with no further medical action. In the expectant management group, 59% (19/32) progressed satisfactorily (relative risk [RR], 1.3; 95% CI, 0.9-1.8). Consequently, almost 60% of patients benefited from therapeutic abstention and from avoiding MTX, a potentially hazardous drug. According to the study authors, the main limitation was that no placebo group was included. Later, we will describe newer evidence that solves this bias risk.

Ylöstalo conducted a prospective study and found that approximately 20% of all tubal ectopic pregnancies will resolve spontaneously by tubal abortion into the abdominal cavity or by necrosis and cell reabsorption (Ylöstalo et al. 1992). The key is to clearly identify patients who will be cured with no pharmacologic or surgical intervention, in short, the group whose ectopic pregnancies are much less active. The problem, however, is that no pathognomonic signs exist to help select these patients. In view of the literature described and other recent articles (Mavrelos et al. 2013), expectant management is a safe, acceptable, and effective treatment option of tubal ectopic pregnancy in cases of very less active ectopic pregnancies that can be defined using the following criteria:

- Clinical stability with no or minimal abdominal pain,
- No evidence of significant hemoperitoneum on ultrasound scan,
- Ectopic pregnancy measuring < 30 mm in mean diameter with no evidence of embryonic cardiac activity,
- Serum β-human chorionic gonadotropin (β-hCG) < 1500 IU/L, and
- Patient consent

For the first time, RCOG guidelines included in 2019, expectant management as a new approach to selected patients (Webster et al. 2019).

In 2015, a Brazilian group published the first randomised trial comparing MTX to expectant management with placebo (Silva et al. 2015). Inclusion criteria were similar to the previous studies mentioned above: hemodynamic stability, initial serum β-hCG concentration < 2,000 mIU/mL, declining titers of β-hCG 48 h prior to treatment, visible tubal pregnancy without cardiac activity or signs of tubal rupture on transvaginal ultrasound < 5.0 cm and fertility desire. Patients with contraindications for MTX were excluded 10 patients were allocated to the MTX group and 13 to the placebo group. Successful treatment with negative titers of β-hCG was achieved in 9 cases (90.0%) within the treatment group and in 12 (92.3%) within the control group ($p > 0.999$). No difference between time for β-hCG value to become undetectable was observed (22 ± 15.4 days for MTX vs 20.6 ± 8.4 days for placebo ($p = 0.80$)).

Jurkovic et al. published a multicenter randomised controlled trial that took place between 2005 and 2014 in the UK. It is to date, the largest published clinical trial that compares expectant management with medical treatment (D Jurkovic et al. 2017). Inclusion criteria were clinically stable women with a conclusive ultrasound diagnosis of a tubal ectopic pregnancy with absence of both an embryonic heartbeat and hemoperitoneum, presenting with a low serum β-hCG level of < 1500 IU/L and no contraindications to MTX administration. Women were assigned randomly to a single systemic injection of either 50 mg/m2 MTX (42 patients) or placebo (38 patients). The primary outcome of the study was the resolution of clinical symptoms and decline in level of serum β-hCG to < 20 IU/L or a negative urine pregnancy test. The rates of success were 89% for methotrexate and 74% for placebo. The difference in success rate was not statistically significant ($\chi2 = 2.4$; $P = 0.12$). The authors emphasize the success rate when baseline serum β -hCG level is 1000–1500 IU/L. In this subgroup the difference noted was a 33% success in expectant management compared with 62% in those receiving MTX, again not statistically significant. Higher successful rates were observed in the study by Silva et al. since a particular inclusion criteria was the declining titers of β-hCG 48 h prior to treatment which already means involution of pregnancy (Silva et al. 2015).

As shown, recent bibliography highlights the absence of difference in success rates between expectant management and MTX in very selected patients. Benefits of choosing this option include: low cost, lower complication rates and avoidance of use of MTX; the latter usually seems an attractive advantage to women desiring future pregnancies. When choosing this strategy, patients must be informed that, although uncommon, complication features like tubal rupture may happen. If women experience abdominal pain or heavy bleeding, they must be urged to seek medical assistance immediately. Thus, patients that are unable to be assisted by a practitioner in a relatively short period of time are not encouraged to choose this treatment option.

Follow-up: Some clinicians believe that expectant management of ectopic pregnancy is linked to a longer follow-up period until β-hCG is negative compared to medical treatment. No difference in the duration of the follow-up has been reported in the studies previously presented. In a retrospective study of 158 women with diagnosis of tubal ectopic pregnancy that were managed expectantly, a median length of follow-up until resolution of 18 days was expected (Mavrelos et al. 2015). During follow-up, a decrease of more than a 15% of β-hCG in 3 consequent measurements is needed to keep this strategy. Afterwards, weekly measurements of β-hCG until it is undetectable. If after 10 weeks of weekly controls, β-hCG is still positive, a single dose of MTX is recommended. If a woman cannot comply with this strict and close follow-up, expectant management must be discouraged.

RCOG recommends β-hCG check on days 2,4, and 7 after the initial test. If levels drop by >15% on days 2,4, and 7, weekly monitoring is required until a negative result is obtained. When β-hCG titers do not fall by more than 15%, maintain their levels or rise, expectant management should be consequently abandoned (Webster et al. 2019).

Medical Treatment

At present, medical treatment of ectopic pregnancy is synonymous with MTX. MTX is a folic acid antagonist that selectively inhibits the enzyme dihydrofolate reductase, thus preventing folates from being reduced to tetrahydrofolates. This metabolic event is not the only inherent event of the drug, as the agent also exerts an antiproliferative cellular effect via the polyglutamate chain. It acts by inhibiting thymidylate synthetase, stopping reactions key to de novo synthesis of purine and pyrimidine nucleotides and thus interrupting DNA and RNA synthesis. Because syncytiotrophoblast cells have strong metabolic activity, MTX has a trophic action on such cells and the drug works well, due to rich perfusion in the region.

MTX crosses the cell membrane weakly and requires a specific, active, and saturable transport mechanism to reach the cell cytoplasm. It leads to partial destruction of phase S populations inside the trophoblastic cell and is much more effective for logarithmic growth phases. This mechanism of action is responsible for regression of ectopic pregnancy. The drug is readily absorbed in the gastrointestinal tract at low doses, but incompletely at higher doses, in which case parenteral administration is recommended. A total of 40% to 90% is excreted in urine as parent drug within 48 hours.

The toxic effects of MTX mainly affect the gastrointestinal tract and bone marrow and are usually reversible, although severe symptoms have been described. Obvious lesions in the intestinal epithelium will lead to nausea, abdominal pain, and bloody diarrhea. Bone marrow degeneration is seen in the circulating blood as pronounced leukopenia. There have also been reports of stomatitis, elevated liver enzymes, and at higher doses, anorexia, progressive weight loss, depression, and coma (Stika 2012).

One of the key aspects in medical treatment for ectopic pregnancy is to identify the ideal candidate to receive MTX. An ideal patient for MTX would meet the following criteria (Bachman and Barnhart 2012) (Table 1):

- Hemodynamic stability and no severe or persistent abdominal pain
- Low initial β-hCG concentration (<5000 IU/l)
- Small mass (< 4 cm) by transvaginal ultrasonography
- Unruptured mass
- No embryonic cardiac activity

- Certainty that there is no intrauterine pregnancy
- Willingness for follow-up
- No known sensitivity to MTX
- Normal baseline liver and renal function test results

Table 1. Selection of appropriate candidates for medical management of ectopic pregnancy

Good Candidate	Poor Candidate	Contraindicated
Hemodynamically stable	High HCG (>5000 IU/L)	Intrauterine pregnancy
No severe or persistent abdominal pain	Large mass (<4 cm)	Evidence of immunodeficiency
Low β-HCG (< 5000 IU/L)	Embryonic cardiac activity present	Moderate to severe anemia, leucopenia or thrombocytopenia
Small mass (< 4 cm)	Significant abdominal pain	Sensitivity to MTX
Unruptured mass	Refusal to accept blood transfusion	Active pulmonary disease
No embryonic cardiac activity	Inability to participate in follow-up	Active peptic ulcer disease
Certainty that there is no intrauterine pregnancy		Clinically important liver impairment
Willingness for follow-up		Clinically important renal impairment
No known sensitivity to MTX		Breastfeeding

Bachman and Barhhart 2012, Pfeifer et al. 2013.

When the patient to be treated with MTX is adequately selected, the success rate has been reported as 63% to 96.7% of cases (Capmas, Bouyer, and Fernandez 2014) and according to the Practice Committee of the American Society for Reproductive Medicine ("Medical Treatment of Ectopic Pregnancy: A Committee Opinion." 2013) MTX represents first-line therapy for unruptured ectopic pregnancy that is diagnosed early. Comparably to expectant management, close monitoring after injection of MTX is needed. Women must be able to attend posttreatment follow-up appointments and have access to emergency medical services within a reasonable timeframe in case of symptoms of tubal rupture.

Once MTX treatment has been decided, the ideal dose, follow-up, and route of administration must be defined.

MTX Dose

Three MTX treatment regimens are commonly used at present: multiple, double and single dose (Table 2).

- The multiple-dose protocol includes folinic acid (leucovorin) to attenuate the toxicity of chemotherapy. At present, the regimen used most often consists of four doses, which involve four MTX injections of 1 mg/kg/day, alternating every 24 hours with 0.1 mg/kg of leucovorin. Treatment is considered successful when β-hCG levels drop at least 15% from previous levels. β-hCG levels should be monitored weekly thereafter, until the results are negative (Bachman and Barnhart 2012).
- The single-dose protocol consists of 50 mg/m^2 body surface area of intramuscular MTX as a single dose, eliminating leucovorin rescue therapy. Treatment success is defined as a drop of at least 15% in β-hCG levels between days 4 and 7, with patient follow-up thereafter consisting of weekly β-hCG testing until levels are undetectable. If the expected reduction is not achieved between day 4 and 7, the MTX dose should be repeated (Bachman and Barnhart 2012).
- The double-dose protocol was introduced to achieve a balance between the benefits of higher success rates of multiple-dose protocol, the inconvenients of its side effects and the strict follow-up schedule of the single-dose protocol (Barnhart et al. 2007). It consists of a 50mg /m^2 body surface area of intramuscular MTX in days 0 and 4. Treatment success definition is equal to the single-dose regimen. Unless there is a >15% drop in β-hCG levels between days 4 and 7, a third dose should be administered on day 7. β-hCG will again be tested on day 11. Again, if we do not see a >15% drop, a fourth dose MTX must be dispensed. If levels have not decreased by day 14th, surgical treatment must be considered. If treatment succeeds, then weekly determination must be followed.

Later, the 2007 Cochrane Database System Review (Hajenius et al. 2007) included two clinical trials with a total of 159 patients diagnosed with ectopic pregnancy, in which the results showed no significant differences between single and multiple dose treatment groups (OR, 0.89; 95% CI, 0.32-2.5). Mean serum β-hCG concentrations varied between 2230 to 2973 IU/L in the single-dose group (50 mg/m^2) and 2180 to 2244 IU/L in the multiple dose group (1 mg/kg). At present, the Practice Committee of the American Society for Reproductive Medicine (ASRM, 2013) again recommends the multiple-dose protocol, as it has a lower failure rate than the single-dose MTX protocol.

Table 2. Methotrexate regimens used to treat ectopic pregnancy, modified from Bachman et al.

Protocol (Dose)	MTX Dose	Regimen	β-hCG Measurement	Treatment Success	When to Administer Additional Dose
Multiple	1 mg/kg and 0.1 mg/kg leucovorin	Alternate daily doses of each	Days 0, 1, 3, 5, 7	β-hCG drops 15% from previous value	Second, third, or fourth dose given if β-hCG does not drop 15% from previous value. Maximum of 4 doses
Single	50 mg/m^2	Day 0	Days 0, 4, 7	β-hCG declines 15% between days 4 and 7	Second dose on day 7 if β- hCG does not drop 15%
Double	50mg/m^2	Day 0 and 4	Days 0, 4, 7 If necessary, 11 and 14	β-hCG declines 15% between days 4 and 7 or 7 and 11; or 11 and 14	Repeat dose on day 7, 11 and 14 if β-hCG does not drop 15%

In 2017, a systematic review of 6 controlled clinical trials (table 3) that compared the effectiveness and safety between different dosages of MTX was performed (Yang et al. 2017). The study design followed the PRISMA statement guidelines. The risk of bias of the included studies was moderate-high. The studies' eligibility criteria included those randomized controlled trials performed in patients diagnosed with ectopic pregnancy comparing single-dose vs. double-dose or multiple-dose MTX. The main outcomes were the overall success events and the side-effects. The overall-success was defined as a higher than 15% reduction of β-hCG between day 4 and day 7 (single- and double-dose group). For multiple-dose protocol, the treatment success was defined as a 15% decrease of β-hCG in 48h or after administration of four doses of MTX. Comparing single and double-dose, a non-significant trend towards a higher success after the second option was found (RR 1.09, 95% CI 0.98 to 1.20, I 2 = 0%).

Regarding the side effects, a non-significant higher trend was observed after the administration of double-dose MTX (RR 1.33, 95% CI 0.92 to 1.94, I2 = 0%). Double-dose regimen was found to be more efficient in women with a baseline β-hCG between 3600-5500 IU/L or a mass diameter between 2,7 and 3,5cm. Between single and multiple-dose protocols, both success rates were similar (RR 1.07, 95% CI 0.99 to 1.17, I2 = 0%). In contrast, side-effects observed in the second group were significantly higher (RR 1.64, 95% CI 1.15 to 2.34, P = 0.006; I2 = 0%). ACOG recommendations issued in 2018 state that the single-dose protocol may be used in patients with a relatively low initial β-hCG level or a plateu in its values, while the double-dose regimen may be considered in women with an initial high β-hCG value. Unfortunately, no precise thresholds of β-hCG values to choose between one or another regimen have been indicated.

Route of Administration

Over time, a wide variety of MTX dosing routes have been tested, although all recent studies use the intramuscular route, either for a single, double or multiple-dose regimen. Oral route may be a reasonable alternative with similar outcomes to intramuscular route, but scarcely used. Local injection of the drug in the gestational sac has major advantages, as elevated MTX concentrations are achieved inside the ectopic pregnancy and general toxicity is reduced. If a laparoscopic approach is chosen (Jamal and Amarin 2001), then the patient also runs the inherent risks of both this technique and the fluoroscopy-guided vaginal route (Gervaise et al. 2003), which makes it essential to locate the sac accurately. Additionally, the operator must have sufficient experience and adequate instruments. MTX instillation via hysteroscopic fallopian tube catheterization has also been tested but requires skilled gynecologists (Goldenberg et al. 1992).

Table 3. Main characteristics of the studies included in systematic review by Yang et al. comparing doses of MTX

Study	Study design	Treatment		Inclusion criteria	Exclusion criteria	Main outcomes
		Single-dose group	Double/multiple-dose group			
Hamed et al., 2012	RCT	50mg/m^2 MTX day 0 (n=78)	50mg/m^2 MTX days 0 and 4 (n=79)	<4cm, β-hCG <15000IU/L, no cardiac activity, haemodynamic stability	Non-adnexal ectopic pregnancy, clinically or by ultrasound suspected tubal rupture, contraindications of MTX use	Succes rate, side effects, treatment duration
Saadati et al., 2016	RCT	50mg/m^2 MTX day 0 (n=38)	50mg/m^2 MTX days 0 and 4 (n=38)	β-hCG <15000IU/L, no cardiac activity, haemodynamic stability	Contraindications of MTX use	Succes rate, side effects
Song et al., 2016	RCT	50mg/m^2 MTX day 0 (n=46)	50mg/m^2 MTX days 0 and 4 (n=46)	<4cm, β-hCG <15000IU/L, no cardiac activity, haemodynamic stability, tubal pregnancy except interstitial location	Heterotopic pregnancy, persistence of ectopic pregnancy, clinically or by ultrasound suspected tubal rupture, contraindications of MTX use	Succes rate, side effects, treatment satisfaction, cost, days off work
Alleyassin et al., 2006	RCT	50mg/m^2 MTX day 1 (n=54)	1 mg/kg MTX, days 1,3,5,7 PLUS leucovorin 0,1 mg/kg days 2,4,6,8 (n=54)	<3,5cm, β-hCG <15000IU/L, no cardiac activity, haemodynamic stability	Clinically or by ultrasound suspected tubal rupture	Succes rate, side effects
Guvendag Guven et al., 2010	RCT	50mg/m^2 MTX day 1 (n=62)	1 mg/kg MTX, days 1,3,5,7 PLUS leucovorin 0,1 mg/kg days 2,4,6,8 (n=58)	<3,5 cm, β-hCG reaching plateau, no history of tubal surgery, haemodynamic stability	Liver or kidney disease	Succes rate, side effects
Tabatabaii Bafghi et al., 2012	RCT	50mg/m^2 MTX day 1 (n=35)	1 mg/kg MTX, days 1,3,5,7 PLUS leucovorin 0,1 mg/kg days 2,4,6,8 (n=35)	<4cm, β-hCG <15000IU/L, no cardiac activity, haemodynamic stability	Bleeding shown by ultrasound or LPS surgery	Succes rate, side effects, fertility

RCT: randomized controlled trial.

Other Pharmacologic Strategies

The next pharmacologic strategies that will be presented are hypothetically intended to enhance MTX efficacy and increase the percentage of ectopic pregnancies that can be safely treated medically, thus avoiding surgery. According to Jurkovic and Wilkinson, MTX has a limited role because not more than 25% to 30% of ectopic pregnancies meet the criteria to be safely treated using a medical strategy (Davor Jurkovic and Wilkinson 2011). Therefore, any new therapeutic agent able to raise the success rate would increase the percentage of ectopic pregnancies cured with no need for surgery.

These new drugs (mifepristone and gefitinib) would be indicated in hemodynamically stable patients with active ectopic pregnancies when the fallopian tube is not yet ruptured but the risk is high. Patients could benefit if they do not fully meet the treatment criteria for MTX (eg, ectopic pregnancies with very high β-hCG levels, very large ectopic pregnancies, or live embryos), in short, if they have signs indicating that an ectopic pregnancy is in progress.

At present, there is considerably more experience with mifepristone. Molecularly, this drug selectively occupies and competes with the endogenous progesterone receptor, thus destroying trophoblastic and decidual tissue, lowering luteinizing-hormone levels, and blocking the corpora lutea, which leads to embryo necrosis and abortion. It plays an important role as MTX co-adjuvant in the treatment of unruptured tubal ectopic pregnancy in patients with elevated progesterone levels (>10 ng/mL), given its luteolytic effect.

During 2013 and 2014, various research groups focused their investigation lines in gefitinib. It is a small molecule that selectively inhibits tyrosine kinase in the epidermal growth factor receptor. Epidermal growth factor (EGF) is a protein substance that, together with hormones and neurotransmitters, plays an important role in intercellular communication and stimulates cell proliferation by regulating the cell cycle, maintaining cell survival, stimulating cell migration, cell differentiation, and even apoptosis. Placental tissue has been found to strongly express EGFR compared to other nonmalignant tissues. Moreover, its activation promotes cytotrophoblastic mobility, blocks programmed trophoblastic cell death, and rescues the placenta from apoptosis when exposed to hypoxia or toxic stimuli. By blocking EGF, gefitinib hypothetically induces cell death of ectopic trophoblastic tissue. Since October 2013, reasearchers are developing an open-label study to determine the safety, tolerability, and efficacy of gefitinib plus MTX to treat ectopic pregnancy. Skubiz et al. included 28 patients with stable tubal ectopic pregnancy that received a single dose of intramuscular MTX plus seven daily tablets of gefitinib (Skubisz et al. 2018). This combination successfully resolved 86% of larger tubal ectopic pregnancies (hCG 1000–10,000 IU/L) without the need for 'rescue' surgery. The authors compared these results to a control group treated with single dose of MTX, taken from a contemporaneous cohort. A non-significative trend could be seen between both groups; however authors blame this fact to the lack of power in this study (success rates of MTX only 66% vs. MTX + gefitinib 86%, $p = 0.08$). Authors are currently beginning a phase III clinical trial, to allow this new pharmacological strategy to be used in the clinic.

In conclusion, the range of therapeutic options for ectopic pregnancy is extremely broad and varied. The right decision for each case will depend on the individual characteristics of each patient, each gynecologist, and each facility.

Surgical Treatment

Conservative Surgery (Salpingotomy)

Surgical treatment is reserved for either ruptured or about to rupture ectopic pregnancies in hemodynamically unstable patients or if the use of medical treatment is contraindicated ("ACOG Practice Bulletin No. 193: Tubal Ectopic Pregnancy." 2018). The decision to perform conservative or radical surgery is usually made during the procedure and depends mainly on the patient's history (salpingectomy is indicated in the case of ipsilateral recurrence), the appearance and condition of the contralateral fallopian tube, and the presence of any bleeding. If the fallopian tube is ruptured, radical surgery should not be routinely performed unless hemostasis is expected to be difficult. Fallopian tube removal will most certainly be the best choice than a tube-sparing procedure if it is in poor condition (Capmas, Bouyer, and Fernandez 2014).

In both conservative and radical surgery, the surgical approach is not usually questioned. Laparoscopy is clearly the treatment of choice compared to laparotomy, and its advantages include a shorter hospital stay, lower costs, decreased morbidity (mainly postoperative pain), shorter surgical time, more limited blood loss during surgery, and fewer postoperative adhesions (Hsu et al. 2004). Laparoscopic surgery is safe even in cases of hypovolemic shock, provided that there is adequate laparoscopic material, a skilled nursing team, and surgeons with advanced laparoscopic skills. Most importantly, the surgeon must be familiar with the latest laparoscopic techniques and exercise clinical judgment in choosing the best management strategy and understanding one's limitations. Patients must be stabilized before surgery, if necessary by intravenous colloid infusion or blood transfusion. A bladder catheter should be inserted, and diuresis and vital signs should be monitored, possibly by invasive hemodynamic techniques. Once the patient is stable, the surgery can begin. It is crucial for the anesthesiologist to agree on the surgeon's choice to undertake laparoscopic surgery (Togas Tulandi and Kabli 2006). It has been speculated that in the case of active bleeding, creation of pneumoperitoneum with a Verres needle could lengthen the time to hemostasis control. Several classic studies (Byron, Markenson, and Miyazawa 1993) showed that entry via direct trocar insertion is possible without a higher number of major complications and with a shorter time for the entry technique (2.2 minutes versus 5.9 minutes for the direct insertion and Verres needle techniques, respectively). Therefore, in patients with bleeding ectopic pregnancy where time is critical, direct entry with the trocar may be recommended. The next point to consider in cases of hemoperitoneum is pelvic organ visualization. Consequently, routine placement of an intrauterine manipulator (except in cases of heterotopic pregnancy) will facilitate fallopian tube exposure and help identify the bleeding site, although increased intra-abdominal pressure from pneumoperitoneum could falsely occlude the bleeding point. It is essential to have appropriate material available, particularly a bipolar electrocoagulation system and a 10-mm suction-irrigation system (Togas Tulandi and Kabli 2006). In view of all these recommendations, laparoscopy is safer than laparotomy, even in critical situations.

Laparoendoscopic single-site surgery (LESS) requires a single abdominal incision at the umbilicus where multiport trocars can be inserted. This access device allows multiple instruments to be introduced simultaneously through a single incision, and ensures that pneumoperi-toneum is maintained regardless of whether these instruments are inserted or not. The laparoscopic instruments used were similar to those employed in conventional laparoscopy; however, the instruments are straight and stiff, which may hinder the visual field during surgery and could result in them crossing. Since 1970, it has been widely used in gynecology, traditionally for tubal ligation procedures. In the last 20 years, with the introduction of multichannel single port systems and articulating instruments it has gained popularity among gynaecologists and has successfully been used even in oncologic procedures. Gasparri et al. compared surgical outcomes of ectopic pregnancies with conventional laparoscopy versus LESS (Gasparri et al. 2018). 5 comparative studies with a total of 450 patients were included. 194 (43.1%) patients underwent LESS, whereas 256 (56.9%) underwent conventional LPS. They found no difference between duration of hospitalization, operating time, mean haemoglobin drop, number of patients requiring blood transfusion, and number of intra- and post-operative complications between the two techniques. Its main limitation is that this single-port technique requires both time for surgeon training and sufficient surgical skill.

The surgical technique begins with evacuation of hemoperitoneum to avoid hindering endoscopic vision, and preventive hemostasis must be achieved by instilling a vasoconstrictor agent at the site of the ectopic pregnancy and at the two ends of the vascular hila below the fallopian tube to prevent both intraoperative and postoperative bleeding. The fallopian tube is then approached and salpingotomy is performed by electrosection (scissors could also be used to prevent tissue damage), making a millimetric, longitudinal incision at the antimesenteric border of the fallopian tube, with the incision made at the junction of the inner third with the outer two thirds of the hematosalpinx. The trophoblast is then aspirated through the salpingotomy. The suction tube diameter must be large enough to exert proper traction and allow complete removal of the material. Traction must be progressive to avoid breaking up the trophoblast. The intervention is completed with hemostasis control of the fallopian tube; slight pressure on the fallopian tube is simplest, as it is agreed that electrocoagulation (even when bipolar) should be avoided to prevent irreversible fallopian tube lesions. Salpingotomy suture is not necessary. Adequate lavage of the region is necessary to remove any trophoblastic residue in the abdominal cavity. The procedure does not require specialized surgical material, but it is extremely important to use a large-diameter aspirator and unipolar electrocautery unit. The Triton multipurpose device invented by Manhes combines electrocoagulation, aspiration, and lavage in the same instrument, a tool that is highly advisable but not essential (T Tulandi and Guralnick 1991).

Five factors are decisive when choosing between conservative and radical surgery: surgical morbidity, risk of failure, desire for pregnancy, prognosis of fertility, which includes the probability of intrauterine pregnancy and the risk of recurrence of ectopic pregnancy and costs (Stock and Milad 2012).

Surgical Morbidity

As we explained previously, both techniques can be safely performed with adequate laparoscopic equipment, a skilled nursing team, and surgeons with advanced laparoscopic skills. Firstly, the surgeon must consider the ectopic pregnancy site: in interstitial ectopic pregnancies, medical treatment with MTX is recommended but conservative treatment must be avoided if surgery is needed. Secondly, hemostasis is a major consideration, as salpingectomy becomes essential if vasoconstrictors are not available or bleeding cannot be controlled. Thirdly, the fallopian tube must be in good condition, and salpingectomy is preferable if the fallopian tube is unlikely to heal properly (Maymon et al. 1995).

A group of Egyptian gynecologists described a novel technique during laparotomy, which allowed the control of bleeding from the internal surface of the tube after removal of trophoblastic tissue (Shazly et al. 2019). The main objective was to devascularize blood supply coming from the ascending arterioles under the tube. Two to three simple horizontal sutures were taken just below the lower border of the tube making a continuous line along the affected segment. Even if the study only included 5 patients, successful control of bleeding was achieved in all of them.

Risk of Failure

The persistence of ectopic trophoblastic tissue is one of the main complications of conservative surgery and the main reason why a second operation is sometimes needed. Incomplete trophoblast ablation will lead to progressive encysted hematocele with persistently elevated β-hCG levels. The first case of trophoblast persistence was described in 1979 (Kelly, Martin, and Strickler 1979), and later literature contains many reports. A meta-analysis (Hajenius et al. 2007) of randomized clinical trials showed that laparoscopic salpingostomy is associated with a high probability of persistence of trophoblastic tissue (3%-20% of cases). Similar data have been recently reported by the ESEP study (Femke Mol et al. 2014), an open-label, multicenter randomized controlled trial designed to determine if fertility outcomes improve after salpingotomy versus salpingectomy. This trial reported trophoblast persistence in 7% (14/215) of patients who underwent conservative surgery, compared with < 1% (1/231) in the radical surgery group, a difference that was significant. In addition, 2% (5/215) of patients required repeat laparoscopy and salpingectomy due to trophoblast persistence. Based on these findings, the technique should be abandoned and salpingectomy should be performed if any of the risk factors for persistence are present: 1) large ectopic pregnancy (Kayatas et al. 2014), which requires salpingectomy (the reports vary, but conservative treatment is generally not recommended for a diameter >3-5 cm); 2) poor fallopian tube access, with salpingostomy not recommendable in cases of obesity or peritubal adhesions;

3) β-hCG levels >8000 IU/L, making salpingostomy not advisable (Milad, Klein, and Kazer 1998); and 4) poor condition of the fallopian tube, with salpingectomy usually indicated when the fallopian tube is significantly injured. These are recommendations only, however, and not absolute contraindications. The surgeon should assess each individual carefully and decide based on these criteria and his or her experience.

Desire for Offspring

If pregnancy is not desired, then radical treatment with salpingectomy, possibly associated with contralateral sterilization, is clearly indicated (Pouly et al. 1991).

Costs

An economic evaluation of cost-effectiveness of salpingotomy and salpingectomy was conducted alongside the ESEP study (F Mol et al. 2015). Salpingotomy is less cost effective than salpingectomy as a surgical procedure for tubal pregnancy, as its costs are higher without a better ongoing pregnancy rate while risks of persistent trophoblast are higher.

Persistence of Ectopic Pregnancy

Persistence of ectopic pregnancy (PEP) results from incomplete removal of trophoblastic tissue that may complicate medical or surgical treatment of ectopic pregnancy. Diagnose is made by worsening of clinical symptoms or detection of rising/plateauing values of postoperative β-hCG. PEP after salpingectomies is quite rare, which is why scarce information about its incidence is available. NICE guidelines suggest performing a urine pregnancy test 3 weeks after surgery and following up for care if it is positive (NICE, 2019). If salpingostomy is performed, an estimated 5-29% of all cases may develop PEP. Preoperative prediction or early postoperative detection of these patients would be desirable. There are some features that may help us to predict PEP: short duration of amenorrhoea, high progesterone levels, small size of ectopic pregnancy, tubal bleeding, surgeon's inexperience, removal of the gestational tissue in fragments, and trophoblasts infiltrating deeply into the tubal wall. Lund et al. looked for other perioperative variables to determine which ones could have clinical use in the daily practice in a retrospective cohort of 417 patients treated by salpingotomy for ectopic pregnancy (Lund et al. 2002). 48 (11.5%) patients were diagnosed with PEP. Higher values of preoperative hCG levels were found to be significant in patients with PEP compared with those treated successfully. No other specific preoperative variables were able to predict the risk of PEP.

In a large cohort of 854 women that underwent laparoscopic salpingostomy for ectopic pregnancy removal, 794 (93%) required no further treatment (successes), while 60 (7.0%) developed PEP (Morse et al. 2018). The authors developed a simple calculation to triage patients at the risk of developing PEP using the first two postoperative measurements of b-HCG with a negative predictive value of 99% and positive predictive value of 88%. The ratio consists of the following calculation:

HCG1*HCG2/HCG1 (being HCG1 10 to 72h postoperatively and HCG2 72 to 120h postoperatively; both separated by a minimum of 48h).

Depending on the ratio, authors proceed as follow:

a) ratio >0.75: negative predictive value for PEP 99%. Consider follow-up with HCG at routine post-operative visit.
b) ratio ≤ 0.2: positive predictive value for PEP 88%. Consider treatment with intramuscular methotrexate unless contraindicated.
c) 0.2 > ratio ≥0.75: positive predictive value for PEP 6.3%. Consider following HCG every 2–3 days until the diagnosis is more apparent.

In order to minimize the possibility of trophoblast persistence after salpingostomy, the option of associating systemic MTX after surgery has been repeatedly considered, although routine use is still debated. A clinical trial in 129 patients who underwent linear salpingostomy was presented in 1997. This trial included two groups: a control group of 62 women who underwent surgery alone and a prophylaxis group of 54 women treated with a single dose of MTX 1 mg/kg intramuscularly within 24 hours after surgery. Persistent ectopic pregnancy was defined as a rise in serum β-hCG levels or a decline of less than 20% between two consecutive measurements taken three days apart. Ten women had persistent ectopic pregnancy, one (1.9%) in the prophylaxis group and nine (14.5%) among the controls, a difference that was statistically significant ($P < .05$). The RR of developing persistent ectopic pregnancy after prophylactic MTX was 0.13 (95% confidence interval 0.02, 0.97). Mild side effects were reported by three (5.5%) women after MTX, but resolved spontaneously.

Based on these results, the authors concluded that the incidence of persistent ectopic pregnancy was significantly reduced after a single prophylactic dose of systemic MTX administered postoperatively. This regimen is safe and can be used to decrease the extent of postoperative monitoring after conservative treatment of unruptured ectopic pregnancy (Graczykowski and Mishell 1997). However, due to the high risk of adverse reactions with MTX, the Cochrane Database System Review (Hajenius et al. 2007) authors do not recommend the routine use of systemic MTX after laparoscopic salpingostomy; the adverse effects reported are mainly asymptomatic elevation of liver enzymes, with rare cases of drug-induced hepatitis (1%). The DEMETER study also confirmed that postoperative MTX injection significantly reduces the persistence of trophoblast. In 2013, the Practice Committee of the American Society for Reproductive Medicine (ASRM, 2013) concluded that postoperative, prophylactic, single-dose systemic MTX may reduce the incidence of persistent ectopic pregnancy after salpingostomy. Therefore, the issue of whether routine postoperative MTX injection is safe and cost-effective still requires a definitive answer, particularly when MTX use could simplify the subsequent follow-up necessary. Because the likelihood of failures is very low, β-hCG levels can be tested one month later (Capmas, Bouyer, and Fernandez 2014).

The surgical treatment of PEP often involves salpingectomy in order to remove all trophoblastic tissue within the tube wall. Conservative surgery plus postoperative monitoring is only justified if fertility is better preserved compared with salpingectomy. The use of MTX may be indicated in three different approaches: a) routinely administer MTX prophylactically; b) administer prophylactic MTX only if there are concerns over spill or incomplete removal of tissue during surgery; c) use MTX only in women whose hCG levels do not normalize after surgery. The American College of Obstetricians and Gynecologists ("ACOG Practice Bulletin No. 193: Tubal Ectopic Pregnancy." 2018) considers administration of a single prophylactic dose of MTX if there are any concerns about a possible incomplete resection.

Comparison between Medical Treatment (MTX) in a Single-Dose Regimen and Conservative Surgery

Success Rates

A combination of three clinical trials (H Fernandez et al. 1998; McLaren et al. 2009; Saraj et al. 1998) conducted in hemodynamically stable patients with small, unruptured ectopic pregnancies showed that a single dose of systemic MTX (50 mg/m^2 or 1 mg/kg IM) was significantly less successful than laparoscopic salpingostomy (RR, 0.82; 95% CI, 0.72-0.94). However, it is important to understand the indications for each therapeutic modality, and the ASRM has concluded that post-treatment success rates are comparable for medical therapy and conservative surgical treatment (ASRM, 2013). Therefore, both conservative surgery and medical therapy may be viewed as appropriate first-line therapies in many early unruptured ectopic pregnancies.

Recovery Time

Recovery time is the time to negative serum β-hCG levels after ectopic pregnancy and varies from 20 to 31 days. Because medical treatment can fail due to trophoblast persistence after salpingostomy (particularly if MTX is not administered postoperatively), β-hCG levels must be monitored until the result is < 2 IU/L (Capmas, Bouyer, and Fernandez 2014). Several clinical trials have compared the recovery time after conservative surgery and MTX. In 1998, Saraj et al. presented a prospective randomized clinical trial that evaluated resolution of serum β-hCG and progesterone levels in patients (n = 75) with ectopic pregnancy who received single-dose intramuscular MTX (n = 38) and compared it to patients undergoing laparoscopic salpingostomy (n = 37) (Saraj et al. 1998). The mean time for β-hCG concentrations to drop to < 15 mIU/mL was significantly shorter for laparoscopic salpingostomy than for MTX: 20.2 ± 2.7 and 27.2 ± 2.3 days, respectively (P < .05). Colarcurci et al. conducted a similar study; in which group 1 included 15 patients treated with linear salpingostomy and group 2 included 15 patients treated with MTX (Colacurci et al. 1998). The time to resolution was 33.6 ± 6.6 days in group 1 and 31 5 ± 7.8 days in group 2, differences that were not statistically meaningful. Therefore, the authors concluded that the outcomes were comparable to those seen with laparoscopic treatment and suggested that β-hCG becomes negative regardless of type of treatment and residual trophoblast. The DEMETER study (Hervé Fernandez et al. 2013) also found that the recovery time is shorter in the conservative surgery group plus MTX than the group that received MTX alone, and that the differences were statistically significant. These studies appear to demonstrate that recovery time is shorter in patients who have undergone laparoscopic surgery; however, in my opinion, it is even more important to monitor β-hCG levels until they are negative.

Cost

In 2001, Sowter et al. presented a study that compared the direct and indirect costs of single-dose systemic MTX with laparoscopic surgery for unruptured ectopic pregnancy (Sowter et al. 2001). These authors performed a cost minimization study performed with a randomized trial and included 62 women with ectopic pregnancy randomized to either a single-dose MTX (50 mg/m^2) or laparoscopic surgery. The economic evaluation showed systemic MTX therapy in eligible ectopic pregnancy patients led to significantly reduced direct costs. Most likely, indirect costs to women and their caregivers were lowered only when pretreatment serum β-hCG levels were 1500 IU/L. Recently, the Practice Committee of the American Society for Reproductive Medicine (ASRM, 2013) also concluded that medical therapy seems to be more cost-effective than surgery except when initial β-hCG level are high or an embryo heartbeat is observed.

Radical Surgery (Salpingectomy)

Similar to conservative surgery, the hemoperitoneum should be aspirated if necessary to achieve satisfactory exposure of the affected fallopian tube and assess the ectopic pregnancy and entire pelvic cavity (size, rupture or nonrupture, presence of adhesions, condition of contralateral fallopian tube, etc.), with adhesiolysis performed, if necessary. The procedure is started by clamping the fallopian tube in place at its isthmic portion at a distance of 1.5 cm from the uterine horn, thus achieving good exposure of the fallopian tube isthmus and mesosalpinx. Bipolar electrocoagulation is used to coagulate the mesosalpinx and its posterior cut, until the proximal portion of the fallopian tube is reached (at a distance of 1-2 cm from the uterine horn). The fallopian tube is then electrocoagulated with bipolar energy and cutting. Once the fallopian tube is sectioned, the tube must be extracted either by an endoscopic sac introduced over a 12-mm trocar or by direct removal through one of the suprapubic routes, size permitting. The surgery is completed once hemostasis has been confirmed and the abdominal and pelvic cavity has been carefully washed. The indications, advantages and disadvantages of this technique have already been discussed in the previous section. In Table 4 we review the main indications to help practitioners decide between choosing a conservative or radical surgical treatment.

Table 4. Clinical scenarios to decide between salpingectomy and salpingostomy

Strong consideration of salpingectomy	Possible consideration of salpingotomy	Strong consideration of salpingostomy
Future fertility not desired	Presence of normal contralateral tube	Desired future fertility and history of infertility
Repeat ectopic pregnancy in same tube	Diameter of tubal pregnancy >3.35cm	Impaired or absent contralateral tube
Tubal rupture	Fetal cardiac activity	Risk factors for bilateral tubal damage
Tubal damage with healthy contralateral tube	Unwilling or unable to return to close follow-up	Unwilling or unable to consider IVF for future fertility
Isthmic tubal pregnancy		
Heterotopic pregnancy		
Contraindication to, or unwilling to consider MTX		
Sustained bleeding		

Adapted from (Ozcan, Wilson, and Frishman 2021)

References

"ACOG Practice Bulletin No. 193: Tubal Ectopic Pregnancy." 2018. *Obstetrics and Gynecology* 131 (3): e91–103. https://doi.org/10.1097/AOG.0000000000002560.

Bachman, Emelia Argyropoulos, and Kurt Barnhart. 2012. "Medical Management of Ectopic Pregnancy: A Comparison of Regimens." *Clinical Obstetrics and Gynecology* 55 (2): 440–47. https://doi.org/10.1097/GRF.0b013e3182510a73.

Barnhart, Kurt, Amy C Hummel, Mary D Sammel, Seema Menon, John Jain, and Nahida Chakhtoura. 2007. "Use of '2-Dose' Regimen of Methotrexate to Treat Ectopic Pregnancy." *Fertility and Sterility* 87 (2): 250–56. https://doi.org/10.1016/j.fertnstert.2006.06.054.

Byron, J W, G Markenson, and K Miyazawa. 1993. "A Randomized Comparison of Verres Needle and Direct Trocar Insertion for Laparoscopy." *Surgery, Gynecology & Obstetrics* 177 (3): 259–62.

Capmas, Perrine, Jean Bouyer, and Hervé Fernandez. 2014. "Treatment of Ectopic Pregnancies in 2014: New Answers to Some Old Questions." *Fertility and Sterility* 101 (3): 615–20. https://doi.org/10.1016/j.fertnstert.2014.01.029.

Chang, Jeani, Laurie D Elam-Evans, Cynthia J Berg, Joy Herndon, Lisa Flowers, Kristi A Seed, and Carla J Syverson. 2003. "Pregnancy-Related Mortality

Surveillance--United States, 1991--1999." *Morbidity and Mortality Weekly Report. Surveillance Summaries (Washington, D.C. : 2002)* 52 (2): 1–8.

Colacurci, N, P De Franciscis, R Zarcone, N Fortunato, M Passaro, A Mollo, and G Russo. 1998. "Time Length of Negativization of HCG Serum Values after Either Surgical or Medical Treatment of Ectopic Pregnancy." *Panminerva Medica* 40 (3): 223–25.

"Ectopic Pregnancy Mortality - Florida, 2009-2010." 2012. *MMWR. Morbidity and Mortality Weekly Report* 61 (6): 106–9.

Egarter, C, H Kiss, and P Husslein. 1991. "Prostaglandin versus Expectant Management in Early Tubal Pregnancy." *Prostaglandins, Leukotrienes, and Essential Fatty Acids* 42 (3): 177–79. https://doi.org/10.1016/0952-3278(91)90154-w.

Fernandez, H, S C Yves Vincent, S Pauthier, F Audibert, and R Frydman. 1998. "Randomized Trial of Conservative Laparoscopic Treatment and Methotrexate Administration in Ectopic Pregnancy and Subsequent Fertility." *Human Reproduction (Oxford, England)* 13 (11): 3239–43. https://doi.org/ 10.1093/humrep/13.11.3239.

Fernandez, Hervé, Perrine Capmas, Jean Philippe Lucot, Benoit Resch, Pierre Panel, and Jean Bouyer. 2013. "Fertility after Ectopic Pregnancy: The DEMETER Randomized Trial." *Human Reproduc-tion (Oxford, England)* 28 (5): 1247–53. https://doi.org/10.1093/humrep/det037.

Gasparri, Maria Luisa, Michael D Mueller, Katayoun Taghavi, and Andrea Papadia. 2018. "Conventional versus Single Port Laparoscopy for the Surgical Treatment of Ectopic Pregnancy: A Meta-Analysis." *Gynecologic and Obstetric Investigation* 83 (4): 329–37. https://doi.org/10.1159/ 000487944.

Gervaise, Amélie, Sylvie Capella-Allouc, François Audibert, Catherine Rongières-Bertrand, Yves Vincent, and Hervè Fernandez. 2003. "Methotrexate for the Treatment of Unruptured Tubal Pregnancy: A Prospective Nonrandomized Study." *JSLS : Journal of the Society of Laparoendoscopic Surgeons* 7 (3): 233–38.

Goldenberg, M, D Bider, G Oelsner, D Admon, and S Mashiach. 1992. "Treatment of Interstitial Pregnancy with Methotrexate via Hysteroscopy." *Fertility and Sterility* 58 (6): 1234–36. https://doi.org/10.1016/ s0015-0282(16)55575-7.

Graczykowski, J W, and D R Jr Mishell. 1997. "Methotrexate Prophylaxis for Persistent Ectopic Pregnancy after Conservative Treatment by Salpingostomy." *Obstetrics and Gynecology* 89 (1): 118–22. https://doi.org/ 10.1016/s0029-7844(96)00370-5.

Hajenius, P J, F Mol, B W J Mol, P M M Bossuyt, W M Ankum, and F van der Veen. 2007. "Interventions for Tubal Ectopic Pregnancy." *The Cochrane*

Database of Systematic Reviews 2007 (1): CD000324. https://doi.org/10.1002/14651858.CD000324.pub2.

Hsu, Senzan, Mohamed F Mitwally, Ashraf Aly, Mazin Al-Saleh, Ronald E Batt, and John Yeh. 2004. "Laparoscopic Management of Tubal Ectopic Pregnancy in Obese Women." *Fertility and Sterility* 81 (1): 198–202. https://doi.org/10.1016/j.fertnstert.2003.05.025.

Jamal, H S, and Z Amarin. 2001. "Laparoscopic Methotrexate Instillation in Unruptured Tubal Pregnancy--Is It Worthwhile?" *Journal of Obstetrics and Gynaecology : The Journal of the Institute of Obstetrics and Gynaecology* 21 (4): 402–4. https://doi.org/10.1080/01443610120068644.

Jurkovic, D, M Memtsa, E Sawyer, A N A Donaldson, A Jamil, K Schramm, Y Sana, et al. 2017. "Single-Dose Systemic Methotrexate vs Expectant Management for Treatment of Tubal Ectopic Pregnancy: A Placebo-Controlled Randomized Trial." *Ultrasound in Obstetrics & Gynecology : The Official Journal of the International Society of Ultrasound in Obstetrics and Gynecology* 49 (2): 171–76. https://doi.org/10.1002/uog.17329.

Jurkovic, Davor, and Helen Wilkinson. 2011. "Diagnosis and Management of Ectopic Pregnancy." *BMJ (Clinical Research Ed.)* 342 (June): d3397. https://doi.org/10.1136/bmj.d3397.

Kayatas, Semra, Oya Demirci, Pinar Kumru, Didar Mahmutoglu, Bahar Saribrahim, and Sevcan Arzu Arinkan. 2014. "Predictive Factors for Failure of Salpingostomy in Ectopic Pregnancy." *The Journal of Obstetrics and Gynaecology Research* 40 (2): 453–58. https://doi.org/10.1111/jog.12187.

Kelly, R W, S A Martin, and R C Strickler. 1979. "Delayed Hemorrhage in Conservative Surgery for Ectopic Pregnancy." *American Journal of Obstetrics and Gynecology* 133 (2): 225–26. https://doi.org/10.1016/0002-9378(79)90483-6.

Korhonen, J, U H Stenman, and P Ylöstalo. 1996. "Low-Dose Oral Methotrexate with Expectant Management of Ectopic Pregnancy." *Obstetrics and Gynecology* 88 (5): 775–78. https://doi.org/10.1016/0029-7844(96)00293-1.

Lund, Claus Otto, Lisbeth Nilas, Nannie Bangsgaard, and Bent Ottesen. 2002. "Persistent Ectopic Pregnancy after Linear Salpingotomy: A Non-Predictable Complication to Conservative Surgery for Tubal Gestation." *Acta Obstetricia et Gynecologica Scandinavica* 81 (11): 1053–59. https://doi.org/10.1034/j.1600-0412.2002.811110.x.

LUND, J. 1955. "Early Ectopic Pregnancy; Comments on Conservative Treatment." *The Journal of Obstetrics and Gynaecology of the British Empire* 62 (1): 70–76.

Mavrelos, D, M Memtsa, S Helmy, G Derdelis, E Jauniaux, and D Jurkovic. 2015. "β-HCG Resolution Times during Expectant Management of Tubal Ectopic

Pregnancies." *BMC Women's Health* 15 (May): 43. https://doi.org/10.1186/s12905-015-0200-7.

Mavrelos, D, H Nicks, A Jamil, W Hoo, E Jauniaux, and D Jurkovic. 2013. "Efficacy and Safety of a Clinical Protocol for Expectant Management of Selected Women Diagnosed with a Tubal Ectopic Pregnancy." *Ultrasound in Obstetrics & Gynecology : The Official Journal of the International Society of Ultrasound in Obstetrics and Gynecology* 42 (1): 102–7. https://doi.org/10.1002/uog.12401.

Maymon, R, A Shulman, R Halperin, A Michell, and I Bukovsky. 1995. "Ectopic Pregnancy and Laparoscopy: Review of 1197 Patients Treated by Salpingectomy or Salpingotomy." *European Journal of Obstetrics, Gynecology, and Reproductive Biology* 62 (1): 61–67. https://doi.org/10.1016/0301-2115(95)02165-4.

McLaren, Janet F, Richard O Burney, Amin A Milki, Lynn M Westphal, Michael H Dahan, and Ruth B Lathi. 2009. "Effect of Methotrexate Exposure on Subsequent Fertility in Women Undergoing Controlled Ovarian Stimulation." *Fertility and Sterility* 92 (2): 515–19. https://doi.org/10.1016/j.fertnstert.2008.07.009.

"Medical Treatment of Ectopic Pregnancy: A Committee Opinion." 2013. *Fertility and Sterility* 100 (3): 638–44. https://doi.org/10.1016/j.fertnstert.2013.06.013.

Mello, N M van, F Mol, H R Verhoeve, M van Wely, A H Adriaanse, E A Boss, A B Dijkman, et al. 2013. "Methotrexate or Expectant Management in Women with an Ectopic Pregnancy or Pregnancy of Unknown Location and Low Serum HCG Concentrations? A Randomized Comparison." *Human Reproduction (Oxford, England)* 28 (1): 60–67. https://doi.org/10.1093/humrep/des373.

Milad, M P, E Klein, and R R Kazer. 1998. "Preoperative Serum HCG Level and Intraoperative Failure of Laparoscopic Linear Salpingostomy for Ectopic Pregnancy." *Obstetrics and Gynecology* 92 (3): 373–76. https://doi.org/10.1016/s0029-7844(98)00218-x.

Mol, F, N M van Mello, A Strandell, D Jurkovic, J A Ross, T M Yalcinkaya, K T Barnhart, et al. 2015. "Cost-Effectiveness of Salpingotomy and Salpingectomy in Women with Tubal Pregnancy (a Randomized Controlled Trial)." *Human Reproduction (Oxford, England)* 30 (9): 2038–47. https://doi.org/10.1093/humrep/dev162.

Mol, Femke, Norah M van Mello, Annika Strandell, Karin Strandell, Davor Jurkovic, Jackie Ross, Kurt T Barnhart, et al. 2014. "Salpingotomy versus Salpingectomy in Women with Tubal Pregnancy (ESEP Study): An Open-Label, Multicentre, Randomised Controlled Trial." *Lancet (London,*

England) 383 (9927): 1483–89. https://doi.org/10.1016/S0140-6736(14)60123-9.

Morse, Abraham N, Wenyue Si, Shuang Qin, and Huiying Liang. 2018. "Optimal Use of Peri-Operative Human Chorionic Gonadotrophin Concentrations to Identify Persistent Ectopic Pregnancy after Laparoscopic Salpingostomy A Retrospective Cohort Study." *Reproductive Biomedicine Online* 36 (3): 361–68. https://doi.org/10.1016/j.rbmo.2017.12.006.

Ozcan, Meghan C H, Jeffrey R Wilson, and Gary N Frishman. 2021. "A Systematic Review and Meta-Analysis of Surgical Treatment of Ectopic Pregnancy with Salpingectomy versus Salpingostomy." *Journal of Minimally Invasive Gynecology* 28 (3): 656–67. https://doi.org/10.1016/j.jmig.2020.10.014.

Pouly, J L, C Chapron, M Canis, G Mage, A Wattiez, H Manhes, and M A Bruhat. 1991. "Subsequent Fertility for Patients Presenting with an Ectopic Pregnancy and Having an Intra-Uterine Device in Situ." *Human Reproduction (Oxford, England)* 6 (7): 999–1001. https://doi.org/10.1093/oxfordjournals.humrep.a137477.

Saraj, A J, J G Wilcox, S Najmabadi, S M Stein, M B Johnson, and R J Paulson. 1998. "Resolution of Hormonal Markers of Ectopic Gestation: A Randomized Trial Comparing Single-Dose Intramuscular Methotrexate with Salpingostomy." *Obstetrics and Gynecology* 92 (6): 989–94. https://doi.org/10.1016/s0029-7844(98)00324-x.

Shazly, Sherif A, Ahmed G Gayar, Ahmed Y Abdelbadee, Ahmed M Afifi, and Ahmed A Nassr. 2019. "Partial Tubal Devascularisation: A Novel Procedure for Tubal Conservation in Ectopic Pregnancy." *Journal of Obstetrics and Gynaecology : The Journal of the Institute of Obstetrics and Gynaecology* 39 (2): 202–5. https://doi.org/10.1080/01443615.2018.1476472.

Silva, Priscila Matthiesen, Edward Araujo Júnior, Gustavo Nardini Cecchino, Julio Elito Júnior, and Luiz Camano. 2015. "Effectiveness of Expectant Management versus Methotrexate in Tubal Ectopic Pregnancy: A Double-Blind Randomized Trial." *Archives of Gynecology and Obstetrics* 291 (4): 939–43. https://doi.org/10.1007/s00404-014-3513-0.

Skubisz, Monika M, Stephen Tong, Ann Doust, Jill Mollison, Terrance G Johns, Peter Neil, Miranda Robinson, et al. 2018. "Gefitinib and Methotrexate to Treat Ectopic Pregnancies with a Pre-Treatment Serum HCG 1000-10,000 IU/L: Phase II Open Label, Single Arm Multi-Centre Trial." *EBioMedicine* 33 (July): 276–81. https://doi.org/10.1016/j.ebiom.2018.06.017.

Sowter, M C, C M Farquhar, K J Petrie, and G Gudex. 2001. "A Randomised Trial Comparing Single Dose Systemic Methotrexate and Laparoscopic Surgery for the Treatment of Unruptured Tubal Pregnancy." *BJOG : An International*

Journal of Obstetrics and Gynaecology 108 (2): 192–203. https://doi.org/10.1111/j.1471-0528.2001.00038.x.

Stika, Catherine S. 2012. "Methotrexate: The Pharmacology behind Medical Treatment for Ectopic Pregnancy." *Clinical Obstetrics and Gynecology* 55 (2): 433–39. https://doi.org/10.1097/GRF.0b013e3182510a35.

Stock, Laura, and Magdy Milad. 2012. "Surgical Management of Ectopic Pregnancy." *Clinical Obstetrics and Gynecology* 55 (2): 448–54. https://doi.org/10.1097/GRF.0b013e3182510a19.

Tulandi, T, and M Guralnick. 1991. "Treatment of Tubal Ectopic Pregnancy by Salpingotomy with or without Tubal Suturing and Salpingectomy." *Fertility and Sterility* 55 (1): 53–55. https://doi.org/10.1016/s0015-0282(16)54058-8.

Tulandi, Togas, and Nadia Kabli. 2006. "Laparoscopy in Patients with Bleeding Ectopic Pregnancy." *Journal of Obstetrics and Gynaecology Canada : JOGC = Journal d'obstetrique et Gynecologie Du Canada : JOGC*. Netherlands. https://doi.org/10.1016/s1701-2163(16)32157-0.

Webster, Katie, Hilary Eadon, Sarah Fishburn, and Geeta Kumar. 2019. "Ectopic Pregnancy and Miscarriage: Diagnosis and Initial Management: Summary of Updated NICE Guidance." *BMJ (Clinical Research Ed.)* 367 (November): l6283. https://doi.org/10.1136/bmj.l6283.

Wong, J A, and J F Clark. 1968. "Correlation of Symptoms with Age and Location of Gestation in Tubal Pregnancy." *Journal of the National Medical Association* 60 (3): 221–23.

Yang, Chun, Jing Cai, Yuhong Geng, and Ying Gao. 2017. "Multiple-Dose and Double-Dose versus Single-Dose Administration of Methotrexate for the Treatment of Ectopic Pregnancy: A Systematic Review and Meta-Analysis." *Reproductive Biomedicine Online* 34 (4): 383–91. https://doi.org/10.1016/j.rbmo.2017.01.004.

Ylöstalo, P, B Cacciatore, J Sjöberg, M Kääriäinen, A Tenhunen, and U H Stenman. 1992. "Expectant Management of Ectopic Pregnancy." *Obstetrics and Gynecology* 80 (3 Pt 1): 345–48.

Chapter 3

Rising Caesarean Section Rates – An Evolutionary Approach

S. Kirchengast*, PhD

Department of Evolutionary Anthropology,
University of Vienna, Austria

Abstract

Caesarean sections (CS) are one of the most frequently performed surgeries in women of reproductive age. Currently, the average global rate of CS is about 21.1%, the prevalence however, differs markedly between different countries but also between different social strata within a country. Although Caesarean sections are lifesaving procedures which helped to reduce maternal and new-born mortality rates, the worldwide rising rates of C-sections however, are subject to growing concern. The main argument to perform caesarean sections is to reduce maternal and new-born mortality, because human childbirth is still a dangerous experience for many women. Consequently, caesarean sections are nearly exclusively seen from an obstetrical or public health perspective. From the viewpoint of evolutionary anthropology however, we have to ask: why is human childbirth so painful and dangerous making caesarean sections necessary? This is completely uncommon in nature. Therefore, in the present review the problem of human childbirth and the consequently rising rates of caesarean sections are discussed from the viewpoint of evolutionary anthropology.

* Correspoding Author's E-mail: sylvia.kirchengast@univie.ac.at.

In: A Closer Look at Pregnancy and Childbirth
Editor: Louise J. Salgado
ISBN: 978-1-68507-658-0

Keywords: caesarean section, maternal mortality, human evolution, evolutionary medicine

Introduction

Caesarean sections are one of the most frequently performed surgeries among women of reproductive age (Saeed et al. 2017). The dictionary of obstetrics and gynaecology defines caesarean section as the "surgical termination of pregnancy or delivery by operative opening of the uterus." Once introduced in clinical practice as an important innovation and life- saving procedure for mothers as well as offspring (Bertran et al. 2007, 2016), the worldwide escalating caesarean section rates, have turned to a major public health concern and are cause of considerable debate because of possible maternal and new-born risks but also because of increasing costs for the health system and social inequality in the access to this in many cases lifesaving procedure (Henderson et al. 2001; Torloni et al. 2011, Vilar et al. 2007). Today, there is no doubt that caesarean sections are effective in saving maternal and infants lives, but only when necessary by medical reasons such as abnormal child presentation such breech or transverse presentation, cephalon-pelvic disproportion, obstructed labour, foetal distress, twin pregnancy, high blood pressure in the mother, uterine rupture, problems with the placenta or umbilical cord, HIV infection, preeclampsia and some others (Savage 2007, WHO 2007, 2008, 2015). Consequently, today caesarean section is recommended when vaginal delivery might pose a risk to the mother or the foetus. In 1985, the World Health Organization (WHO 1985) stated that there is no justification for any region to have caesarean section rates higher than 10 to 15% because maternal and new-born mortality and morbidity was not reduced when the caesarean section rate was more than 15%. (WHO 1985). More recent studies plead for a caesarean section rate of 19%, because caesarean section rates of 19 per 100 live births were associated with lowest maternal and neonatal mortality (Volpe 2011, Molina et al. 2015). Despite these recommendations, caesarean section rates increased dramatically up to more than 50% in some countries during the past decades.

Caesarean Sections Worldwide

According to recent estimates, the worldwide caesarean section rate is 21.1% ranging from 1.4 to 58.15% (Bertran et al. 2021). Figure 1 demonstrates the caesarean section rates for each continent and for developed, less developed and least developed countries. Highest CS-rates were found for the Americas (39.9%), lowest CS-rates for the African continent. Looking at each continent separately, marked regional differences in CS-rates appear. As to be expected lowest CS rates are found among less developed countries, first of all in Sub-Saharan Africa (5%), where the five countries with the lowest caesarean section rates around the world are located. These countries are the Chad (1.4%), Niger (1.4%), Ethiopia (1.9%), Madagascar (2%) and Cameroon (2.4%) (Bertran et al. 2021). Extremely low CS-rates are also documented for Timor -Leste (3.5%), Papua-New Guinea (3%) and Haiti (5.4%) (Bertran et al. 2021). Highest caesarean section in contrast, are documented for the Americas, in particular for Latin America and the Caribbean (42.8%) (see Figure 2). Especially high caesarean section rates are found in the Dominican Republic (56.4%) and Brazil (55.7%), but also Cyprus (55.3%), Turkey (53.1%), Egypt (51.8%), Iran (47.9%), and Romania (46.9%) (Bertran et al. 2021). In most European countries, the United States and New Zealand the caesarean section rate is about 25 to 35% (Bertran et al. 2021). Comparing the 34 OECD countries, highest CS-rates are found for Turkey (55.3%, Mexico (48.7%), Chile (47.7%) and Korea (45.2%) (OECD 2019). The mean CS-rates for the OECD countries was 28.1%. For a detailed description see Figure 3. Within the European Union, caesarean sections were performed at least 1.4 million times in 2017, however the CS-rates differ markedly between the individual countries of the European Union. Caesarean sections were most frequent in Cyprus (55.3%), followed by Romania (46.9%), Bulgaria (43.1%), Poland (39.3%) and Hungary (37.3%), and the least in Finland (16.5%), Sweden (16.6%), Estonia and Lithuania (both 19.4%) and France (19.7%) (Eurostat 2019).

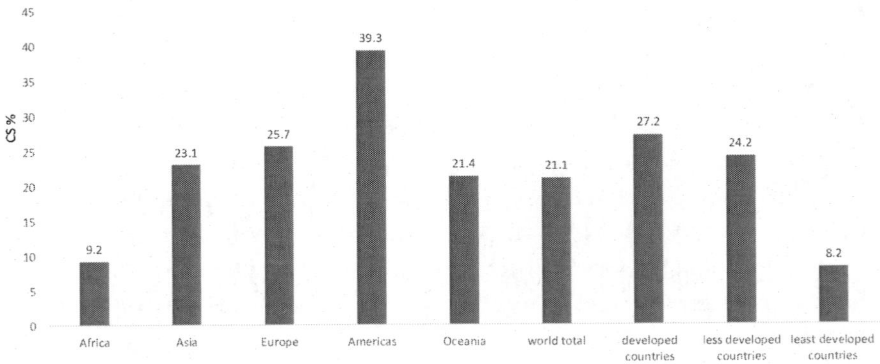

Source: Bertran et al. 2021.

Figure 1. Caesarean section rates according to world region.

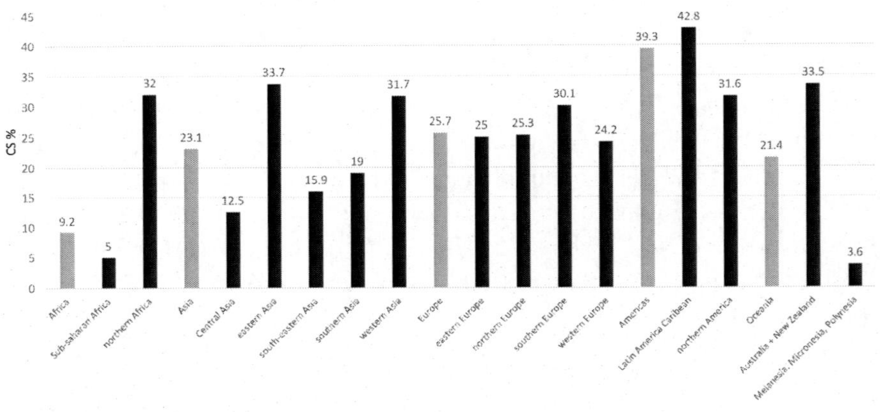

Source: Bertran et al. 2021.

Figure 2. Caesarean section rates according to continent region.

These rates are clearly higher than the recommended ones. During the last 20 years CS-rates increased markedly all over the worlds. Worldwide, CS-rates increased 19.4% (Bertran et al. 2021).

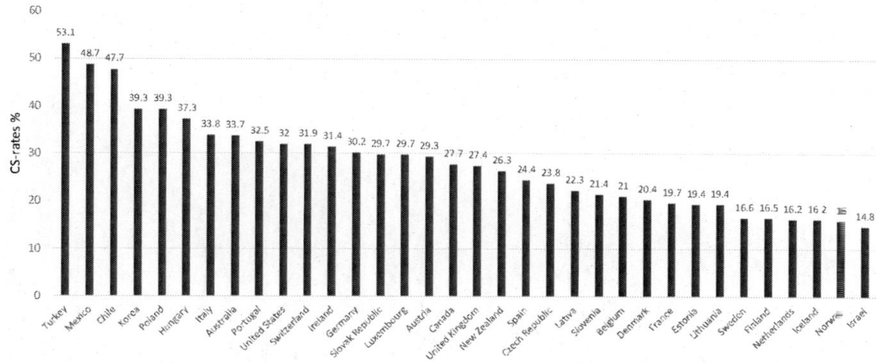

Source: OECD 2019.

Figure 3. Caesarean section rates in the OECD countries.

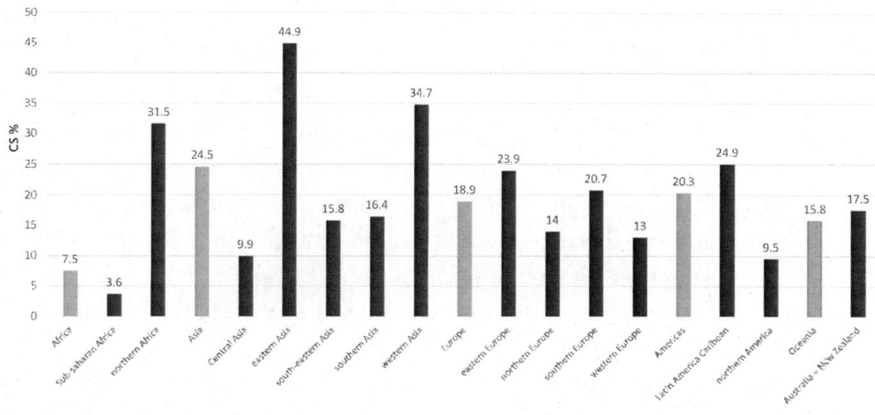

Source: Bertran et al. 2021.

Figure 4. Caesarean section rates increase between 1990 and 2018.

Considering the individual world regions separately, in the increase of CS-rates differed significantly, from 3.5% in sub-Saharan Africa to 44.9% in eastern Asia (Bertran et al. 2021) (see Figure 4). Comparing the situation in developed, less developed and least developed countries, it turned out, that the CS-rates increased highest in less developed countries (22.9%), and lowest in least developed countries (8.6%). In developed countries CS-rates increased steadily 15.1% since 1990 (Betran et al. 2021). This trend is rather worrying because an extraordinary high CS-rate does not reduce maternal mortality, in contrast, it represents an independent risk factor for avoidable morbidity and long-term consequences.

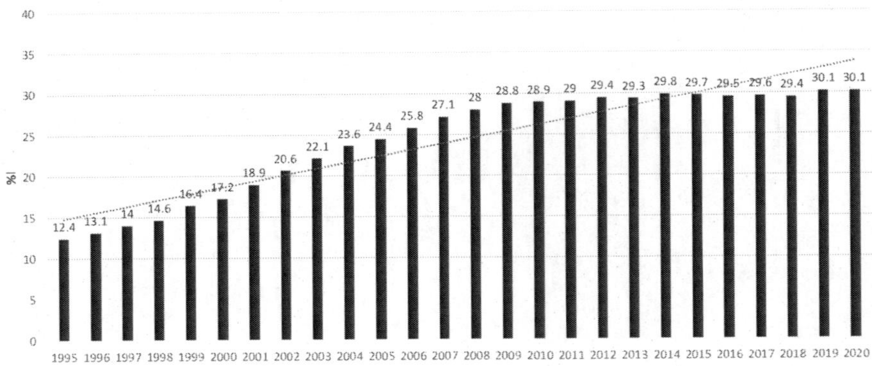

Source: Statistik Austria 2020.

Figure 5. Caesarean section rate in Austria 1995-2020.

If we look at Austria, one of the richest countries of the European Union, for example, we see a steady increase of CS-rates from 12.4% in 1995 to 28.9% in 2010. This is an increase of more than 100% in fifteen years. During the last 10 years the increase of CS-rates continued, however, the dramatic increase in CS rates has flattened significantly over the past 10 years. Between 2010 and 2020, only an increase from 28.9 to 30.1% can be observed. (Statistik Austria 2020) (see Figure 5).

Similar trends are found all over the world with exception of the less developed countries. There are numerous reasons for this trend towards an increasing rate of caesarean sections, which can be interpreted from different viewpoints. There is no doubt, that the extraordinary high CS- rates today – mentioned above - cannot be explained by increased risk or medical indications only (Litorp et al. 2015). Some authors such as Weiner et al. (2008), Michel Odent (2004) and Fischer and Mitteröcker (2015) see high rates of caesarean section as a consequence of the obstetrical dilemma and they speculate that rising caesarean section rates may have implications on the future of human evolution. Consequently, caesarean sections are not only important topics of Gynaecology and Obstetrics or Public Health, but also of Evolutionary Anthropology. The present paper focuses on the rising caesarean section rates from the viewpoint of Evolutionary Anthropology.

The History of Caesarean Sections

Focusing on caesarean sections from an evolutionary perspective, at first, the question arises whether the caesarean section is exclusively a recent phenomenon: Therefore, we have to start with a look back into the history of caesarean section.

The term caesarean section is usually associated with the birth of Julius Caesar in 100 BC. According to Plinius the elder, Caesar was removed from his mother's womb by an abdominal incision. This story however, is highly improbable because Caesar's mother Aurelia delivered after Caesar six further children and died 54BC. It was more than unlikely, that she survived such a surgical procedure for many years at that time. References to caesarean section appear in ancient Egyptian, Hindu, Graecan and Roman folklore. Religious law of Egypt in 3000 BC and of India in 1500 BC required abdominal delivery of a child from its dead mother's womb. In Greek mythology the God Apollo removed his son Asclepius by an abdominal cut from Asclepius's dying mother Coronis (van Dongen 2009).

The King of Rome Numa Pompilius codified Roman law in 715 BC. This Lex Regia, later called Lex Caesarea, made it mandatory to remove the child from its dying mother. even if there was no chance of its own survival. This was done to ensure separate burials of mother and child.

In medieval times, the Catholic Church encouraged the use of caesarean section to save the child and wanted to offer their souls a change of salvation through baptism. To save the mother was not a concern because the Church prohibited the abortion or craniotomy. The first documented successful caesarean section on a living woman was performed by the Swiss sow-gelder Jacob Nufer in 1500. His wife was pregnant for the first time and even 13 midwifes were not able get the foetus out of the womb. Therefore, Nufer decided to perform a caesarean section. Mother and child survived and Nufer's wife gave birth to several children even twins and she died ageing 77 years old. Unfortunately, this case was documented 80 years later, therefore the first documented successful Caesarean section performed on a living woman took place 1610 in Wittenberg, when Jeremias Trautmann performed a CS on Ursula Opitz. Ursula Opitz however died 25 days later from infection, while her child survived until the age of nine years (van Dongen 2009, Todman 2007).

Up to the 19th century caesarean sections have been performed on dying or already dead women only. This was mainly due to the fact, that even during the 19th and early 20th century maternal death rate of caesarean section was almost 100%. The main problems were severe bleedings because only the abdominal wall was closed but not the uterus wall, and on the other hand infections associated with the surgical procedure. The first obstetrician who performed more or less save caesarean sections was Eduardo Porro (1842-1902) who stopped severe bleeding by the removal of the uterus, ovaries, and oviducts after caesarean section, a drastic procedure which saved the life of the mother, however resulted in sterility (Todman 2006). During 20th century, caesarean sections became increasingly safe and maternal mortality caused by caesarean section dropped down markedly. As the risk associated with caesarean sections decreased progressively, the incidence of caesarean sections increased.

Caesarean Section Today

As pointed out above, caesarean sections are one of the most frequently performed operations in women, although the World health organization recommended caesarean section rates of 0 to 15% at population level (WHO 2016). Especially during the last decades caesarean section rates increased nearly all over the world (Bertran et al. 2016, 2021, MacFarlane 2015). Various reasons of this trend have been discussed. On the one hand, caesarean sections are increasingly easier for obstetricians and are more acceptable for patients. Consequently, many obstetricians see a caesarean section as less risky than a vaginal birth and therefore, they recommend it. Furthermore, birth can be perfectly scheduled and does not occur during night or week end (Gabbe and Holzmann 2001). Caesarean section is increasingly seen as a safe surgical technique with many benefits for the foetus such as a reduced risk of trauma, hypoxic encephalopathy and cerebral damage caused by prolonged hypoxic status. Furthermore, caesarean section may reduce the risk of operative vaginal delivery and the damage of the pelvic floor (Gabbe and Holzmann 2001). In addition to caesarean sections forced by obstetricians, caesarean section on patients - mainly maternal - request gain in importance (Litorp et al. 2015, Faas-Fehervary et al. 2005, Tarney 2014). The main reasons for women to request caesarean sections are the fear of childbirth (tocophobia) including the fear of pain, being alone during labour, pelvic floor injury, or losing control. On the other hand, pregnant women wish increasingly to know date and place of birth some months before birth may take place (Ajeet et al. 2011, Meloni et al. 2012). These medical and psychosocial reasons for increasing CS-rates are only one side of the coin, but we have also to consider the biological and especially evolutionary explanations. Therefore, the rising rates of CS-sections should be discussed from the viewpoint of evolutionary anthropology.

Caesarean Section from the Viewpoint of Evolutionary Anthropology

Human Childbirth – A Biological Perspective

At first, we have to state, that from a biological perspective, humans or more correctly *Homo sapiens*, are part of the animal kingdom. As early as 1768, the famous Swedish scientist Carl von Linne classified humans a part of the ordo "primates" together with monkeys and apes (Linne 1768). In contrast to other mammals and even non-human primates however, human females experience painful and dangerous deliveries which takes much longer than in other mammals (Shipman 2013). From a biological perspective, dangerous and long deliveries are rather unexpected. A long, exhausting and maybe risky delivery is clearly a life-threatening event for the mother and the foetus. Furthermore, helplessness of the delivering women might attract predators and mother as well as the foetus are in danger. Maternal and/or new-born death are in clear contradiction to the so called *"biogenetic imperative"* which declares successful reproduction as the ultimate goal of each living being (Markl 1983). Human childbirth is therefore, mainly described as unique in animal kingdom. Humans however, are not the only animals that experience difficulties during childbirth. Some special breed such as Belgian white or blue breed of cattle or dogs such as French or English bulldogs are nearly unable to deliver without caesarean section because of special physical characteristics such as hypermuscularity or large foetal heads in relation to small maternal pelvis. Cattle and bulldogs however, are the result of artificial breeding practice by humans and not natural problems with an evolutionary basis. Nevertheless, among our closest relatives, the non-human primates, problems during delivery have be observed. In general, primates – non-human ones as well humans -are characterized by a large brain size and consequently a large head in relation to body size. This disproportion causes problems during delivery because neonatal heads are close to the size of the maternal bony birth canal

(Rosenberg and Trevathan 2002). Among small-bodies species such as squirrel monkeys, marmosets and macaques, neonatal death resulting from cephalo-pelvic disproportion have been reported (Rosenberg and Trevathan 2002). Our closest relatives the great apes (orangutan, gorilla and chimpanzee) appear to have spacious birth canals and consequently obstructed labour caused by cephalo-pelvic disproportion are quite uncommon (Rosenberg and Trevathan 2002).

In humans as well as in non-human primates, the birth canal has three relevant planes, the inlet, the midplane and the outlet. During delivery the neonate has to pass through these three planes. Among non-human primates all planes of the birth canal are greater in anterior-posterior diameter than in transverse diameter, while the foetal skull is always longer in the sagittal than in the transverse diameter (Rosenberg 1992). The passage through the birth canal is consequently quite simple among non-human primates and does not require significant changes of orientation of the foetus (Trevathan 1993). The neonate is born face first facing the maternal pubic bone with the head in an extended position (Rosenberg and Trevathan 2002). Monkeys and apes generally deliver alone and quite quickly when predators but also group member are least likely to be present (Rosenberg and Trevathan 2002). They need no assistance and birth represents a solitary event. Among humans the situation is quite different: the three planes of the birth canal are not constant in dimensions. The pelvic inlet shows the largest dimensions in transverse diameter, while the pelvic outlet shows the larges dimension in sagittal direction. Therefore, the foetus has to perform a number of movements and alterations of the position of the head the so-called "cardinal movements of labour" to navigate through the birth canal (Rosenberg 1992). The new-born emerges in a posterior position facing the maternal sacrum. Assistance during delivery by group members is obligatory in all human societies.

Considering this specific situation, childbirth mechanism among *Homo sapiens* is characterized by three main features (Rosenberg and Trevathan 2014):

1. Rotation of the foetus
2. Navigation through the three pelvic planes
3. Emergence of the foetus in the occiput anterior position

This complicated birth mechanism seems to be one of the main reasons of birth difficulties and sometimes maternal mortality among *Homo sapiens*. As a consequence, pregnancy and in particular childbirth, increased maternal and offspring mortality and had in this way an important impact on natural selection throughout human evolution and history (Rosenberg 1992, Rosenberg and Trevathan 2018). Even today, several hundred thousand women die on account of pregnancy and childbirth every year and an even larger number of women suffer from long term health complications associated with parturition (Alkema et al. 2016).

Maternal Mortality – In History and Today

As pointed out above, caesarean section in a recent sense was introduced as a life-saving procedure. Consequently, we have to focus on maternal mortality patterns among *Homo sapiens* in this analysis. There is no doubt that pregnancy and especially birth have been and still are dangerous and life-threatening events in female life (Loudon 2000, Chamberlain 2005). The World health organization defines maternal death as the death of a woman while pregnant or within 42 days of termination of pregnancy irrespective of the duration and site of the pregnancy, from any cause related to or aggravated by the pregnancy or its management but not from accidental or incidental causes" (WHO 2016). Birth however, is also a risky process for the foetus and neonatal death rates have been high even in highly industrialized countries up to the post world war II period. Neonatal death is defined as the death of the new-born within 28 days after birth. (WHO 2016).

Bioarchaeological research provided the earliest evidence of maternal death. Looking at skeletal remains from prehistoric and historic cemeteries but also at epitaphs from ancient Greek and Roman area, it turned out, that among women a typical younger age at death - about 5 years younger compared with men - can be observed. The analysis of Later Stone Age foragers of the South African Cape revealed a higher mortality among young women of reproductive age in comparison to males of the same age group (Pfeiffer et al. 2013). Nevertheless, it is not clear that these sex differences emerge from increased female reproduction related mortality. Direct evidence of maternal mortality in skeletal samples from bioarchaeological excavations is still rare. Maternal death is indisputable when a female skeleton is found with a full-term infant in a deformed or obstructed pelvis (Högberg et al. 1987). Additionally, a female skeleton of reproductive age with a foetal skeleton in the pelvis, between the legs or embraced by the woman may be interpreted as maternal death (Högberg et al. 1987). As pointed out by Cruz and Cochina

(2010), archaeological evidence of maternal death is scare and therefore unlikely to reflect the high incidence of mortality during and after delivery. Up to today, only few examples of maternal death in skeletal samples are described. This may be mainly due to the fact that foetal skeletal remains are seldom preserved, on the other hand cultural habits may permitted a common burial of mother and child. The earliest confirmed evidence for a maternal death caused by obstructed labour originates from the Siberian site Lokomotiv near the lake Baikal (Liverse et al. 2015). The burial of a 20 to 25 years old woman dated in early Neolithic times 7000 to 8000 years ago. The skeletal remains indicated that the young woman died during the delivery of twins. It can be assumed that the first twin showed transverse presentation causing obstructed labour, which means that the birth process stopped due to mechanical problems. The first twin was not able to pass the birth canal and consequently, the mother but also both twins died. Another rare example of maternal death during labour originates from an early medieval Anglo-Saxon cemetery in Cambridgeshire dated between 450 to 700 years AD. The excavation yielded the skeleton of a 25 to 30 years old woman with a foetus which lay low and transverse across her pelvis. Consequently, a transverse position of the foetus can be assumed (Sayer and Dickerson 2013). Even today transverse presentation is dangerous and requires a caesarean section.

From historical records it is well known that pregnancy and first of all childbirth were frequently related with female mortality in past populations but also still in many recent societies (Loudon 2000). Even in Europe, everybody knew about death in childbirth and especially pregnant women have been aware about the danger associated with giving birth. Although average life expectancy was short and death rates from many conditions were high at that time, maternal mortality represented a special tragedy because death associated with childbirth affected mostly young more or less healthy women of reproductive age, who had been quite well before becoming pregnant (Chamberlain 2005). Furthermore, maternal death often resulted in a social tragedy. The mother died and left the new-born and maybe other children as orphans and a widowed husband. This scenario was a frequent one (Chamberlain 2005).

Coping Strategies

Consequently, several cultural adaptations or coping strategies have been developed to reduce the risk of delivery since a long time (Rosenberg and

Trevathan 2002, Rosenberg 1992, Trevathan 1993, Buck 2011, Rosenberg and Trevathan 2014). First of all, the companionship of another person, such as relatives, experienced women, midwives or professional obstetricians during labour, had a positive impact on delivery (Rosenberg and Trevathan 2002, Rosenberg 1992, Trevathan 1993, Rosenberg and Trevathan 2014). During the last century, surgical procedures such as caesarean sections gain in importance (Todman 2007). Risky and life- threatening childbirth required the development of coping strategies to reduce the risk of maternal and neonate death. Two different kinds of coping strategies can be distinguished: biological and cultural ones (Buck 2011). From an evolutionary viewpoint the biological consequences are the evolution of a marked sexual dimorphism in pelvic shape and size which enables women to give birth even to large headed infants (Gruss and Schmitt 2015). On the other hand, human life history adapted towards the births of premature helpless new-borns whose brains continue to grow even during infancy and childhood. This secondary altricity of human infants made several changes in life history patterns such as the introduction of the childhood phase but also in biocultural behaviour, in particular alloparenting, necessary (Bogin et al. 2014).

Typical cultural strategies are assisted delivery and the development of midwifery and obstetrics. According to Karen Rosenberg a certain kind of midwifery may be assumed since the Genus *Australopithecus* (Rosenberg 1992). Of course, this assumption cannot be verified but there is some evidence that female *Homo sapiens* seek assistance during the process of birth from prehistory onwards. Midwifery is consequently an old profession in order to protect the mother and her new-born (O'Donnell 2004, Rich 2008). Only since the 18th/19th century midwifery turned increasingly to a medical profession and mainly male obstetricians prevail from this time onwards. The medicalization of child birth resulted in the introduction of new methods in obstetrics such as forceps birth, vacuum extraction and last but not least caesarean section (Van Dongen 2009, Antoine and Young (2021).

Death associated with pregnancy and childbirth reduced female life expectancy dramatically in former times and unfortunately even today maternal mortality rate is unacceptably high, first of all in developing countries (WHO 2016).

Currently, worldwide more than 800 women die from preventable causes related to pregnancy and childbirth every day. The majority of these deaths occur in sub-Saharan Africa but also in southern Asian countries such as

Afghanistan and rural India. The maternal mortality rate in developing countries in 2015 is 239 per 100 000 live births while in developed countries maternal mortality rates is 12 per 100 000 live births only (WHO 2016). There are not only large disparities between countries, but also within countries, depending on socioeconomic factors, income, gender roles, female status in society high and area of living urban versus rural areas. The main reasons of recent maternal deaths are postpartum bleeding (15%), complications from unsafe abortion (15%), hypertensive disorders of pregnancy (10%), postpartum infections (8%), and obstructed labour (6%) (GDP 2013). In former times, puerperal phyrexia was a major killer (Chamberlain 2005). In case of caesarean section rates, obstructed labour is of special importance. Obstructed labour or dystocia means that the foetus is not able to exit the pelvis, although the uterus is contracting normally. The main causes of obstructed labour are abnormally positioned foetus such as breech or transverse position but also a too large foetus often in combination with a small or narrow maternal pelvis and consequently mainly a cephalo-pelvic disproportion (WHO 2008).

Maternal Mortality – A Biological Paradox?

From a biological point of view the high rates of maternal mortality but also long and painful labour are rather unexpected. Long labour and risky deliveries are uncommon among other mammals. In contrast, long labour would increase the risk of attracting predators during a time of highest vulnerability. Among recent *Homo sapiens* labour lasts around 9 hours, while apes and monkeys generally give birth within two hours (Shipman 2013). Furthermore, maternal mortality caused by obstructed labour or haemorrhage is quite uncommon among wild mammals. Consequently, in contrast to other mammals and even non-primates *Homo sapiens* is confronted with exceptionally long labour and difficult and dangerous childbirth. But why is human childbirth so risky and painful?

We can look at the Bible. According to book Genesis, God said to Eve after she had eaten the apple from the tree of the knowledge *"I will greatly multiply your pain in childbirth. In pain you will bring forth children."* For scientists this explanation is clearly not a sufficient one.

Human Childbirth and Caesarean Sections - An Evolutionary Perspective

From the viewpoint of evolutionary biology, it seems paradox that reproduction is associated with an increased risk of death for mother and offspring. Maternal death and foetal or new-born death are clearly fitness disasters. Even if the neonate survives birth, the death of the mother increased the risk of neonatal or infant death dramatically. In particular, during prehistory and preagricultural times the death of the mother due to childbirth killed mostly the new-born too. Even the child survived birth, without breastfeeding by the mother there was no chance to survive because the existence of wet-nurses or "bottle-feeding" among prehistoric societies cannot be assumed as a standard (O'Donell 2004). Consequently, a dangerous and maybe life-threatening childbirth contradicts the biogenetic imperative indicating that reproduction is the ultimate goal of any individual and the motor of evolution. As pointed out above, from the biological viewpoint risky and life-threatening deliveries are a paradox, because a successful reproduction is the motor of evolution. Therefore, an evolutionary approach of the problems associated with human childbirth and consequently th rising CVS-rates should be discussed. As Theodosius Dobzhansky pointed out, the concept of evolution should be applied every natural phenomenon "*Nothing in biology makes sense except in the light of evolution*" (Dobzhansky 1973). Consequently, beside a proximate or physiological approach to explain biological phenomenon, an evolutionary or ultimate explanation for each biological condition is necessary. This is especially true of risky human childbirth and as a consequence of high CS-rates today. In the present analysis two evolutionary approaches to explain the problematic of rising CS-rates should be discussed: on the one hand the concept of the evolutionary dilemma of human childbirth, on the other hand the so-called mismatch hypothesis should be applied.

Human Childbirth – An Evolutionary Dilemma?

The first approach to discuss is the evolutionary dilemma hypothesis. As pointed out above, human birth is difficult and dangerous and therefore as early as 1951 Wilton Krogman described human birth as "a scar of evolutionary history" (Krogman 1951). Sherwood Washburn coined the term "obstetric dilemma" (Washburn 1960). The obstetric dilemma or "bipedalism-encephalization conflict" was /is widely considered as the key ultimate factor underlying high levels of maternal and neonate mortality throughout or history and the obstetrical dilemma hypothesis dominated the evolutionary view of human birth since decades (Rosenberg 1992).

According to the evolutionary dilemma hypothesis, painful and dangerous childbirth results from two counteracting evolutionary trends: On the one hand, bipedy, i.e., the upright locomotion on to legs and encephalization, i.e., increasing brain and skull size on the other hand. Both evolutionary trends are considered as typical of humans. The trend to bipedy appeared first about 5 to 6 million years and became the typical locomotion of the genera Australopithecus and Paranthropus, beside the ability to climb on trees. Genus Homo was obligatory biped. Bipedy required typical adaptations of the pelvis on the demands of upright position and bipedal locomotion. To provide a wide base for upper body support and balance, the pelvis became ovoid in shape, flattened in anterior-posterior position and decreased in height. Furthermore, a narrow pelvis in relation to body height is essential to allow the legs to be close together in order to optimize biomechanics of biped locomotion (Gruss and Schmitt 2015). Unfortunately, remains of female pelvic bones are extremely rare in fossil record, therefore the reconstruction of evolution of human childbirth is quite difficult (Simpson et al. 2008, Franciscus 2009, Weaver and Hublin 2009). The other trend making human childbirth so dangerous is encephalization i.e., the increase in brain size and consequently the trend towards larger foetal heads. Brain size and consequently skull size increased dramatically with the emergence of *Homo erectus* about 2 million years ago (Henke and Hardt 2011) and further with the emergence of *Homo sapiens* about 400 000 years ago (Callaway 2017). The antagonistic interaction of bipedalism and encephalization resulting in narrower pelvis and greater new-born heads makes childbirth more complicated. A large neonate head but also the shoulders have a tight fit as the infant passes through the bony birth canal (Rosenberg and Trevathan 2002, Rosenberg 1992, Trevathan 1993, Rosenberg and Trevathan 2014, Buck 2011).

There is no doubt that brain size and consequently head size increased and pelvic structure changed substantially through hominin evolutionary history and that the tight fit between maternal pelvic dimensions and offspring brain size resulted in a complex and dangerous birth process (Wells 2015), although these two evolutionary trends took place not simultaneously. Biped locomotion evolved much earlier than encephalization. Recently the hypothesis of the obstetrical dilemma was re-evaluated, criticized and a new ecological (Wells 2015, Wells et al. 2012), biocultural (Stone 2016) or energetic approach (Dunsworth and Ecclestone 2015) were presented.

The Mismatch Hypothesis

Another approach to focus on human childbirth and CS-rates provides the concept of evolutionary medicine. Nearly 160 years after the publication of Charles Darwin's fundamental work "On the Origin of Species by Means of Natural Selection" in 1859 (Darwin 1859) and more than 140 years after publication of "The Descent of Man and Selection in Relation to Sex" in 1871 (Darwin 1871)], a Darwinian approach is also established in parts of medical science (Zampieri 2009, Fuller 2011, Harris and Malyango 2005). More than 90 years after Darwin's death, evolutionary or ultimate interpretations may lead a better understanding of various current health care issues. During the early 1990s the concept of evolutionary medicine in a recent sense was formalized by the evolutionary biologist George C. Williams and psychiatrist Randolph Nesse (Williams and Nesse 1991), who tried to understand why natural selection has left the human body so vulnerable to diseases. The first concept of evolutionary medicine based on the assumption, that the physiological basis of many medical conditions that are clearly pathological today have been adaptive in the ancestral environment in which *Homo sapiens* evolved and thus have been selected positively for (Williams and Nesse 1991). On the other hand, evolutionary medicine tries to analyse the impact of recent environments on the emergence of disease and medical problems. According to Williams and Nesse the human body is designed for Stone Age conditions. Modern environments may cause many diseases, such as deficiency syndromes, the effects of excess consumption of normally scare nutrients such as fats or salt but also psychological reactions to recent life circumstances (William and Nesse 1991). Consequently, the effects of changing living conditions initiated by the processes of modernization and acculturation on patterns of health and disease are focused on (Nesse and Williams 1994, Nesse and Stearns 2008, Stearns 1999, Trevathan et al. 1999, Trevathan 2007). This concept is also applicable on the problematic of currently rising CS-rates.

There is no doubt that recent *Homo sapiens* has a long evolutionary history and the well-known difficulties of human childbirth have been attributed to contracting evolutionary trends, associated with skeletal changes associated with biped locomotion and the process of encephalization

(Rosenberg and Trevathan 2002, Rosenberg 1992, Trevathan 1993). These aspects of cephalo-pelvic disproportion have been discussed extensively in many studies (Franciscus 2009, Buck 2011, Wells 2015, Wells et al. 2012, Dunsworth and Eccleston 2015, Blackburn 2007, Warrener et al. 2015, Liston 2003, Trevathan and Rosenberg 2014). High caesarean section rates are therefore seen as a result of these evolutionary trends. Evolutionary medicine and the mismatch hypothesis in particular, may provide another aspect of evolutionary patterns of human birth and caesarean section rates. There is clearly no doubt that human childbirth is risky and that human labour is extraordinary long and painful. Furthermore, high maternal mortality rates cannot be denied. But Caesarean section rates of more than 30% are clearly too high to reflect "normal" reproductive patterns of a primate. Evolutionary medicine focuses on the mismatch between the environment in which our species evolved and recent life circumstances.

All recent people are members of the genus *Homo*, which appeared first about 2.4 million years ago in an Eastern African savanna habitat (Henke and Hardt 2011). All species of the genus *Homo* are characterized by an obligatory bipedal locomotion, rapid encephalisation, advanced hunting technology, the ability of making stone tools. With the appearance of *Homo erectus/ergaster* about 2 million years ago marked changes in social behaviour and dieting habits occurred. Increased brain size and larger body size made increased energy supply essential (Aiello and Wells 2002). Hunting, collecting food, looking for drinking water and shelter made a high degree of physical activity essential for surviving. About 300 000 years ago modern *Homo sapiens* originated in Africa and colonized with the exception of Antarctica the whole world. Modern *Homo sapiens* has adapted to widely different habitats and showed a huge developmental plasticity to survive and reproduce successfully under widely different environmental circumstances. Life style of *Homo sapiens* and his ancestors was characterized by a foraging subsistence based on hunting and gathering, the lack of domesticated animals with the exception of the dog, the use of stone and wooden tools, a mobile (nomadic) life style, and small multi-aged egalitarian groups consisting of 20 to 30 group members.

According to the concept of evolutionary medicine several recent medical conditions are the result of a mismatch between the environment in which our ancestors evolved and the recent living conditions. The evolutionary psychologist Bowlby defined the Palaeolithic period when the genus Homo evolved as the environment of evolutionary datedness (EEA) (Bowlby 1969). According to the concept of the environment of evolutionary adaptedness, human biology has adapted through the process of natural selection to the environmental conditions during Palaeolithic. This view is summarized by the notion that "Human biology is designed for Stone Age conditions" as Williams and Nesse pointed out. Our recent life circumstances however are quite different than those during Palaeolithic times. The typical life style of our hunter gatherer ancestors was a highly mobile one because high levels in daily activity in search of food, water and sleeping sites were necessary. Concerning nutritional habits, it is well documented that diets consisted to a high degree of vegetable food, protein (50 to 80%) and a low-fat content (Eaton and Konner 1985). From a medical point of view, typical non-communicable diseases such as hypertension, heart disease, cancer, diabetes or obesity were rather unknown (Eaton et al. 1986). Female life history was characterized by a late age at menarche, an early age of menopause and as a consequence a quite short reproductive span. Long periods of breastfeeding resulted in prolonged birth intervals. *Homo sapiens* is clearly adapted to a life style like this. This kind of life style however changed dramatically. For the first time about 10 000 years ago with the process of Neolithic transition which resulted in the emergence of agriculture and a complete change in subsistence economy and life circumstances (Larsen 1995). A further marked transition of life circumstances occurred during Industrial revolution at the end of 18th century and during the 19th century.

During the 20th and 21stcentury the circumstances of human existence changed dramatically again, especially during the last few decades. Rapid urbanization, a dramatic decrease of physical activity and rising prevalence of obesity and associated diseases are typical of this transition (Kirchengast 2017). Furthermore, reproductive patterns mainly in developed countries changed dramatically. On the one hand, the mean number of offspring decreased, on the other hand, the age at first birth increased. There is no doubt that living standard and health standard have improved during the 20th and 21rst century. Furthermore, advances in medicine reduced risks during pregnancy and childbirth. As a consequence, maternal mortality but also neonatal and childhood mortality dropped down, life expectancy increased dramatically (Trevathan 2007).

Some of these changes in lifestyle have a profound impact on human birth patterns (Kirchengast and Hartmann 2018). The main reasons of caesarean section (when caesarean section on maternal request are excluded) are obstructed labour, twin pregnancy, high blood pressure of the mother and transverse or breech presentation or foetal distress (Savage 2007). Obstructed labour is mainly caused by foetal-pelvic disproportion and macrosomia or large for gestational age neonates (i.e., a birth weight above 4000g). Macrosomia is positively associated with maternal obesity, maternal diabetes and advanced maternal age (Stotland et al. 2004) Consequently, risk factor for increased caesarean section rates are maternal obesity, maternal diabetes, advanced maternal age and infant macrosomia. All those conditions have been quite unknown in the environment of evolutionary adaptedness. Maternal obesity is a quite new condition in our evolution and history, although there is sufficient evidence for the emergence of obesity on an individual basis since the Upper Palaeolithic. On population level however, obesity was not found before the second half of the 20th century (Haslam 2007). Consequently, we are not adapted on the condition obesity during reproductive age.

Obesity, especially super-obesity i.e., a body mass index above 40 kg/m^2, represents a special problem among women of reproductive age. In the United States more than 50% of women ageing between 20 and 39 years are overweight or obese. Europe seems to follow a similar pattern, albeit with some delay. Currently, one in five pregnant women can be classified as obese in Europe (Denison et al. 2010). Obesity during pregnancy has been associated with both short- and long-term health effects for women and their offspring (Leddy et al. 2008, Vahratian 2009). In general, maternal obesity during pregnancy increases the risk for morbidity and mortality of mother and child (Denison et al. 2010, Nohr et al. 2005, Nelson and Fleming 2007, Bhattacharya et al. 2007, Catalano 2010). Furthermore, obese women are more likely to face induction of labour, caesarean section, but also anaesthetic problems, wound infections and postpartum haemorrhage (Denison et al. 2010, Metwally and Ledger 2007). The worldwide increasing rate of caesarean delivery mirrors the increase in obesity trends. In general, obesity is mentioned as one of the most important maternal risk factors of caesarean delivery (Poobalan 2009, Kirchengast and Hartmann 2017, Chui et al. 2007, Seligman et al. 2006, Siega-Riz 2012, Al-Kubaisy et al. 2014). This is especially true of morbid prepregnancy obesity. An Australian study demonstrated that super-obese mothers - i.e., a body mass index above 50kg/m^2 – have a significantly higher risk of obstetric complications during pregnancy and birth. 51.6% of these super-obese women gave birth via caesarean section (Sullivan et al. 2015). Furthermore, obese pregnant women are confronted with a fourfold increased risk of developing gestational diabetes (GDM), which may result in foetal macrosomia and increase caesarean section rate in this way too. Caesarean sections however, are abdominal surgical processes which are especially risky for obese women leading to an increased risk of intraoperative complications such as infectious morbidity, thromboembolic events (Ledfdy et al. 2008 82) but also postpartum haemorrhage (Fyfe et al. 2012), wound complications (Sullivan et al. 2015, Fyfe et al. 2012, Yamasato et al. 2016) prolonged hospitalization (Catalano 2010). Obesity is often associated with low levels of physical activity. As be discussed above, physical activity levels of our ancestors have been high. Low physical activity as typical of recent life circumstances is also associated with increased caesarean section rates (Domenjoz et al. 2014).

Another recent phenomenon which might affect caesarean section rates is the delay of childbirth (Yoshioka-Maeda et al. 2016). During the last decades, the age at first birth increased continuously in the majority of industrialized countries. In Austria for example, age at first birth increased from 23.8 years in 1984 to 30.0 years in 2020 (Statistik Austria 2020). Furthermore, the percentage of mothers older than 40 years nearly doubled from 2.6% in 2004 to 4.3% in 2020 in Austria (Statistik Austria 2020). According to an Australian study advanced maternal age (< 35 years) is associated with a twofold increased likelihood of caesarean section (Dunn et al. 2017). This trend of delaying childbirth and the increasing number of older mothers increase caesarean section rates, too (Kirchengast and Hartmann 2018).

Neither obesity and diabetes nor advanced maternal age are conditions that were frequently found among our evolutionary ancestors. All these conditions are quite new and we are still not fully adapted to these new patterns of lifestyle, weight status and reproductive patterns. The high rates of CS-sections in developed and less developed countries may be therefore a result of the mismatch between our recent life circumstances or environmental conditions and our evolutionary heritage, shaped by life circumstances typical of the environment of evolutionary adaptedness.

Conclusion

Recent trends such as increasing rates of obesity and diabetes among women of reproductive age but also new-born macrosomia and advance maternal age increase caesarean section rates in recent populations. Obesity, diabetes and resulting macrosomia but also delayed childbirth are quite new phenomenon in our evolutionary history. Currently, increasing CS rates may therefore be interpreted as a consequence of a mismatch between our evolutionary heritage and recent life circumstances.

References

Aiello, L. C., and Wells, J. C. K. (2002). Energetics and the evolution of the genus Homo. *Annual Reviews Anthropology* 2002, 31: 323-338.

Ajeet, S., Jaydeep, N., Nandkishore, K., and Nisha, R. (2011). Women's knowledge, perceptions and potential demand towards caesarean section. *National Journal of Community Medicine* 2: 244-248.

Al-Kubaisy, W., Al-Rubaey, M., Al-Naggar, R. A., Karim, B., and Noor, N. A. (2014). Maternal obesity and its relation with caesarean section: a hospital based cross sectional study in Iraq. *Pregnancy and Childbirth*; 14: 235-239.

Antoine, C., and Younbg, B. K. (2021). Cesarean section one hundred years 1920-2020: The Good, the Bad and the Ugly. *Journal of Perinatal Medicine* 49: 5-16.

Bertran, A. P., Merialdi, M., and Lauer, J. A. (2007). Rates of caesarean section: analysis of global, regional, and national estimates. *Paediatric and Perinatal Epidemiology* 21: 98-113.

Bertran, A. P., Ye, J., Moller, A. B., Zhang, J., Gülmezoglu, A. M., and Torloni, M. R. (2016). The increasing trend, in caesarean section rates: global, regional and national estimates 1990-2014. *PLOS one* 11: e0148343.

Bertran, A. P., Ye, J.-, Moller, A. B., Souza, J. P., Zhang, J. (2021), Trends and projections of caesarean section rates: global and regional estimates. *BMJ Global Health* 6: e005671.

Bhattacharya, S., Campbell, D. M., Liston, W. A., and Bhattacharya, S. (2007). Effect of body mass index on pregnancy outcomes in nulliparous women delivering singleton babies. *Public Health* 7: 168-176.

Blackburn Wittmann, A., and Wall LL. (2007). The evolutionary origin of obstructed labor: bipedalism, encephalization and the human obstetric dilemma. *Obstetrics and Gynecology Survey* 62: 739-748.

Bogin, B., Bragg, J., and Kuzawa, C. (2014). Humans are not cooperative breeders but practice biocultural reproduction. *Annals of Human Biology* 41: 368-380.

Bowlby, J. (1969). *Attachment and loss. Basic Books*, New York.

Buck, S. (2011). The evolutionary history of the modern birth mechanism: looking at skeletal and cultural adaptations. *University of West Ontario Journal of Anthropology* 19: 1-12.

Callaway, E. (2017). Oldest *Homo sapiens* fossil claim rewrites our species' history. *Nature* https://doi.org/10.1038/nature.2017.22114.

Catalano, P. M. (2010). Obesity, insulin resistance, and pregnancy outcome. *Reproduction* 140: 365-371.

Chamberlain, G. (2005). British maternal mortality in the 19th and early 20th century. *Journal of the Royal Society of Medicine* 99: 559-563.

Chui, S. Y., Kim, S. Y., Schmid, C. H., Dietz, P. M., Callaghan, W. M., Lau, J., and Curtis, K. M. (2007). Maternal obesity and rik of caesarean delivery: a meta-analysis. *Obesity Reviews* 8: 385-394.

Cruz, C. B., and Codinha, S. (2010) Death of mother and child due to dystocia in 19th century Portugal. *International Journal of Osteoarcheology* 20: 491-496.

Darwin, C. (1859) *On the Origin of Species by means of natural selection*. John Murray, London.

Darwin, C. (1871). *The Descent of Man and Selection in Relation to Sex*. John Murray, London.

Denison, F. C., Roberts, K. A., Barr, S. M., and Norman, J. E. (2010). Obesity, pregnancy, inflammation and vascular function. *Reproduction* 140: 373-385.

Domenjoz, I., Kayser, B., and Boulvain, M. (2014). Effect of physical activity during pregnancy on mode of delivery. *American Journal of Obstetrics and Gynecology* 211: 401–411.

Dobzhansky, T. (1973). Nothing in Biology makes sense except in the light of evolution. *The American Teacher* 35: 125-129.

Dunn, L., Kumar, S., and Beckmann, M. (2017) Maternal age is a risk factor for caesarean section following induction of labor. *Australian and NewZealand Journal of Obstetrics and Gynecology* 57, 426–431.

Dunsworth, H., and Eccleston, L. (2015). The evolution of difficult childbirth and helpless hominin infants. *Annual Review Anthropology* 44: 55-69.

Eaton, S. B, and Konner, M. (1985). Paleolithic nutrition: a consideration of its nature and current implications. *New England Journal of Medicine* 312, 283-289.

Eaton, S. B., Konner, M., and Shostak, M. (1988). Stone agers in the fast lane; chronic degenerative diseases in evolutionary perspective. *American Journal of Medicine* 84, 739-749.

Eurostat (2019). *Large differences in share of caesarean births*. https://ec.europa.eu/eurostat/web/products-eurostat-news/-/ddn-20191217-1.

Faas-Fehervary, P., Schwarz, K., Bauer, L., and Melchert, F. (2005). Caesarean section on demand: Influence of personal birth experience and working environment on attitude of German gynecologists. *European Journal of Obstetric and Gynecology Reproductive Biology* 122: 162-166.

Fischer, B., and Mitteröcker, P. (2015). Covariation between human pelvic shape, stature and head size alleviates the obstetric dilemma. *PNAS* 112, 5655-5660.

Franciscus, R. G. (2009). When did modern human pattern of childbirth arise? New insights from an old Neanderthal pelvis. *PNAS* 106: 9125-9126.

Fuller, J. (2011), Darwinian Medicine: The past and present state of medicine's unifying Science. *UTMJ* 88, 209-214.

Fyfe, E. M., Thompson, J. M. D., Anderson, N. H., Groom, K. M., and McCowan. LM. (2012). Maternal obesity and postpartum haemorrhage after vaginal and caesarean delivery among nulliparous women at term: a retrospective cohort study. *Pregnancy andChildbirth* 12:112.

Gabbe, S., and Holzmann, G. (2001), Obstetricians' choice of delivery. *Lancet* 357: 722-723.

GBD. Mortality and Causes of Death, Collaborators (2013). "Global, regional, and national age-sex specific all-cause and cause-specific mortality for 240 causes of death, 1990-2013: a systematic analysis for the Global Burden of Disease Study 2013." *Lancet* 385: 117–71.

Gruss, L. T., and Schmitt, D. (2015) The evolution of the human pelvis: changing adaptations to bipedalism, obstetrics and thermoregulation. *Philosophical Trans Royal Society B* 370: 20140063.

Harris, E. E., and Malyango, A. A. (2005). Evolutionary explanations in medical and health profession courses: are you answering your students "why" questions? *BMC Med Education,* 5: 16-23.

Haslam, D. (2007) Obesity: a medical history. *Obestrics Reviews* 8, 31-36.

Henderson, J., McCandish, R., Kumiega, L., and Petrou, S. (2001), Systematic review of economic aspects of alternative modes of delivery. *British Journal of Obstetrics and Gynecology,* 108: 49-57.

Henke, W., and Hardt, T. (2011). The genus Homo: origin, speciation and dispersal, in: S. Condemi, G.-C. Weniger (Eds.), *Continuity and Discontinuity in the peopling of Europe: One hundred fifty years of Neanderthal study, Vertebrate Paleobiology and Paleoanthropology*. Springer Press, New York, pp. 17-43.

Högberg, U., Iregren, E., Siven, C. H., and Diener, L. (1987). Maternal deaths in medieval Sweden: an osteological and life table analysis. *Journal of Biosocial Science* 19: 495-503.

Kirchengast, S. (2017). Diabetes and obesity – an evolutionary perspective. *AIMS Medical Science* 4: 28-51.

Kirchengast, S., and Hartmann, B. (2017). Maternal obesity increases the risk of primary as well as secondary caesarean section. *Annals Obesity Disorders* 2: 1017-1021.

Kirchengast, S., and Hartmann, B. (2018) Recent lifestyle parameters are associated with increasing caesarean section rates among singleton term births in Austria. *International Journal of Environmental Research and Public Health.* 21;16(1). pii: E14. doi: 0.3390/ijerph160 10014.

Krogman, W. M. (1951). The scars of human evolution. *Scientific American* 184: 54-57.

Larsen, C. (1995) Biological changes in human populations with agriculture. *Annual Review Anthropology* 24, 185-213.

Leddy, M. A., Power, M. L., and Schulkin, J. (2008). The impact of maternal obesity on maternal and fetal health. *Reviews Obstetrics and Gynecology* 1: 170-178.

Liston, W. A. (2003). Rising caesarean section rates: Can evolution and ecology explain some of the difficulties of modern childbirth? *Journal Royal Society Medicine* 96: 559-561.

Litorp, H., Mgaya, A., Kidanto, H. L., Johnsdottir, S., and Essen, B. (2015) "What about the mother" Women's and caregivers' perspectives on caesarean birth in a low-resource setting with rising caesarean section rates. *Midwifery* 31: 713-720.

Liverse, A. R., Bazaliiski, V. I., and Weber, A. W. (2015). Death by twins: a remarkable case of dystochic childbirth in early Neolithic Sibiria. *Antiquity* 89: 23-38.

Loudon, I. (2000). Maternal mortality in the past and its relevance to developing countries today. *American Journal Clinical Nutrition* 72: 241-246.

MacFarlane, A. J, Blondel, B., Mohangoo, A. D., Cuttini, M., Nijhuis, J., Novak, Z., Olafsdottir, H. S., and Zeitlin, J. Euro-Peristat Scientific Committee. (2015). Wide differences in mode of delivery within Europe: risk-stratified analyses of aggregated routine data from the Euro-Peristat study. *British Journal Obstetrics Gynecology* doi 10.1111/1471-0528.13284.

Markl, H. (1983). "Wie unfrei ist der Mensch? Von der Natur in der Geschichte." In: Markl H. (ed). *Natur und Geschichte.* München. ["How unfree is man? Of nature in history." In: Markl H. (ed). *Nature and history*.]

Meloni, A., Loddo, A., Martsidis, K., Delana, S. F., Porru, D., Antonelli, A., Marongiu. D., Piras, B., Paoletti, A. M., and Melis, G. B. (2012). The role of caesarean section in modern obstetrics. *Journal Pediatric and Neonatal Individual Medicine* 1: 53-58.

Metwally, M., Li, T. C., Ledger, W. L. (2007) The impact of obesity on female reproductive function. *Obesity Reviews* 8: 515-523.

Molina. G., Weiser, T. G., Lipsitz, S. R., Esquivel, M. M., Uribe-Leitz, T., Azad, T., Shah. N., Semrau, K., Berry, W. R., Gawande, A. A., and Haynes, A. B. (2015) Relationship between caesarean delivery rate and maternal and neonatal mortality. *JAMA* 314: 2263-2270.

Nelson, S. M., and Fleming, R. (2007). Obesity and reproduction: impact and interventions. *Current Opinion Obstetrics Gynecology* 19: 384-389.

Nesse, R. M., and Williams, G. C. (1994). Why we get sick: the new science of Darwinian medicine. *Vintage books*, New York.

Nesse, R. M, and Stearns, S. C. (2008). The great opportunity: Evolutionary applications to medicine and public health. *Evolutionary Applications* 1, 28-48.

Nohr, E. A., Bech, B. H., Davies, M. J., Frydenberg, M., Henriksen, T. B., and Olsen, J. (2005). Prepregnancy obesity and fetal death. *Obstetrics and Gynecology*106: 250-259.

O'Donnell, E. (2004). Birthing in prehistory. *Journal of Anthropology and Archeology* 23: 163-171.

OECD (2019): *Caesarean sections.* www.oecd-ilibrary.org/sites/fa1f7281-en/index.

Odent, M. (2004) *The caesarean*. Free Association books London.

Pfeiffer, S., Doyle, LE. Kurki, H. K., Harrington, L., Ginter, J. K., and Merritt, C. E. (2014). Discernment of mortality risk with childbirth in archeologically derived forager skeleton. *International Journal of Paleopathology* 7: 15-24.

Poobalan, A. S., Aucott, L. S., Gurung, T., Smith, W. C. S., and Bhattacharya, S. (2009). Obesity as an independent risk factor for elective and emergency delivery in nulliparous women – systematic review and meta-analysis of cohort studies. *Obesity Reviews* 10: 28-35.

Rich, S. A. (2008). Midwifery and Neolithic Malta: Interpeting and contextualizing two terracotta figurines. *Journal of Applied Anthropology* 34: 260-268.

Rosenberg, K. R., and Trevathan, W. R. (2002). Birth, obstetric and evolution. *British Journal of Obstetrics and Gynecology* 109: 119-1206.

Rosenberg, K. R. (1992). The evolution of modern human childbirth. *Yearbook American Journal of Physical Anthropology* 35: 89-124.

Rosenberg, K. R, and Trevathan, W. R (2014). Evolutionary obstetrics. *Evolution Medicine Public Health* doi: 10:.1093/e,ph/eou025.

Saeed, K. B. M., Greene, R. A., O'Neill, C. P., and Sinéad, M. (2017). "Incidence of surgical site infection following caesarean section: a systematic review and meta-analysis protocol." *BMJ Open* 7 e013037.

Sayer, D., and Dickinson, S. D. (2013) Reconsidering obstetric death and female fertility in Anglo-Saxon England. *Word Archeology* 45: 285-297.

Savage, W. (2007). The rising Caesarean section rate: a loss of obstetric skill? *Journal Obstetrics Gynaecology* 27: 339–46.

Seligman, L. C., Duncan, B. B., Branchtein, L., Daio, D. S. M., Menguw, S. S., and Schmidt M. I. (2006). Obesity and gestational weight gain: caesarean delivery and labor complications. *Reviews Saude Publica* 2006;40: 457-465.

Siega-Riz, A. M. (2012) Prepregnancy obesity: determinants, consequences and solutions. *Advances in Nutrition* 3: 105-107.

Shipman, P. (2013). Why is Childbirth so painful? *American Scientific* 101:426.

Smid, M. C., Kearney, M. S., and Stamilio, D. M. (2015) Extreme obesity and post-caesarean wound complications in the maternal-fetal medicine unit caesarean registry. *American Journal Perinatology* 32: 1336-1341.

Simpson, S. W., Quade, J., Levin, N. E., Butler, R., Dupont-Nivet, G., Everett, M., and Semaw, S. A. (2008). Female *Homo erectus* pelvis from Gona Ethiopia. *Science* 322: 1089-1092.

Stamilio. D. M., and Scifres, C. M. (2014). Extreme obesity and postcaesarean complications. *Obstetrics and Gynecology* 124: 227-232.

Statistik Austria. (2016). *Demographic Yearbook*. Vienna, Austria.

Stearns, S. (1999), *Evolution in Health and Disease*. Oxford University Press.

Stone. P. K. (2016). Biocultural perspectives on maternal mortality and obstetrical death from the past to the present. *Yearbook American Journal Physical Anthropology* 159: S150-S171.

Stotland, N. E., Hopkins, L. M., and Caughey, A. B. (2004). Gestational weight gain, macrosomia and risk of caesarean birth in nondiabetic nulliparas. *Obstetrics and Gynecolology* 104: 671-677.

Sullivan. E. A, Dickinson, J. E., Vaughan, G. A., Peek, M. J., Ellwood, D., and Homer, C. S. (2015). Knight M, McLintock C, Wang A, Pollock W, Jackson Pulver L, Li Z, Javid N, Denney-Wilson E, Callaway L. Australasian Maternity Outcomes Surveillance System. Maternal super-obesity and perinatal outcomes in Australia: a national population-based cohort study. *BMC Pregnancy Childbirth* 15:322-332.

Tarney, C. M. (2014). When patients request the knife – caesarean delivery on maternal request. *Journal of Women's Health, Issues and Care* 3: 1000130.

Todman, D. (2007). A history of caesarean section: from ancient world to modern area. *Australian and NewZealand Journal of Obsterics and Gynecology*, 47357-361.

Todman, D. Eduardo Porro (1842-1902) and the development of caesarean section: a reappraisal. *International Journal of Gynecology Obstetrics*.

Torloni, M. R., Betran, A. P., Souza, J. P., Widmer, M., Allen, T, Gulmezoglu, M., Merialdi, M. (2011) Classifications for caesarean section: a systematic review. *Plos one*. 6: e14566.

Trevathan, W. R, and Rosenberg, K. R. (2014). Caesarean section. *Evolution Medicine Public Health* doi: 10.1093/emph/eou0311.

Trevathan, W. R. (1993). The evolutionary history of childbirth. *Human Nature* 4: 337-350.

Trevathan, W. R., McKenna, J. J., and Smith, E. O. (1999). *Evolutionary medicine*. Oxford University Press.

Trevathan, W. R. (2007). Evolutionary medicine. *Annual Review Anthropology* 36, 139-154.

Van Dongen, P. W. L. (2009). Caesraean section – etymology and early history. *South African Journal Obstetrics Gynecology* 15: 1-5.

Vahratian, A. (2009). Prevalence of overweight and obesity among women of childbearing age. *Maternal Child Health Journal* 13: 268-273.

Vilar, J., Carroli, G., Zavaleta, N., Donner, A., Wojdyla, D., and Faunders, A. (2007) Maternal and neonatal individual risks and benefits associated with caesarean delivery: multicenter prospective study. *BMJ*; 335: 1025.

Volpe, F. M. (2011). Correlation of caesarean rates to maternal and infant mortality rates: an ecologic study of official international data. *Review Panam Salud Publica* 29: 303-308.

Warrener, A. G., Lewton, K. L., Pontzer, H., and Lieberman, D. E. (2015). A wider pelvis does not increase locomotor cost in humans with implications for the evolution of childbirth. *Plos one* 10: e0118903.

Washburn, S. l. (1960). Tools and human evolution. *Scientific American*, 203: 63-75.

Weaver, T. D., and Hublin, J. J. (2009). Neanderthal birth canal shape and the evolution of human childbirth. *PNAS* 106: 81251-8156.

Weiner, S., Monge, J., and Mann, A. (2008). Bipedalism and parturition: an evolutionary imperative for caesarean delivery. *Clinical Perinatology* 35: 469-478.

Wells, J. C. K. (2015). Between scylla and charybdis: renegotiating resolution of the obstetric dilemma in response to ecological change. *Philosophical Transactions Royal Society B* 370: 20140067.

Wells, J. C. K., DeSilva, J. M., and Stock, J. T (2012).. The obstetric dilemma: An ancient game of Russian roulette or a variable dilemma sensitive to ecology? *Yearbook American Journal Physical Anthropology;* 55: 40-71.

Williams, G. C., and Nesse, R. M. (1991). The dawn of Darwinian medicine. *Quarterly Review Biology* 66, 1-22.

World Health Organization (2015). *WHO statement on Caesrean section rate.* www.who.int/reproductivehealth/publications/maternal_perinatal _health/cs-statement/.

World Health Organization (2016) *Health statistics and information systems: Maternal mortality ratio (per 100 000 live births).* World Health Organization.

World Health Organization (2007). *Recommended interventions for improving maternal and newborn health.* WHO/MPS/07.05 Geneva.

World Health Organization. (2008) *Education material for teachers of midwifery: midwifery education modules* Geneva. pp. 17–36.

World Health Organization. (1985) Appropriate technology for birth. *Lancet* 326: 436-437.

Yamasato, K., Yoshino, K., Chang, A. L., Caughey, A. B., and Tsai, P. J. (2016). Caesarean delivery complications in women with morbid obesity. *Journal Maternal Fetal Neonatal Medicine* 29: 3885-3888.

Yoshioka-Maeda, K., Ota, E., Ganchimeg, T., Kuroda, M., and Mori, R. (2016). Caesarean section by maternal age group among singleton deliveries and primiparous Japanese women: a secondary analysis of the WHO global survey on maternal and perinatal health. *BMC Pregnancy and Childbirth* 16: 39-45.

Zampieri F. (2009) Origins and History of Darwinian Medicine. *Humana Mente* 9, 13-3.

Chapter 4

Non-Tubal Ectopic Pregnancy: Treatment Update

Enrique Achiaga Sánchez[1], MD, Cristina de Miguel López[1], MD, María Teresa Gómez García[2,3,*], PhD, José M. García Cebrián[1], MD, Sergio Rico Cardenal[1], MD and Antonio Nicolás Amezcua Recover[2,3], PhD

[1]Department of Obstetrics and Gynecology,
Complejo Hospitalario Universitario de Albacete, Albacete, Spain
[2]Department of Obstetrics and Gynecology,
Complejo Hospitalario Universitario de Albacete, Albacete, Spain
[3]School of Medicine, Universidad de Castilla La Mancha,
Albacete, Spain

Abstract

Ectopic pregnancy (EP) is defined as a pregnancy implanted at a place other than the endometrial line of the uterine body, mostly the fallopian tube (96%). However, EP can have other locations such as the ovary (3%), interstitial/cornual (2-3%), abdominal (1%), c-section scar (<1%) and cervical (<1%). In these days, EP remains the leading cause of early pregnancy related death. Diagnosis of this condition is usually made via

* Corresponding Author's E-mail: tgomezg67@gmail.com.

In: A Closer Look at Pregnancy and Childbirth
Editor: Louise J. Salgado
ISBN: 978-1-68507-658-0

transvaginal ultrasound (TVUS). Serial serum beta-human chorionic gonadotropin (bHCG) measurement may help to differentiate normal from abnormal pregnancies and rise suspicion of an EP. Non-tubal ectopic pregnancies (NTE) are a very rare entity. Their heterogeneous clinical presentation, diagnostic difficulties and absence of gold-standard treatments cause high rates of morbidity and mortality compared to tubal ectopic pregnancies. In this chapter, our aim is to collect the latest evidence on treatment for non-tubal EP.

Ovarian ectopic pregnancy accounts for cases where embryonic implantation occurs within the ovary. Even though cases are rare, its incidence is increasing due to assisted reproduction techniques. Diagnosis is a challenge, with most of cases being misdiagnosed as corpus luteum, tubal ectopic pregnancy or ovarian tumors. Therefore, patients usuallydebut with intraperitoneal hemorrhage and laparoscopic partial or total oophorectomy is the management of choice. Methotrexate (MTX) may be an option in high-risk patients or persistent residual trophoblast.

Interstitial pregnancies implant in the proximal tubal segment that lies within the muscularuterine wall. Insertion on the round ligament is the characteristic anatomic finding. Regarding its low incidence, no clear criteria for medical treatment have been assessed and surgical management is based on cornual resection.

Abdominal pregnancy is implanted within the peritoneal cavity. Diagnosis is usually sonographic and drugs such as MTX have had minimal success on its treatment, so surgery is always the first option once this entity is confirmed.

C-section scar pregnancies are located in the myometrium at the site of a previous uterine c-section. Cases have risen lately and they are supposed to increase slowly. Optimal management is still unknown. Expectant, medical, and surgical approaches have been used. Surgical approach either using hysteroscopy, laparoscopy, suction curettage or open surgery has the highest success rate and lowest complication rates. Clinical and sonographicfeatures, gestational age at diagnosis, complication rates, desire of the patient and the physician's experience should be considered when choosing between treatments.

Cervical pregnancy involves implantation in the cervical canal. It seems like its incidence has been rising lately due to ART. Diagnosis is based on symptoms and TVUS. Because of its oddity, there are no clear criteria for medical treatment, although MTX is usually the first-line therapy.

Keywords: non-tubal ectopic pregnancy, treatment, update

Introduction

Ectopic pregnancy (EP) is defined as a pregnancy implanted at a place other than the endometrial line of the uterine body. It occurs in the fallopian tube the vast majority of times -around 96%-, which is known as tubal ectopic pregnancy (TEP), but there are other places where the blastocyst can become implanted and this is known as non-tubal ectopic pregnancy (NTEP) [1]. A population-based study of 1800 surgically treated cases by Bouyer J (2002) showed that 3.2% of EP are located at the ovary, 2.4% at the uterine horn (also known as interstitial pregnancy) and 1,3% are abdominal pregnancies [2].

We must not forget about uterine ectopic sites of implantation such as the cervix (<1%), a histerotomy scar (1/2216 pregnancies) [3] or the miometrium.

Cervical Pregnancy

Cervical pregnancy (CP) is defined as the implantation of the blastocyst in the endocervical canal. It is a rare condition which affects approximately 1 in 9,000 pregnancies.

It has gained relevance over the past few years because it is related to assisted reproductive technologies (ART), particularly in-vitro fertilization (IVF). Since the beginning of the 90s, CP had been believed to represent 3,7% of IVF ectopic gestations [4]. However, recent studies, such as an analysis of 91,067 pregnancies achieved by ART published by Matorras (2020) showed a smaller proportion (around 2%) [5]. The authors suggest this is due to a technical improvement in IVF techniques. In addition, they highlight several risk factors of CP in ART, such as a history of at least two pregnancies, miscarriages, at least one curettage and smoking.

CP usually presents as profuse vaginal bleeding which can be life-threatening. Pain is not a very typical symptom, as it only occurs in about a third of patients [6].

As for diagnosis, transvaginal ultrasound (TVUS) is a worthwhile technique which can detect up to 87,5% of cases and several diagnostic criteria were proposed by Kung (2004) [7] (Figure 1):

1. The presence of the gestational sac or placental texture dominantly within the cervix.
2. No evidence of intrauterine pregnancy.

3. Visualization of an endometrial stripe.
4. Hourglass uterine shape with ballooned cervical canal.
5. A sac with active cardiac motion below the internal os for viable pregnancy.

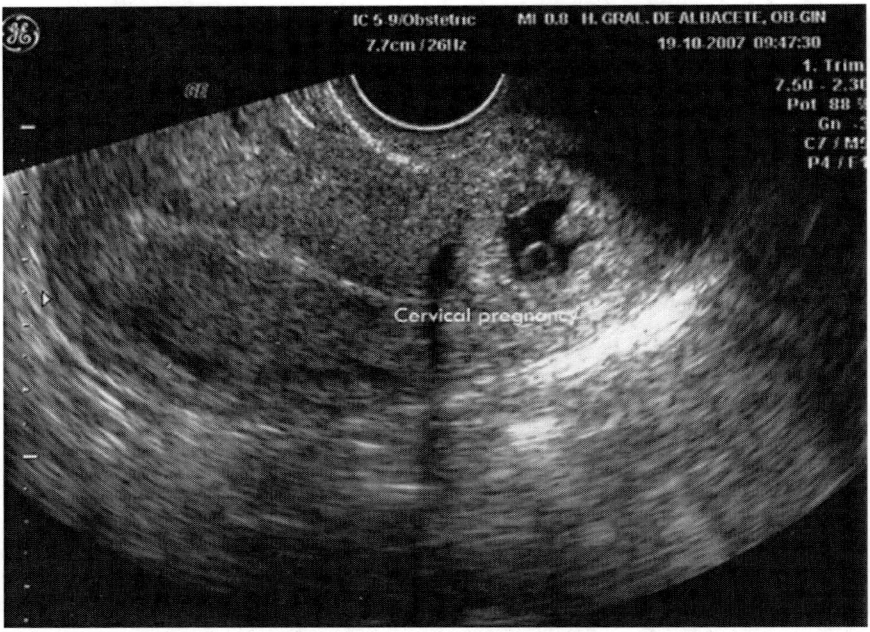

Figure 1. Cervical pregnancy. From Gómez et al. [16].

Serum BHCG levels will support TVUS in order to reach a correct diagnosis. Serum BHCG levels over 3150 mIU/mL usually represent an important threshold because in 99% of intrauterine pregnancies we will find a gestational sac. However, some authors propose 1500 mIU/mL (a gestational sac will be found in 80% of the cases) or 2000 mIU/mL (a gestational sac will be found in 91% of the cases) [8].

Improvements and technical advances in TVUS and laboratory findings have allowed a much earlier diagnosis of CP and this is the reason why its treatment and prognosis have changed within the past few decades.

Cervical pregnancy's low incidence makes it hard to establish a standard treatment and our knowledge is limited to case reports and case series. However, we must highlight the importance of conservative treatment when the patient is hemodynamically stable because a surgical approach can lead to hysterectomy if there is uncontrolled bleeding [9].

Medical treatment with MTX is recommended as the first-line option when the embryo does not present cardiac activity. Administration of MTX can follow a single-dose pattern or a multidose pattern, as it has been described in multiple cases, and it can be injected systemically (intramuscular route) and/or locally (intra-sac route) [10].

When the embryo presents cardiac activity, several authors have proposed the administration of intra-amniotic potassium chloride (KCl) [11]. To perform KCl injection, a 20 to 22 gauge needle is advanced transvaginally into the gestational sac and fetal thorax under direct ultrasound visualization using a needle guide attachment. When the tip of the needle is in the embryo, KCl (1 to 5 mL of 20 percent KCl solution) is injected until there is cessation of cardiac activity [12].

In view of what has been exposed above, there is a wide variety of regimes for medical treatment in CP. Some cases have been treated with a single-dose regime of MTX, others were resolved after a multi-dose regime and both options have been described with or without the combination of intra-sac administration of KCl and/or MTX. Anyways, we can conclude conservative medical approach leads to resolution of CP in the vast majority of cases and side effects will depend on the dose of MTX used and each patient's susceptibility to this drug.

We must not forget the mifepristone/MTX regime as another treatment option which has been used and described within the past decades. The mechanism of action of the two-drug combination in resolving a CP is unclear. It has been speculated that the trophoblastic effect of MTX is enhanced by antidecidual-like action of mifepristone, which would lead to cervical trophoblast destruction [13]. In 2002, Sexton and Sharp presented the first clinical description of a patient diagnosed with a cervical ectopic pregnancy successfully treated with methotrexate and mifepristone. The management initially consisted of MTX, but oral mifepristone 400 mg was added on the third day due to a low response. The measure was actually rescue therapy for the failed monotherapy, but the successful outcome suggested that this could be another type of safe, effective treatment for these unusual pregnancies [14]. This theory was also supported by De Greef et al. in 2005: they described a case in which the association of MTX and mifepristone had a crucial effect on resolution of ectopic pregnancy. After four repeated doses of methotrexate over 1 week, cardiac activity persisted and mifepristone administration was necessary to confirm an undetectable embryo heartbeat [15]. The authors proposed that the combination of mifepristone with a prostaglandin used for therapeutic termination of an intrauterine pregnancy could theoretically be an alternative in ectopic cervical pregnancy, but a search of the literature to date found no articles on the issue. Later on, in 2012, Gómez García presented a series of CP cases treated successfully with a methotrexate/mifepristone combination. In one of the cases, intravaginal misoprostol was used in order to achieve the elimination of the gestational sac and to complete the treatment [16].

Other forms of treatment include intracervical dilation and curettage, which has been the traditional approach, but we can not forget there is a risk of severe hemorrhage which can lead to hysterectomy.

That's why some authors like Ishikawa H et al. (2016) have proposed measures such as intracervical administration of vasopressin before curettage: they injected diluted vasopressin transvaginally into the cervix surrounding the gestational sac, but not directly into the gestational sac, and/or the lower segment of the uterine body under transvaginal ultrasonographic guidance. After cessation of fetal heartbeats, they aspirated the conceptus by performing suction curettage. They injected additional vasopressin into the gestational sac in cases with a viable fetus after the initial injection. Forced contraction of the cervical smooth muscle facilitated removal of the conceptus with minimal blood loss during curettage. The uterus was successfully preserved without any complications in all patients [17].

Other authors have presented studies in which they performed a selective uterine artery embolization (UAE) before curettage in order to prevent excessive bleeding, like Hu J et al. (2016): nineteen patients underwent selective UAE. None of the 19 patients reported any further vaginal bleeding after the UAE procedure. Curettage was performed within the first 24–72 hours after UAE. None of the 19 patients required a hysterectomy for CP. No severe side effects related to UAE were observed. No further treatment was needed after curettage [18].

We have also found a series of CP cases presented by Scutiero G et al. (2013) treated via hysteroscopy resection after UAE. No vaginal bleeding or other side effects were observed throughout and after the treatment, all women recovered without complications, and no subsequent treatment was needed [19].

Finally, hysterectomy is the last step of CP's treatment and it is restricted to those patients in which bleeding is uncontrolled and life-threatening. Although it might be an option for those patients who do not desire to get pregnant in the future, we must not forget this is a major surgery and it shouldn't be performed as a first-line treatment option.

Hysterotomy/Cesarean Scar Pregnancy

Hysterotomy scar pregnancy or cesarean scar pregnancy (CSP) refers to placental implantation within the scar of a previous cesarean delivery [1]. It was first described by Larsen JV back in 1978 [20] and it is believed its incidence might have increased significantly due to the increase of cesarean birth rates worldwide. CSP occurs in about 1 out of 2000 pregnancies [21] and it is known to represent up to 6% of ectopic pregnancies in patients with a prior cesarean delivery [3]. Around 52% of CSP will appear in women with just one previous cesarean scar [22] and it seems prior c-sections indicated due to breech presentation are more likely to increase the risk of CSP [23]. No published data exist regarding an association between hysterotomy closure technique and CSP.

CSP has been classified depending on the characteristics of the place of implantation. In this way, we will find endogenic CSP in which the embryo implants on the scar or exogenic CSP in which the embryo implants within a dehiscent scar. It is worth mentioning that endogenic CSPs usually have a better outcome and prognosis than exogenic ones [24].

There is a wide variety of clinical presentations for CSP. In a review by Rotas et al. (2006) they included 59 articles. Four of those articles were case series that included 8, 12, 15, and 18 cases, respectively. The total number of cases reported was 112. All selected publications provided information on clinical presentation and diagnosis, with emphasis on success, failure, and complications of different treatments. It was observed that the majority of women who reported symptoms had vaginal bleeding and/or abdominal pain while the rest remained asymptomatic and were diagnosed by transvaginal ultrasound (TVUS) [3].

Diagnostic criteria for CSP were first proposed by Vial et al. in 2000 [25], but several modifications have been added within the past few years, so nowadays, TVUS criteria are the following, according to the Society for Maternal-Fetal Medicine:

1. An empty uterine cavity and endocervix.
2. Placenta, gestational sac, or both embedded in the hysterotomy scar.

3. A triangular (at 8 weeks of gestation and earlier) or rounded or oval (after 8 weeks of gestation) gestational sac that fills the scar "niche" (the shallow area representing a healed hysterotomy site).
4. A thin (1-3 mm) or absent myometrial layer between the gestational sac and bladder.
5. A prominent or rich vascular pattern at or in the area of a cesarean scar.
6. An embryonic or fetal pole, yolk sac, or both with or without fetal cardiac activity [26].

CSP can be difficult to distinguish from other clinical entities which have similar echogenic characteristics, such as cervical pregnancy, spontaneous miscarriage in transit or eutopic gestation with a low implantation. This was shown in a review of 751 cases of CSP by Timor-Tritsch (2012) in which they observed 13,6% of CSP were misdiagnosed [27].

As for treatment, no optimal approach has been published and most of the existing information proceeds from case reports and series of cases. However, it seems clear that expectant management is never an option when the embryo presents cardiac activity due to the high risk of severe maternal morbidity, as it has been described in several series of cases and reviews, such as the one made by Cali G (2018), which concluded there is a considerable risk of severe hemorrhage, early uterine rupture, hysterectomy and severe abnormally invasive placenta. Otherwise, expectant management could be a feasible option in those cases in which the embryo does not present cardiac activity [28]. The need for measuring these patients 'myometrial thickness has been assessed by Kaelin Agten A et al. (2017) and they concluded women with a <2mm myometrium containing an exogenic CSP were at high risk of undergoing hysterectomy [24].

In the case of mothers who do not give their consent to terminate pregnancy, an exhaustive counseling should be performed and potential maternal risks should be discussed. After this, a cesarean birth should be performed between 34+0 and 35+6 weeks and antenatal corticosteroid therapy for fetal maturation prior to the surgery should be taken into consideration if necessary. The birth should take place in a facility which is provided with equipment and professionals capable of managing massive hemorrhage [29].

In hemodynamically stable women who desire a future pregnancy, wedge resection (transvaginal or via laparotomy or laparoscopy) and TVUS-guided aspiration curettage have been performed with high success rates. One of the advantages of resection is that the uterine scar can be excised and repaired in that moment, but it is not known whether this technique prevents CSP in the future [30]. As for sharp curettage, it is not recommended due to its high rates of complications and needs for a second intervention [26].

Quick recovery after surgery and the lack of need for future interventions make this approach the most recommendable amongst patients who desire future pregnancy.

As far as medical treatment is concerned, MTX has shown to be a feasible option. However, many studies recommend against the use of systemic MTX alone due to its high risk of side effects. In a literature review by Cheung (2015) they determined the outcome of using ultrasound-guided local methotrexate injection as the first-line treatment of CSP and they concluded it is effective in 73,9% of patients when used alone and in 88,5% of patients when an additional dose of systemic MTX was used. This approach seemed to be useless in those patients whose BHCG serum's level was above 100.000 IU/L [31].

TVUS-guided intra-gestational administration of KCl has been described in the management of heterotopic CSP because exposure to MTX can be hazardous for the intrauterine cotwin. This technique has shown encouraging results [32].

Medical treatment's main disadvantage, particularly for those women who desire future pregnancy, is that it can take weeks for the CSP to be absorbed.

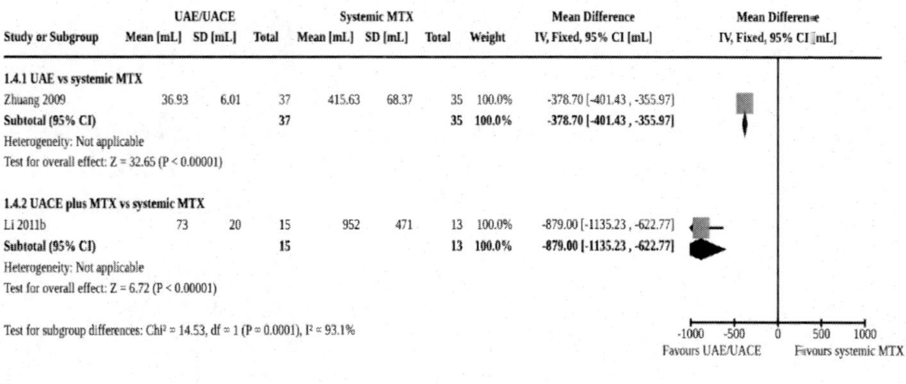

Figure 2. UAE/UACE versus systemic MTX, both + suction curettage, Outcome: Blood loss. From Long Y et al. [33].

As for additional techniques such as uterine artery embolization (UAE), in 2020, The Cochrane Library published a review on interventions for NTEP in which they included five randomized clinical trials reporting CSP. Two compared UAE or uterine arterial chemoembolization (UACE) plus methotrexate (MTX) versus systemic MTX and subsequent dilation and suction curettage; one compared UACE plus MTX versus ultrasonography-guided local MTX injection; and two compared suction curettage under hysteroscopy versus suction curettage under ultrasonography after UAE/UACE.

The quality of evidence ranged from moderate to very low. The main limitations were imprecision, multiple comparisons with a small number of trials, and insufficient data available to assess heterogeneity.

The authors were not able to conclude whether UAE/UACE was able to improve the success rates or minimize complications in CSP treatment. However, it seemed there was a smaller blood loss in those cases in which UAE/UACE was performed instead of or besides systemic MTX alone prior to suction curettage (Figure 2).

As far as hysteroscopy-guided suction curettage vs. TVUS-guided suction curettage is concerned, the authors were not able to conclude which approach improved the success rates or minimized complications in CSP treatment [33].

Several studies have shown there is a considerable risk of recurrence of CSP in women who have undergone conservative management. Rates range between 5% and 40% depending on the series of cases, so patients should always be informed about the risk of a subsequent CSP [34-36].

Abdominal Pregnancy

Abdominal pregnancy (AP) occurs when the products of conception implant in the peritoneal cavity, but not the fallopian tubes nor the miometrium [1]. It is known as a rare condition affecting 1 in 10,000 pregnancies and that is the reason why the vast majority of the evidence we have got on AP comes from case reports or series of cases [37]. Many locations have been described over the past decades, including the broad ligament, omentum, uterine serosa or even other abdominal organs such as spleen or liver.

Clinical presentation of AP is varied because the embryo or fetus can be implanted at different places. For example, those pregnancies implanted at the bowel may be coincident with prominent digestive symptoms such as nausea and vomiting. On the other hand, some cases of AP can remain unnoticed until term and debut as fetal movements perception [38]. In a few cases, patients present with a shock after a massive intra-abdominal hemorrhage due to placental implantation in large blood vessels or intraabdominal viscera [37].

Because of all these characteristics exposed above, there is not a gold-standard test nor specific algorithm to reach diagnosis of abdominal pregnancy. As for BHCG serum level, it apparently matches gestational age such as in eutopic pregnancies and unlike tubal ectopic pregnancies, in which speed of rise is lower [39]. This can make it even harder to diagnose this condition.

As far as treatment is concerned, it is always recommended to interrupt pregnancy when a diagnosis of AP is reached and we can find many management options amongst the wide variety of cases published within the past years.

Firstly, we must not forget that therapeutic options depend on the place of implantation of the AP, the moment of diagnosis (first trimester or second/third trimester) and whether the fetus is above the lower limit of viability of pregnancy or not.

When AP is found during the first trimester, laparoscopy is often performed in order to treat this condition and to determine the exact place of implantation [40]. If placental implantation involves a large blood vessel, additional techniques such as selective arterial embolization have been proposed with encouraging results. However, when this happens, the risk of severe hemorrhage increases and that is why a laparotomy should be performed [41].

As for medical treatment, administration of MTX has been attempted in extremely few cases, leading to poor results. Due to this, no further research has been done and, therefore, it is not recommended [42]. However, we have found few cases in which intra-gestational administration of MTX and KCl has been successful [43, 44].

When AP is diagnosed during the second/third trimesters, management becomes automatically more complex because placental tissue is more developed and vascularised and the implantation area is larger, which can lead to further organic compromise and complications at the time of placental extraction. What is more, it will be necessary to individualize an appropriate obstetrical approach depending on the fetus 'gestational age in case the mother does not give her consent for the interruption of pregnancy.

Once obstetrical management has been decided, the main concern will be the path to follow when it comes to placental extraction. Throughout the literature, we mainly find two ways of dealing with this problem. However, it seems clear that the first step must involve cutting off placental blood supplies [45].

On the one hand, some authors have presented cases in which they attempted to remove the placenta when its location made it possible, i.e., it is not implanted in vital abdominal organs or main blood vessels. This has usually been achieved thanks to a multidisciplinary implication of healthcare staff and several techniques have been described, such as selective arterial embolization. In order to plan the surgery, an imaging technique such as a magnetic resonance (MRI scan) will be helpful [46].

On the other hand, several series of cases propose a conservative management after ligating placental vessels when extraction does not seem feasible. After several months or even years, serum BHCG levels decrease and the placenta is absorbed. However, leaving the placenta inside the patient's abdomen leads to necrosis and this has been related to a greater risk of intraabdominal infection, sepsis, fistula and/or obstruction. If conservative management is chosen, it will be necessary to monitor serum BHCG levels until they become undetectable [38, 47].

Methotrexate is known to inhibit DNA synthesis, repair and cellular replication. Due to this, it does not sound reasonable to attempt medical management of AP with MTX after surgery because placental tissue will be mitotically inactive [48]. However, some authors have suggested the use of MTX in patients whose serum BHCG level remains stable.

Some studies have proved the best approach is to remove as much placental tissue as possible in order to avoid some of the complications described above.

As for the use of mifepristone as part of conservative medical management, no studies showing encouraging results have been published within the past years.

Postoperative reproductive outcomes after treating an AP have not been studied properly yet, but we must not forget this is a heterogeneous clinical condition whose symptoms range from mild to severe and remission can take years, so it is hard to determine the effect that AP can have on future pregnancies accurately.

Interstitial Pregnancy

Interstitial pregnancy (IP) refers to those pregnancies implanted in the proximal tubal segment that lies within the muscular uterine wall. This kind of ectopic pregnancy was traditionally known as cornual pregnancy, but this term is not correct because cornual pregnancy accounts for those pregnancies implanted in the horns of uteri with müllerian anomalies [1]. IP represents 2-4% of all EP cases and its death rates have remained stable within the past decades: while EP mortality rate has moved from 72%-90% by the end of the 19th century to 0,14% in 1990, IP still has a death rate of around 2,5% [49,50]. This is probably because IP can easily be misdiagnosed as an eutopic pregnancy with an eccentric implantation. Risk factors for IP were described in a summary elaborated by Tulandi (2004), which highlighted ipsilateral salpingectomy, previous ectopic pregnancy and in vitro fertilization [51].

IP usually presents as a typical TEP (abdominal pain and vaginal bleeding), but what makes it different to TEP is the gestational age at presentation (8-10 weeks) and, subsequently, the incidence of rupture (20-50% of cases) [52].

Diagnosis can be reached via TVUS (Figure 3) and several criteria have been proposed, such as eccentric location of the gestational sac or myometrial thickness under 5mm. However, according to Ackerman et al. (1993), these findings are not very specific of IP and they proposed another ultrasound marker, which they called interstitial line: an echogenic line extending into the cornual region and abutting the midportion of the interstitial mass or gestational sac. They found no false positives in their study and they established the interstitial line as the marker we should pay attention to when an IP is suspected [53].

As for treatment, due to the delay in diagnosis and the high risk of rupture, there will be a considerable proportion of patients undergoing a surgical approach because of hemodynamic instability.

Conservative medical treatment has been described in several case reports and series of cases. Authors have proposed local MTX injection with encouraging results. Besides, local KCl injection has been performed in substitution of MTX (particularly in heterotopic pregnancies) or when the embryo presents cardiac activity [54].

In a series of cases presented by Gómez et al. (2012), they treated 2 cases of IP with mifepristone and systemic MTX successfully and no rescue therapy was needed. Both patients stayed in the hospital for two days, it took 35 and 49 days for the BHCG serum level to be undetectable and they recovered their normal menstrual periods after 25 and 30 days, respectively [16].

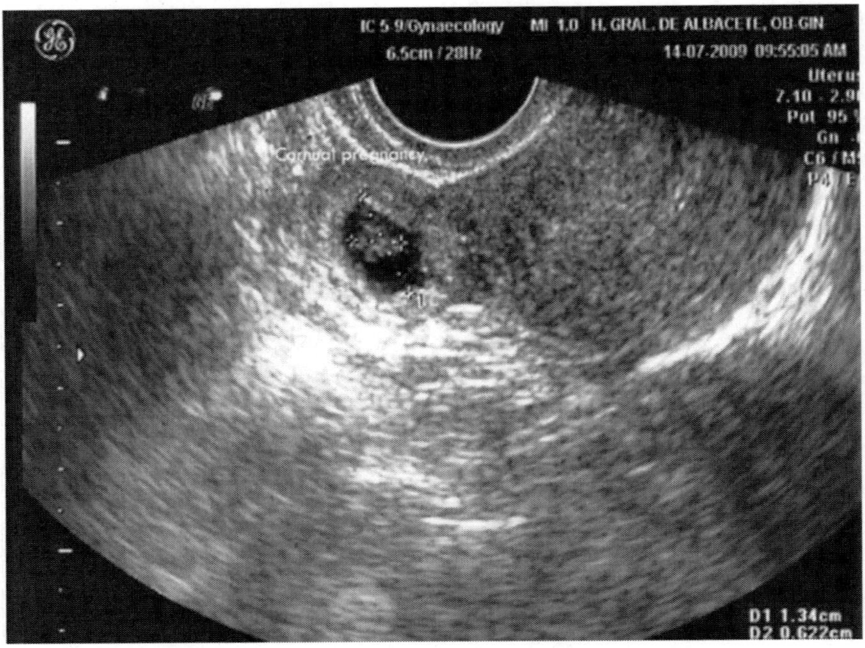

Figure 3. Interstitial pregnancy. From Gómez et al. [16].

As far as surgical approach is concerned, it traditionally consisted of hysterectomy or cornual resection. However, other techniques have been proposed within the past years such as laparoscopic cornuotomy [55]. According to the prestigious online database UpToDate, the procedure for laparoscopic cornuostomy is as follows: dilute intramyometrial vasopressin is injected into the cornual myometrium at the commencement of the operation to minimize blood loss and improve visibility. Alternatively, hemostasis can be achieved by ligating the ascending branches of the uterine vessels. If a cornuostomy is planned, the products of conception can be removed with hydrodissection, grasping forceps, aspiration, or gentle curettage. Hydrodissection is preferred to flush out the gestational products, as it helps to ascertain complete removal of trophoblast [56].

In a comparison made by Lee MH et al. (2017) they studied the difference between performing laparoscopic cornual resection and cornuotomy in patients with IP. They analysed 75 women and discovered both techniques had similar clinical results, although cornuotomy seemed to reduce the surgical time. What's more, the incidence of subsequent IP did not differ between the 2 surgery groups. Four patients developed IP out of the 53 patients initially managed by cornual resection, while IP was diagnosed in 1 patient out of the 22 patients managed by cornuotomy [57].

Other options such as combined hysteroscopic and laparoscopic approach have been reported with encouraging results (Katz 2003), although authors warned of the potential limitations of this technique: they reported women must be hemodynamically stable and the possibility that an ectopic pregnancy located in the distal portion of the interstitial segment of the fallopian tube may not be amenable to hysteroscopic therapy [58].

The outcomes of surgical approach for IP involve higher risks of cesarean delivery and uterine rupture in subsequent pregnancies [59]. On the other hand, we do not have information about the fertility and pregnancy outcomes after medical conservative treatment [60].

Ovarian Pregnancy

Ovarian pregnancy (OP) accounts for those pregnancies implanted in the ovary [1]. It's incidence ranges from 0,5-3% of all ectopic pregnancies, depending on the studies [2]. It is known as a rare condition and that is the reason why the vast majority of the evidence we have got on OP comes from case reports or series of cases. Although OP has been traditionally thought to be related to the use of certain contraceptive methods such as intrauterine devices (IUD), recent publications have shown to deny this evidence because women carrying IUDs will always be less likely to get pregnant than women who are not carrying them. However, IUDs reduce eutopic implantations by 99,5% and tubal implantation by 95%, as it was shown in Lehfeldt's multiple case review (1970) [61-64].

Clinical manifestations of OP are non-specific and can easily be mistaken for other kinds of EP. This is the reason why diagnosis is still a challenge nowadays and it is often reached intraoperatively when patients undergo surgery because of a tubal ectopic pregnancy or tubal miscarriage. Back in 1878, Spielberg established several surgical criteria in order to make an accurate diagnosis of OP, which are:

1. fallopian tubes, including fimbria, must be intact and separate from the ovary.
2. the pregnancy must occupy the normal position of the ovary.

3. the ovary must be attached to the uterus through the uteroovarian ligament.
4. there must be ovarian tissue attached to the pregnancy in the specimen [65].

However, there are several studies trying to throw light on ultrasound characteristics of OP, such as a thick echogenic ring which is more echogenic than the ovary around the gestational sac [66].

Treatment is based on surgery. The usual technique involves an ovarian wedge resection in order to remove the EP and preserve the rest of the organ. However, this may not be possible in certain cases in which the location of the OP compels the surgeon to remove the whole ovary.

The introduction of laparoscopy as the treatment of choice has not shown improvement when it comes to blood loss, or maternal mortality, but it is known that performance of laparoscopy is related to a faster recovery and, thereby, a diminishment of postoperative hospitalization days.

When it comes to medical management of OP, there are no official guidelines recommending it, although several cases in which they administered methotrexate after an OP diagnosis have been reported. In all of these cases, an early diagnosis was made and it was based on BHCG serum levels and transvaginal ultrasound, which revealed a gestational sac with or without a yolk sac, but never a fetal node. After the administration of MTX, BHCG levels became negative and ovaries restored their normal morphology. Post treatment periods were uneventful [67].

As for postoperative reproductive outcomes in patients with OP, a retrospective cases analysis (Wong CH, 2021) showed encouraging results when it came to spontaneous eutopic pregnancy. Besides, no cases of recurrent ectopic pregnancy were found [68-70].

Heterotopic Pregnancy

Heterotopic pregnancy (HP) accounts for those pregnancies in which, simultaneously, there are two places of implantation. Usually, one of the pregnancies is intrauterine and the other extrauterine (Figure 4), rather than two extrauterine locations at a time [1]. It was first described by Duverney (1706) and it affects around 1 out of 30,000 pregnancies [71]. However, several risk factors have been described such as ART and it has been suggested that incidence in this group of patients may reach 1.5 out of 1,000 ART pregnancies [72].

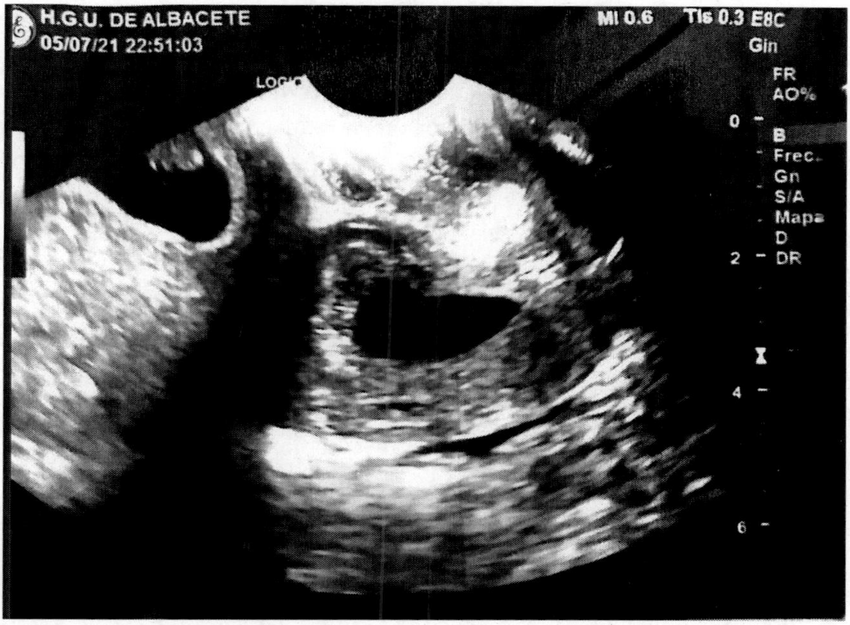

Figure 4. Heterotopic cervical pregnancy diagnosed at our center (2021) in a patient who underwent ART. Outcome is yet to be published as the pregnancy is still in its first trimester.

Clinical presentation is similar to classical tubal pregnancy the vast majority of times, but there is an important delay in the diagnosis because EP is usually discarded when an intrauterine pregnancy is visualized via TVUS. Therefore, there is a considerable risk of rupture in this kind of EP. As for the intrauterine pregnancy, there is a higher rate of spontaneous abortion than in an isolated eutopic pregnancy [73].

When it comes to treatment, most of the evidence we have got on HP comes from case reports or series of cases due its rare nature.

Our approach will depend on the patient's clinical condition and their hemodynamic stability and the location of the ectopic pregnancy. For those HP with a tubal extrauterine implantation, options are discussed in the chapter Tubal Ectopic Pregnancy: Treatment Update. However, it is mandatory to mention that if the intrauterine pregnancy is to be conserved, systemic therapy should be avoided because of the potential effects it may have on the embryo.

When HP is non-tubal, we can find several published cases with different management options.

In 2019, in a patient with a cervical HP, Rubattu A et al. performed a hysteroscopic excision of the cervical gestational sac to preserve the intrauterine pregnancy. The procedure was performed under a general anaesthesia using a 3.5 mm bipolar hysteroscope which was introduced in the cervix without the use of a speculum or cervical dilators. The entire procedure was performed under transabdominal ultrasound guidance. Saline solution was used as the distention medium and the tip of the hysteroscope was not advanced beyond the internal cervical os. After an incision was made in the gestational sac of the CP, the cervical embryo was coagulated with bipolar forceps. The b-hCG level after the hysteroscopic surgery was 35,933 mIU/mL. The intraoperative and postoperative bleeding was minimal. An ultrasound performed on post-operative day number one confirmed a viable intrauterine pregnancy without any evidence of residual pregnancy in the cervix. The intrauterine pregnancy continued without complications and the follow-up ultrasounds were unremarkable [74].

As another example, in 2004 in a patient with a twin intrauterine pregnancy and a CSP, Hsieh BC et al. performed an embryo aspiration of the CSP. After the introduction of the needle into the gestational sac, they aspirated the contents of the gestational sac under vaginal sonography, resulting in the disappearance of the sac. The patient tolerated the procedure well. She was observed overnight and discharged the following day. Ultrasound was repeated 2 weeks later and revealed that the gestational sac in the Caesarean scar had shrunk to a small echogenic area. Six weeks later, transvaginal ultrasound showed normal uterine anatomy with complete disappearance of the gestational sac [75].

To sum up, HP is an infrequent and heterogeneous clinical condition because of its multiple possible locations and those will play a crucial role on the prognosis and outcome. Several ways of management have been proposed and it will always be essential to individualize each case.

References

[1] Hoffman, Barbara L., and J Whitridge Williams. 2016. *Williams Gynecology*. New York: Mcgraw-Hill Education. (Hoffman 2016, 161-176).

[2] Bouyer, J., Coste J., Fernandez H., Pouly J. L., and Job-Spira N. 2002. "Sites of Ectopic Pregnancy: A 10 Year Population-Based Study of 1800 Cases." *Human Reproduction (Oxford, England)* 17 (12): 3224–30. https://doi.org/10.1093/HUMREP/17.12.3224.

[3] Rotas, Michael A., Shoshana Haberman, and Michael Levgur. 2006. "Cesarean Scar Ectopic Pregnancies." *Obstetrics & Gynecology* 107 (6): 1373–81. https://doi.org/10.1097/01.aog.0000218690.24494.ce.

[4] Karande, V. C., J. T. Flood, N. Heard, L. Veeck, and S. J. Muasher. 1991. "Analysis of Ectopic Pregnancies Resulting from In-Vitro Fertilization and Embryo Transfer*." *Human Reproduction* 6 (3): 446–49. https://doi.org/10.1093/oxfordjournals.humrep.a137356.

[5] Matorras, Roberto, Adriana Zallo, Rafael Hernandez-Pailos, Marcos Ferrando, Fernando Quintana, José Remohi, Iker Malaina, Lucía Laínz, and Antonia Exposito. 2020. "Cervical Pregnancy in Assisted Reproduction: An Analysis of Risk Factors in 91,067 Ongoing Pregnancies." *Reproductive BioMedicine Online* 40 (3): 355–61. https://doi.org/10.1016/j.rbmo.2019.12.011.

[6] Vela, Gerardo, and Togas Tulandi. 2007. "Cervical Pregnancy: The Importance of Early Diagnosis and Treatment." *Journal of Minimally Invasive Gynecology* 14 (4): 481–84. https://doi.org/10.1016/j.jmig.2006.11.012.

[7] Kung, Fu-Tsai, Hao Lin, Te-Yao Hsu, Chih-Yang Chang, Hsuan-Wei Huang, Li-Ying Huang, Yin-Jou Chou, and Kuan-Hui Huang. 2004. "Differential Diagnosis of Suspected Cervical Pregnancy and Conservative Treatment with the Combination of Laparoscopy-Assisted Uterine Artery Ligation and Hysteroscopic Endocervical Resection." *Fertility and Sterility* 81 (6): 1642–49. https://doi.org/10.1016/j.fertnstert.2003.11.034.

[8] Connolly, AnnaMarie, David H. Ryan, Alison M. Stuebe, and Honor M. Wolfe. 2013. "Reevaluation of Discriminatory and Threshold Levels for Serum β-HCG in Early Pregnancy." *Obstetrics & Gynecology* 121 (1): 65–70. https://doi.org/10.1097/aog.0b013e318278f421.

[9] Kim, Tae Jin, Seok Ju Seong, Keum Jung Lee, Je Hoon Lee, Joong Sik Shin, Kyung Taek Lim, Hwan Wook Chung, et al. 2004. "Clinical Outcomes of Patients Treated for Cervical Pregnancy with or without Methotrexate." *Journal of Korean Medical Science* 19 (6): 848. https://doi.org/10.3346/jkms.2004.19.6.848.

[10] Kirk, E., G. Condous, Z. Haider, A. Syed, K. Ojha, and T. Bourne. 2006. "The Conservative Management of Cervical Ectopic Pregnancies." *Ultrasound in Obstetrics and Gynecology* 27 (4): 430–37. https://doi.org/10.1002/uog.2693.

[11] Doubilet, Peter M., Carol B. Benson, Mary C. Frates, and Elizabeth Ginsburg. 2004. "Sonographically Guided Minimally Invasive Treatment of Unusual Ectopic Pregnancies." *Journal of Ultrasound in Medicine* 23 (3): 359–70. https://doi.org/10.7863/jum.2004.23.3.359.

[12]"*Cervical Pregnancy - UpToDate.* n.d. Accessed July 14, 2021. https://www.uptodate.com/contents/cervical-pregnancy?search= ectopic pregnancy&topicRef=5465&source=see_link#H6.

[13] Heikinheimo, Oskari, Arto Leminen, Bruno Cacciatore, Eeva-Marja Rutanen, and Pauli Kajanoja. 2004. "Advanced Cervical Pregnancy: Uterus-Sparing Therapy Initiated with a Combination of Methotrexate and Mifepristone Followed by Evacuation and Local Hemostatic Measures." *Acta Obstetricia et Gynecologica Scandinavica* 83 (2): 211–12. https://doi.org/10.1111/j.0001-6349.2004.0077a.x

[14] Sexton, Christopher, and Nicholas Sharp. 2002. "Cervical Pregnancy Successfully Treated with a Sequential Combination of Methotrexate and Mifepristone." *The Australian and New Zealand Journal of Obstetrics and Gynaecology* 42 (2): 211–13. https://doi.org/10.1111/j.0004-8666.2002.210_2.x.

[15] De Greef, Ingrid, Patrick Berteloot, Dirk Timmerman, Jan Deprest, and Frederic Amant. 2005. "Viable Cervical Pregnancy with Levonorgestrel Containing Intrauterine Device, Treated Successfully with Methotrexate and Mifepristone." *European Journal of Obstetrics & Gynecology and Reproductive Biology* 120 (2): 233–35. https://doi.org/10.1016/j.ejogrb.2004.11.008.

[16] Gómez García, María Teresa, Guadalupe Aguarón Benitez, Beatriz Barberá Belda, Carmen Callejón Rodríguez, and Gaspar González Merlo. 2012. "Medical Therapy (Methotrexate and Mifepristone) Alone or in Combination with Another Type of Therapy for the Management of Cervical or Interstitial Ectopic Pregnancy." *European Journal of Obstetrics & Gynecology and Reproductive Biology* 165 (1): 77–81. https://doi.org/10.1016/j.ejogrb.2012.06.024.

[17] -Ishikawa, Hiroshi, Youichi Unno, Akiko Omoto, and Makio Shozu. 2016. "Local Injection of Diluted Vasopressin Followed by Suction Curettage for Cervical Ectopic Pregnancy." *European Journal of Obstetrics & Gynecology and Reproductive Biology* 207 (December): 173–77. https://doi.org/10.1016/j.ejogrb.2016.11.004.

[18] -Hu, J., X. Tao, L. Yin, and Y. Shi. 2016. "Successful Conservative Treatment of Cervical Pregnancy with Uterine Artery Embolization Followed by Curettage: A Report of 19 Cases." *BJOG: An International Journal of Obstetrics & Gynaecology* 123 (September): 97–102. https://doi.org/10.1111/1471-0528.14005.

[19] Scutiero, Gennaro, Lugi Nappi, Maria Matteo, Silverio Balzano, Luca Macarini, and Pantaleo Greco. 2013. "Cervical Pregnancy Treated by Uterine Artery Embolisation Combined with Office Hysteroscopy." *European Journal of Obstetrics & Gynecology and Reproductive Biology* 166 (1): 104–6. https://doi.org/10.1016/j.ejogrb.2012.10.013.

[20] Larsen JV, Solomon MH. Pregnancy in a uterine scar sacculus: an unusual cause of postabortal hemorrhage. A case report. *S Afr. Med. J.* 1978; 53:142–3.

[21] Seow, K.-M., L.-W. Huang, Y.-H. Lin, M. Yan-Sheng Lin, Y.-L. Tsai, and J.-L. Hwang. 2004. "Cesarean Scar Pregnancy: Issues in Management." *Ultrasound in Obstetrics & Gynecology: The Official Journal of the International Society of Ultrasound in Obstetrics and Gynecology* 23 (3): 247–53. https://doi.org/10.1002/uog.974.

[22] Jurkovic, D., K. Hillaby, B. Woelfer, A. Lawrence, R. Salim, and C. J. Elson. 2003. "First-Trimester Diagnosis and Management of Pregnancies Implanted into the Lower Uterine Segment Cesarean Section Scar." *Ultrasound in Obstetrics and Gynecology* 21 (3): 220–27. https://doi.org/10.1002/uog.56

[23] Maymon, R., R. Halperin, S. Mendlovic, D. Schneider, and A. Herman. 2004. "Ectopic Pregnancies in a Caesarean Scar: Review of the Medical Approach to an Iatrogenic Complication." *Human Reproduction Update* 10 (6): 515–23. https://doi.org/10.1093/humupd/dmh042.

[24] Kaelin Agten, Andrea, Giuseppe Cali, Ana Monteagudo, Johana Oviedo, Joanne Ramos, and Ilan Timor-Tritsch. 2017. "The Clinical Outcome of Cesarean Scar Pregnancies Implanted 'on the Scar 'versus 'in the Niche.'" *American Journal of Obstetrics and Gynecology* 216 (5): 510.e1–6. https://doi.org/10.1016/j.ajog.2017.01.019.

[25] Vial, Y., P. Petignat, and P. Hohlfeld. 2000. "Pregnancy in a Cesarean Scar." *Ultrasound in Obstetrics & Gynecology: The Official Journal of the International Society of Ultrasound in Obstetrics and Gynecology* 16 (6): 592–93. https://doi.org/10.1046/j.1469-0705.2000.00300-2.x.

[26] Miller, Russell, Ilan E. Timor-Tritsch, and Cynthia Gyamfi-Bannerman. 2020. "Society for Maternal-Fetal Medicine (SMFM) Consult Series #49: Cesarean Scar Pregnancy." *American Journal of Obstetrics and Gynecology* 222 (5): B2–14. https://doi.org/10.1016/j.ajog.2020.01.030.

[27] Timor-Tritsch, Ilan E., and Ana Monteagudo. 2012. "Unforeseen Consequences of the Increasing Rate of Cesarean Deliveries: Early Placenta Accreta and Cesarean Scar Pregnancy. A Review." *American Journal of Obstetrics and Gynecology* 207 (1): 14–29. https://doi.org/10.1016/j.ajog.2012.03.007.

[28] Calì, G., I. E. Timor-Tritsch, J. Palacios-Jaraquemada, A. Monteaugudo, D. Buca, F. Forlani, A. Familiari, G. Scambia, G. Acharya, and F. D'Antonio. 2018. "Outcome of Cesarean Scar Pregnancy Managed Expectantly: Systematic Review and Meta-Analysis." *Ultrasound in Obstetrics & Gynecology* 51 (2): 169–75. https://doi.org/10.1002/uog.17568.

[29] "Committee Opinion No. 713." 2017. *Obstetrics & Gynecology* 130 (2): e102–9. https://doi.org/10.1097/aog.0000000000002237.

[30] Birch Petersen, Kathrine, Elise Hoffmann, Christian Rifbjerg Larsen, and Henriette Svarre Nielsen. 2016. "Cesarean Scar Pregnancy: A Systematic Review of Treatment Studies." *Fertility and Sterility* 105 (4): 958–67. https://doi.org/10.1016/j.fertnstert.2015.12.130.

[31] Cheung, Vincent Y. T. 2015. "Local Methotrexate Injection as the First-Line Treatment for Cesarean Scar Pregnancy: Review of the Literature." *Journal of Minimally Invasive Gynecology* 22 (5): 753–58. https://doi.org/10.1016/j.jmig.2015.04.008.

[32] Ugurlucan, Funda Gungor, Ercan Bastu, Murat Dogan, Ibrahim Kalelioglu, Sebnem Alanya, and Recep Has. 2012. "Management of Cesarean Heterotopic Pregnancy with Transvaginal Ultrasound–Guided Potassium Chloride Injection and Gestational Sac Aspiration, and Review of the Literature." *Journal of Minimally Invasive Gynecology* 19 (5): 671–73. https://doi.org/10.1016/j.jmig.2012.05.006.

[33] Long, Ying, Huili Zhu, Yuanyuan Hu, Licong Shen, Jing Fu, and Wei Huang. 2020. "Interventions For Non-Tubal Ectopic Pregnancy". *Cochrane Database Of Systematic Reviews*. doi:10.1002/14651858.cd011174.pub2.

[34] Sadeghi, Homayoun, Thomas Rutherford, Beth Rackow, Katherine Campbell, Christina Duzyj, Marsha Guess, Pinar Kodaman, and Errol Norwitz. 2009. "Cesarean Scar Ectopic Pregnancy: Case Series and Review of the Literature." *American Journal of Perinatology* 27 (02): 111–20. https://doi.org/10.1055/s-0029-1224874.

[35] Wang, Qiao, Hong-Ling Peng, Lei He, and Xia Zhao. 2015. "Reproductive Outcomes after Previous Cesarean Scar Pregnancy: Follow up of 189 Women." *Taiwanese Journal of Obstetrics and Gynecology* 54 (5): 551–53. https://doi.org/10.1016/j.tjog.2015.08.006.

[36] Grechukhina, Olga, Uma Deshmukh, Linda Fan, Katherine Kohari, Sonya Abdel-Razeq, Mert Ozan Bahtiyar, and Anna K. Sfakianaki. 2018. "Cesarean Scar Pregnancy, Incidence, and Recurrence." *Obstetrics & Gynecology* 132 (5): 1285–95. https://doi.org/10.1097/aog.0000000000002940.

[37] Atrash, H. K., Friede A., Hogue C. J. Abdominal pregnancy in the United States: frequency and maternal mortality. *Obstet Gynecol.* 1987 Mar;69(3 Pt 1):333-7.

[38] Rahman, M. S., Al-Suleiman S. A., Rahman J., Al-Sibai M. H. Advanced abdominal pregnancy--observations in 10 cases. *Obstet Gynecol.* 1982 Mar;59(3):366-72. PMID: 7078883.

[39] Daya, Salim. 1987. "Human Chorionic Gonadotropin Increase in Normal Early Pregnancy." *American Journal of Obstetrics and Gynecology* 156 (2): 286–90. https://doi.org/10.1016/0002-9378(87)90269-9.

[40] Gerli, Sandro, Dario Rossetti, Gabriela Baiocchi, Graziano Clerici, Vittorio Unfer, and Gian Carlo Di Renzo. 2004. "Early Ultrasonographic Diagnosis and Laparoscopic Treatment of Abdominal Pregnancy." *European Journal of Obstetrics & Gynecology and Reproductive Biology* 113 (1): 103–5. https://doi.org/10.1016/s0301-2115(03)00366-x.

[41] Cardosi, R. J., Nackley A. C., Londono J., and Hoffman M. S. 2002. "Embolization for Advanced Abdominal Pregnancy with a Retained Placenta. A Case Report." *The Journal of Reproductive Medicine* 47 (10): 861–63. https://pubmed.ncbi.nlm.nih.gov/12418072/.

[42] Zinger, M. and Rosenfeld D. 2001. "Failed Treatment of Abdominal Pregnancy with Methotrexate. A Case Report." *The Journal of Reproductive Medicine* 46 (4): 392–94. https://pubmed.ncbi.nlm.nih.gov/11354843/.

[43] Shippey, Stuart H., Snehal M. Bhoola, Anthony B. Royek, and Mary E. Long. 2007. "Diagnosis and Management of Hepatic Ectopic Pregnancy." *Obstetrics & Gynecology* 109 (2): 544–46. https://doi.org/10.1097/01.aog.0000247293.32523.c3.

[44] Mitra, Avick G., and Mark H. LeQuire. 2003. "Minimally Invasive Management of 14.5-Week Abdominal Pregnancy without Laparotomy." *Journal of Ultrasound in Medicine* 22 (7): 709–14. https://doi.org/10.7863/jum.2003.22.7.709.

[45] Varma, R., L. Mascarenhas, and D. James. 2003. "Successful Outcome of Advanced Abdominal Pregnancy with Exclusive Omental Insertion." *Ultrasound in Obstetrics and Gynecology* 21 (2): 192–94. https://doi.org/10.1002/uog.25.

[46] Lockhat, F., P. Corr, S. Ramphal, and J. Moodley. 2006. "The Value of Magnetic Resonance Imagingin the Diagnosis and Management of Extra-Uterine Abdominal Pregnancy." *Clinical Radiology* 61 (3): 264–69. https://doi.org/10.1016/j.crad.2005.10.013.

[47] Cetinkaya, Mehmet B., Arif Kokcu, and Tayfun Alper. 2005. "Follow up of the Regression of the Placenta Left in Situ in an Advanced Abdominal Pregnancy Using the Cavalieri Method." *Journal of Obstetrics and*

Gynaecology Research 31 (1): 22–26. https://doi.org/10.1111/j.1447-0756.2005.00236.x.

[48] Fox, Karin A., Alireza A. Shamshirsaz, Daniela Carusi, Angeles Alvarez Secord, Paula Lee, Ozhan M. Turan, Christopher Huls, et al. 2015. "Conservative Management of Morbidly Adherent Placenta: Expert Review." *American Journal of Obstetrics and Gynecology* 213 (6): 755–60. https://doi.org/10.1016/j.ajog.2015.04.034.

[49] Lau, Susie, and Togas Tulandi. 1999. "Conservative Medical and Surgical Management of Interstitial Ectopic Pregnancy." *Fertility and Sterility* 72 (2): 207–15. https://doi.org/10.1016/s0015-0282(99)00242-3.

[50] Lurie, Samuel. 1992. "The History of the Diagnosis and Treatment of Ectopic Pregnancy: A Medical Adventure." *European Journal of Obstetrics & Gynecology and Reproductive Biology* 43 (1): 1–7. https://doi.org/10.1016/0028-2243(92)90235-q.

[51] Tulandi, Togas, and Dania Al-Jaroudi. 2004. "Interstitial Pregnancy: Results Generated from the Society of Reproductive Surgeons Registry." *Obstetrics & Gynecology* 103 (1): 47–50. https://doi.org/10.1097/01.aog.0000109218.24211.79.

[52] *UpToDate*. n.d. Www.uptodate.com. Accessed July 14, 2021. https://www.uptodate.com/contents/ectopic-pregnancy-clinical-manifestations-and-diagnosis?search=ectopic%20pregnancy&topicRef=5465&source=see_link#H28.

[53] Ackerman, T. E., C. S. Levi, S M Dashefsky, S. C. Holt, and D. J. Lindsay. 1993. "Interstitial Line: Sonographic Finding in Interstitial (Cornual) Ectopic Pregnancy." *Radiology* 189 (1): 83–87. https://doi.org/10.1148/radiology.189.1.8372223.

[54] Monteagudo, A., V. K. Minior, C. Stephenson, S. Monda, and I. E. Timor-Tritsch. 2005. "Non-Surgical Management of Live Ectopic Pregnancy with Ultrasound-Guided Local Injection: A Case Series." *Ultrasound in Obstetrics and Gynecology* 25 (3): 282–88. https://doi.org/10.1002/uog.1822.

[55] Moawad, Nash S., Sangeeta T. Mahajan, Michelle H. Moniz, Sarah E. Taylor, and William W. Hurd. 2010. "Current Diagnosis and Treatment of Interstitial Pregnancy." *American Journal of Obstetrics and Gynecology* 202 (1): 15–29. https://doi.org/10.1016/j.ajog.2009.07.054.

[56] *UpToDate*. n.d. Www.uptodate.com. Accessed July 14, 2021. https://www.uptodate.com/contents/ectopic-pregnancy-surgical-treatment?search=cornuostomy&source=search_result&selectedTitle=1~1&usage_type=default&display_rank=1#H1551137940.

[57] Lee, Myoung-Hwa, Seung-Yeon Im, Min-Kyoung Kim, So-Young Shin, and Won I. Park. 2017. "Comparison of Laparoscopic Cornual Resection and Cornuotomy for Interstitial Pregnancy." *Journal of Minimally Invasive Gynecology* 24 (3): 397–401. https://doi.org/10.1016/j.jmig.2016.11.015.

[58] Katz, David L., John P. Barrett, Joseph S. Sanfilippo, and David M. Badway. 2003. "Combined Hysteroscopy and Laparoscopy in the Treatment of Interstitial Pregnancy." *American Journal of Obstetrics and Gynecology* 188 (4): 1113–14. https://doi.org/10.1067/mob.2003.258.

[59] Liao, Chi-Yuan, Jessica Tse, Shu-Yi Sung, Shu-Hui Chen, and Wen-Huei Tsui. 2016. "Cornual Wedge Resection for Interstitial Pregnancy and Postoperative Outcome." *Australian and New Zealand Journal of Obstetrics and Gynaecology* 57 (3): 342–45. https://doi.org/10.1111/ajo.12497.

[60] Svenningsen, Rune, Anne Cathrine Staff, Anton Langebrekke, and Erik Qvigstad. 2019. "Fertility Outcome after Cornual Resection for Interstitial Pregnancies." *Journal of Minimally Invasive Gynecology* 26 (5): 865–70. https://doi.org/10.1016/j.jmig.2018.08.017.

[61] Lehfeldt, Hans, Christopher Tietze, and Fred Gorstein. 1970. "Ovarian Pregnancy and the Intrauterine Device." *American Journal of Obstetrics and Gynecology* 108 (7): 1005–9. https://doi.org/10.1016/0002-9378(70)90443-6.

[62] Melcer, Y., Smorgick N, Vaknin Z, Mendlovic S, Raziel A, and Maymon R. 2015. "Primary Ovarian Pregnancy: 43 Years Experience in a Single Institute and Still a Medical Challenge." *The Israel Medical Association Journal : IMAJ* 17 (11): 687–90. https://pubmed.ncbi.nlm.nih.gov/26757565/.

[63] Li, Cheng, Wei-Hong Zhao, Chun-Xia Meng, Hua Ping, Guo-Juan Qin, Shu-Jun Cao, Xiaowei Xi, Qian Zhu, Xiao-Cui Li, and Jian Zhang. 2014. "Contraceptive Use and the Risk of Ectopic Pregnancy: A Multi-Center Case-Control Study." Edited by Marcia E. L. Consolaro. *PLoS ONE* 9 (12): e115031. https://doi.org/10.1371/journal.pone.0115031.

[64] Sivin, I, 1991. "Dose- and Age-Dependent Ectopic Pregnancy Risks with Intrauterine Contraception." *Obstetrics and Gynecology* 78 (2): 291–98. https://pubmed.ncbi.nlm.nih.gov/2067778/.

[65] Goyal, Lajya Devi, Rimpy Tondon, Poonam Goel, and Alka Sehgal. 2014. "Ovarian Ectopic Pregnancy: A 10 Years 'Experience and Review of Literature." *Iranian Journal of Reproductive Medicine* 12 (12): 825–30. https://www.ncbi.nlm.nih.gov/pmc/articles/PMC4330663/.

[66] Comstock, Christine, Kathleen Huston, and Wesley Lee. 2005. "The Ultrasonographic Appearance of Ovarian Ectopic Pregnancies." *Obstetrics & Gynecology* 105 (1): 42–45. https://doi.org/10.1097/01.aog.0000148271.27446.30.

[67] "Diagnosis and Management of Ectopic Pregnancy." 2016. *BJOG: An International Journal of Obstetrics & Gynaecology* 123 (13): e15–55. https://doi.org/10.1111/1471-0528.14189.

[68] Wong, Chian-Huey, Yeou-Lih Wang, and Jian-Pei Huang. 2021. "Postoperative Reproductive Outcomes in Women with Ovarian Pregnancy: A Retrospective Analysis." *Taiwanese Journal of Obstetrics and Gynecology* 60 (2): 295–98. https://doi.org/10.1016/j.tjog.2021.01.007.

[69] Di Luigi, G., Patacchiola F, La Posta V, Bonitatibus A, Ruggeri G, and Carta G. 2012. "Early Ovarian Pregnancy Diagnosed by Ultrasound and Successfully Treated with Multidose Methotrexate. A Case Report." *Clinical and Experimental Obstetrics & Gynecology* 39 (3): 390–93. https://pubmed.ncbi.nlm.nih.gov/23157054/.

[70] Birge, Ozer, Mustafa Melih Erkan, Ertugrul Gazi Ozbey, and Deniz Arslan. 2015. "Medical Management of an Ovarian Ectopic Pregnancy: A Case Report." *Journal of Medical Case Reports* 9 (1). https://doi.org/10.1186/s13256-015-0774-6.

[71] Reece, E.Albert, Roy H. Petrie, Meredith F. Sirmans, Mieczyslaw Finster, and W.Duane Todd. 1983. "Combined Intrauterine and Extrauterine Gestations: A Review." *American Journal of Obstetrics and Gynecology* 146 (3): 323–30. https://doi.org/10.1016/0002-9378(83)90755-x.

[72] Clayton, Heather B., Laura A. Schieve, Herbert B. Peterson, Denise J. Jamieson, Meredith A. Reynolds, and Victoria C. Wright. 2007. "A Comparison of Heterotopic and Intrauterine-Only Pregnancy Outcomes after Assisted Reproductive Technologies in the United States from 1999 to 2002 the Findings and Conclusions in This Article Are Those of the Authors, and Do Not Necessarily Represent the Views of the Centers for Disease Control and Prevention, Atlanta, Georgia." *Fertility and Sterility* 87 (2): 303–9. https://doi.org/10.1016/j.fertnstert.2006.06.037.

[73] Barrenetxea, Gorka, Lorea Barinaga-Rementeria, Arantza Lopez de Larruzea, Jon Ander Agirregoikoa, Miren Mandiola, and Koldo Carbonero. 2007. "Heterotopic Pregnancy: Two Cases and a Comparative Review." *Fertility and Sterility* 87 (2): 417.e9–15. https://doi.org/10.1016/j.fertnstert.2006.05.085.

[74] Rubattu, Antonio, Valentina Corda, Iside Derosas, Maria Carla Monni, Cristina Nocco, Ambra Iuculano, Giangavino Peppi, Nadia Rosas, Giovanni Ruiu, and Giovanni Monni. 2019. "Successful Hysteroscopic Treatment of a Cervical Heterotopic Pregnancy: Case Report and Literature Review." *Journal of Obstetrics and Gynaecology* 40 (4): 580–81. https://doi.org/10.1080/01443615.2019.1607269.

[75] Hsieh, B.-C. 2004. "Heterotopic Caesarean Scar Pregnancy Combined with Intrauterine Pregnancy Successfully Treated with Embryo Aspiration for Selective Embryo Reduction: Case Report." *Human Reproduction* 19 (2): 285–87. https://doi.org/10.1093/humrep/deh080.

Chapter 5

Risk Score Model for Venous Thromboembolism Prophylaxis for Caesarean Section

Choi Wah Kong*, Wing Yi Lok and William W. K. To
Department of Obstetrics and Gynaecology,
United Christian Hospital, Hong Kong, China

Abstract

The relative risk of venous thromboembolism (VTE) in pregnancy is increased four-to six-fold and is further increased postpartum particularly after caesarean section. VTE, although rare, is a major cause of maternal mortality and morbidity in developed countries. Recommendations for VTE prophylaxis from authoritative guideline for women undergoing caesarean delivery differed significantly. The Royal College of Obstetricians and Gynaecologists (RCOG) and the Council of the Society of Obstetric Medicine Australia and New Zealand (SOMANZ) recommend pharmacological prophylaxis by low molecular weight heparin (LMWH) for all the women undergoing emergency caesarean sections and in women with risk factors undergoing elective caesarean sections.

* Corresponding Author's E-mail: melizakong@gmail.com.

In: A Closer Look at Pregnancy and Childbirth
Editor: Louise J. Salgado
ISBN: 978-1-68507-658-0

The American College of Chest Physicians (ACCP) is less stringent and recommends pharmacological prophylaxis in post caesarean section patients having one major or two or more minor risk factors. The American College of Obstetricians and Gynecologists (ACOG) guidelines, in contrast, recommends postpartum pharmacological prophylaxis for only a small group of particularly high-risk women with thrombophilia or prior VTE event. There is a lack of standardization among the international guidelines, and the recommendations are largely based on expert opinion rather than from randomised controlled trials or meta-analyses.

Giving pharmacological prophylaxis to a large proportion of women undergoing caesarean delivery would lead to significant financial costs and also increase in bleeding complications. We have developed a modified risk score model adapted from the RCOG guidelines of VTE prophylaxis for caesarean section in Chinese women. Our risk score model resulted in around 12.7% of women undergoing caesarean section requiring mechanical prophylaxis and around 3.3% women required additional pharmacological prophylaxis in our cohort. In contrast, applying the RCOG guidelines to our cohort, 75.6% women would receive LMWH compared with no women under the ACOG guidelines, while all would require mechanical thromboprophylaxis. There was no VTE in our cohort. Our risk score model appears to be a more reasonable recommendation, balancing clinical risks and cost-effectiveness.

Local VTE prophylaxis guideline for women undergoing caesarean section is recommended based on the incidence of VTE in that locality. This guideline should be safe, easy to apply, rational and financially practical.

Keywords: caesarean section, venous thromboembolism, risk, prophylaxis

Introduction

The natural physiological changes favouring thrombosis during late pregnancy and the postpartum period logically imply that the peripartum period should be a target for venous thromboembolism (VTE) prophylaxis [1]. Deep vein thrombosis (DVT) can predispose to pulmonary thromboembolism (PE) in the acute phase, and troublesome post-thrombotic syndrome months after the acute episode. The relative risk of VTE in pregnancy is increased four-to six-fold [2] and is further increased postpartum [3, 4].

VTE, although rare, is a major cause of maternal mortality and morbidity in developed countries [5, 6]. PE remains a leading direct cause of maternal death in the United Kingdom. A significant fall in the maternal mortality rate from PE from 1.56 per 100 000 maternities in 2003-2005 to 0.70 per 100 000 maternities in 2006-2008 had been observed in the United Kingdom after the publication of the first Royal College of Obstetricians and Gynaecologists (RCOG) guidelines for VTE prophylaxis during pregnancy and the puerperium in 2004 [7]. It had been attributed to increased VTE prophylaxis and the widespread success in the implementation of national guidelines [8]. A previous study to determine whether opportunities to decrease maternal mortality and morbidity by employing post caesarean thromboembolism prophylaxis are being missed, showed that among 1,263,205 women who underwent cesarean delivery in the United States between 2003 and 2010, 75.7% received no thromboembolism prophylaxis, 22.1% received mechanical prophylaxis alone, 1.3% received pharmacologic prophylaxis, and 1.0% received combination prophylaxis. The rate of prophylaxis increased from 8.4% in 2003 to 41.6% in 2010. Medical risk factors for thromboembolism were associated with only modest increases in prophylaxis. The authors concluded that despite the increasing trends, VTE prophylaxis is still underused and represents a major opportunity to reduce maternal morbidity and mortality [9].

Recommendations from International Guidelines

International guidelines agree that pregnant women at risk should be considered for thromboprophylaxis but there is lack of standardization among them with regard to which risk factors should be included and how these should be used in the assessment. Most of the authoritative obstetric VTE guidelines in developed counties, including the American College of Chest Physicians (ACCP) [10] and the Council of the Society of Obstetric Medicine of Australia and New Zealand (SOMANZ) [11] are similar to the RCOG and would recommend LMWH for a large proportion of postpartum women, including most that are delivered by caesarean section [12, 13], though the selection criteria for such pharmacological prophylaxis differs quite widely between different guidelines and appear variable and arbitrary [14].

The recommended duration of postpartum pharmacological prophylaxis may also be different. Similar to the RCOG, the SOMANZ recommends postpartum thromboprophylaxis for all emergency caesarean sections and risk score is used to stratify high risk cases of elective caesarean sections. However, the recommended duration of of 5 days of postpartum thromboprophylaxis is shorter compared to at least 10 days in the RCOG [11]. Other guidelines select patients with caesarean section for postpartum pharmacological prophylaxis based on the presence of additional risk factors. These risk factors differ in different guidelines and they may also be weighed differently. For example, the ACCP guideline recommended pharmacological prophylaxis in post caesarean section patients having one major risk factor or having two or more minor risk factors, which is less stringent compared with the RCOG guideline [10]. BMI >30 kg/m2 is considered to be a minor risk factor in ACCP guidelines but a major risk factor under the SOMANZ. On the other hand, postpartum haemorrhage over 1000 ml is a major risk factor in ACCP guideline but a minor risk factor under the SOMANZ guideline. Under the RCOG guidelines, delivery by caesarean section in labour itself already qualifies the use of postpartum LMWH. Women who had elective caesarean with one additional risk factor also need postpartum LMWH prophylaxis.

It can be seen that these authoritative guidelines would imply including substantially proportions of women who would receive post caesarean pharmacological prophylaxis. However, the RCOG recommendations are largely based on expert opinion with no evidence from randomized controlled trials or meta-analyses [12]. Many of the risk parameters included in the guidelines are based on case control studies reporting relative risks of VTE in women with various risk factors and screening studies that reported asymptomatic DVT, while prospective evidence validating the protocol or evaluating its efficacy were lacking in the literature [13]. The American College of Obstetricians and Gynaecologisits (ACOG) guidelines, in contrast, have not adopted this stance and recommends postpartum pharmacological prophylaxis for only a small group of particularly high-risk women with thrombophilia or prior VTE event. The wide differences in the recommendations reflected the empirical nature of these guidelines. The guidelines for VTE prophylaxis for caesarean delivery of RCOG [15] and ACOG [16] are shown in Table 1.

Table 1. Summary of international society guidelines for obstetric thromboembolic prophylaxis after caesarean delivery

RCOG
Anti-embolism stockings post caesarean section for all
HIGH RISK - At least 6 weeks' postnatal prophylactic LMWH
Any previous VTE
Anyone requiring antenatal LMWH
High-risk thrombophilia
INTERMEDIATE RISK - At least 10 days' postnatal prophylactic LMWH
Low-risk thrombophilia + Family history
Caesarean section in labour
BMI > 40 kg/m2
Readmission or prolonged admission (≥3 days) in the puerperium
Any surgical procedure in the puerperium except immediate repair of the perineum
Medical comorbidities e.g., cancer, heart failure, active SLE, IBD or inflammatory polyarthropathy, nephrotic syndrome, type I DM with nephropathy, sickle cell disease, current intravenous drug user
Age >35 years
INTERMEDIATE RISK (Two or more risk factors)- At least 10 days' postnatal prophylactic LMWH
LOWER RISK (Fewer than two risk factors)- Early mobilization and avoidance of dehydration
Obesity (BMI ≥ 30 kg/m2)
Parity ≥ 3
Smoker
Elective caesarean section
Family history of VTE
Low-risk thrombophilia
Gross varicose veins
Current systemic infection
Immobility, e.g., paraplegia, pelvic girdle pain, long distance travel
Current pre-eclampsia
Multiple pregnancy
Preterm delivery in this pregnancy (<37 weeks)
Stillbirth in this pregnancy
Mid-cavity rotational or operative delivery
Prolonged labour (>24 h)
PPH > 1 L or blood transfusion
ACOG
Placement of pneumatic compression devices before caesarean delivery is recommended for al women
Prophylactic anticoagulation (LMWH or UFH) in the postpartum period
- women with history of unprovoked VTE
- women with history of single provoked VTE if have additional risk factors
- high-risk thrombophilia
- low risk thrombophilia if have history of VTE or have family history of VTE or have other additional risk factors

ACOG = American Congress of Obstetricians; BMI = Body Mass Index; DM = diabetes mellitus; IBD = inflammatory bowel disease; LMWH = low molecular weight heparin; PPH = postpartum haemorrhage; RCOG = Royal College of Obstetricians and Gynaecologists; SLE = systemic lupus erythematous; UFH = unfractionated heparin; VTE =Venous thromboembolism.

Low Molecular Weight Heparin as a Prophylactic Agent

LMWH is the agent of choice for thromboprophylaxis during pregnancy. It has a half-life ranging from three to seven hours if renal function is normal and is most commonly administrated subcutaneously. When given prophylactically after delivery, doses are based on types of LMWH used and adjusted for maternal weight, usually in once daily regimen (e.g., enoxaparin 40 mg daily for women weighing 50-90 kg). LWMH is initiated after caesarean section when bleeding is controlled and at least 4 h after use of spinal anaesthesia or after the epidural catheter has been removed [15]. The optimal duration of postpartum prophylactic anticoagulant is not established and guidelines are inconsistent in their recommendations, from 5 days to 10 days or not providing a specific time frame. As the duration seldom exceeds 6 weeks and warfarin administration frequently requires 1-2 weeks to attain a target range, many women opt to continue LMWH instead of switching to warfarin [16]. Apart from direct financial implications, the use of LMWH also has inherent clinical risks. The Cochrane review reported conflicting results in the risks resulting from anticoagulation prophylaxis. In one trial of 580 women on prophylaxis for VTE after caesarean section, it was shown that women receiving unfractionated heparin (UFH) and physiotherapy were more likely to have bleeding complications than women receiving physiotherapy alone (RR 5.03; 95% CI 2.49 - 10.18), while in two additional trials, that compared LMWH with placebo, no differences between groups were detected in bleeding episodes [17]. On the other hand, a Swedish study that compared women with a personal history of previous VTE who received antepartum and postpartum LMWH prophylaxis with control women showed that LMWH was associated with an absolute increase in haematomata of 2.1% ($P < 0.001$) [18].

Currently, most protocols would choose LMWH as the way of pharmacological prophylaxis as it has the advantages of not requiring monitoring and is safe in breastfeeding. However, parental administration of LMWH can still be inconvenient and painful to the patient and its incidence of allergic skin reactions was reported to be 1.8% (95% CI 1.34-2.37) [19]. It is also obvious that there would also be financial concerns in using pharmacological prophylaxis in a large proportion of women. In a retrospective study in the United Kingdom, implementation of the RCOG guidelines on thromboembolic disease in pregnancy would increase the hospital annual expenditure on LMWH by a factor of 17 [20].

While most protocols used preset standard dosages for VTE prophylaxis, subprophylactic, and supraprophylactic anti-factor Xa levels in these women have also been shown to occur frequently. In a review of 321 anti-factor Xa levels in 77 patients from one centre, all patients were administered LMWH that subsequently was adjusted based upon serial assessment of peak plasma (at 4 hours post-injection) anti-factor Xa levels at less than 36 weeks gestation. Targeted prophylactic range of peak plasma anti-factor Xa level was 0.2–0.4 units/mL. It was found that only 59% of anti-Xa concentrations were in the prophylactic range, whereas 26% were subprophylactic, and 15% were supraprophylactic. Anti-Xa values were not more likely to be in prophylactic range in early compared with late pregnancy, obese compared with nonobese patients, or in patients receiving a weight based minimal dose compared with patients receiving less than a weight-based minimal dose. Anti-factor Xa levels did not correlate with maternal age, weight, body mass index, or gestational age, but there was a positive correlation with the percent of the minimal weight-based dose. As most prophylactic protocols do not routinely monitor anti-factor Xa levels, the assumed efficacy of such prophylaxis may be overstated. [21].

In a recently published multicenter retrospective cohort study evaluating complications associated with early postpartum therapeutic anticoagulation, it was found that in 232 consecutive women treated with therapeutic anticoagulation within 96 hours postpartum, 91 received UFH, 138 received LMWH and three received other anticoagulants. Using a primary composite outcome that included major hemorrhagic complications (requiring transfusion, hospitalization, volume resuscitation, transfer to intensive care unit, or surgery) and major wound complications, it was demonstrated that adverse outcome occurred in 7 of 83 (8.4%) for cesarean deliveries and 9 of 149 (6.0%) for vaginal deliveries. Total complications (including major and minor hemorrhagic and wound complications) occurred in 13 of 83 (15.7%) for cesarean deliveries compared with 9 of 149 (6.0%) for vaginal deliveries (P = 0.016). When comparing cases associated with and without complications, the median delay before resuming anticoagulation was significantly shorter for both cesarean (12 vs 33 hours) and vaginal deliveries (6 vs 19 hours, P=0.006). For cesarean deliveries, 7 of 21 (33.3%) of women experienced complications compared with 6 of 62 (9.7%) if anticoagulation was started before or after 15.1 hours. Despite the anticoagulation treatment, two (0.9%) episodes of VTE occurred within 6 weeks postpartum. This study clearly demonstrates that major complications could occur with early therapeutic anticoagulation, particularly with early resumption of therapy [22].

However, as this study focused on therapeutic anticoagulation, it could be expected that the complication rates associated with prophylactic anticoagulation should be somewhat lower.

The Use of Mechanical Thromboprophylaxis

Both RCOG and ACOG recommend mechanical thromboprophylaxis for all caesarean sections. Elastic stockings or intermittent pneumatic compression alone or in combination with pharmacological thromboprophylaxis have proven efficacy in non-obstetric populations [23]. Although not implemented in a randomized trial setting, it has been demonstrated that universal mechanical prophylaxis with pneumatic compression devices after caesarean delivery in a large United States hospital system was associated with a reduction in fatal PE (7 of 458 097 versus 1 of 465 880) [24]. In an earlier study to evaluate the cost-effectiveness of thromboprophylaxis at caesarean delivery with intermittent pneumatic compression, a decision tree model using Markov analysis was developed to compare two approaches to perioperative care at the time of cesarean delivery: 1) no use of perioperative thromboprophylaxis and 2) the use of intermittent pneumatic compression for thromboprophylaxis at the time of cesarean delivery. Post-caesarean DVT was estimated to occur in 0.7% of patients (75% of whom were asymptomatic), and result in a 9% chance of post-thrombotic syndrome. Mechanical prophylaxis was assumed to decrease the risk of DVT by 70%. Using the assumptions based on probability of morbidity and mortality of VTE as well as anticoagulation, it was demonstrated that routine thromboprophylaxis for caesarean delivery cost US $39,545 per quality-adjusted life year. One-way sensitivity analysis revealed that as long as the incidence of post-caesarean DVT was at least 0.68%, intermittent pneumatic compression reduced the incidence of DVT by at least 50%, or the cost of intermittent pneumatic compression was less than $180, the cost-effectiveness of mechanical prophylaxis did not exceed $50,000 per quality-adjusted life year. It was concluded that mechanical thromboprophylaxis should be a cost-effective strategy under a wide range of circumstances [25]. However, the assumed incidence of post caesarean VTE of 6.8 per 1000 patients is apparently higher than the incidence in many centres, including our locality. Therefore, 100% mechanical prophylaxis as proposed by the RCOG and ACOG model may not be necessary and will lead to high costs in our local practice. As explained in the latter part of this chapter, our local risk score model would utilize mechanical prophylaxis for around 10% of patients, and appears to be a more reasonable recommendation, balancing clinical risks and cost-effectiveness.

Controversies on Existing International Thromboembolic Prophylaxis Protocols

The clinical benefits of using LMWH for thromboprophylaxis in a high proportion of women in the postpartum period has been seriously questioned in several critical aspects. In an elaborate review of the current protocols, it was concluded that there were major oversights on such recommendations. In particular, the prediction models were often based on studies that report asymptomatic deep vein thrombosis; the risk estimates were not adjusted for time exposure; and the harm caused by heparin had been overlooked. The benefits of heparin were exaggerated and its harms are underappreciated. Estimates of the numbers-needed-to-treat and harm were universally lacking [13].

The risk threshold at which pharmacologic prophylaxis of VTE is warranted remains unknown. For certain high risk subgroups of women, such as those with previous VTE, those tested positive for high risk thrombophilias, those with low-risk thrombophilia delivered by caesarean section, or those diagnosed with antiphospholipid antibody syndrome, recommendations from available guidelines are consistent in recommending postpartum pharmacologic prophylaxis [26]. The main discrepancy among current guidelines concerns pharmacologic prophylaxis for women with no history of VTE and no inherited or acquired thrombophilia. A study of 293 patients delivered by caesarean section found that if recommendations from RCOG were followed, 85.0% of women undergoing cesarean deliveries would be candidates for postpartum pharmacologic prophylaxis, compared with 1.0% under ACOG guidelines and 34.8% under ACCP guidelines [27]. The risk-benefit ratio of pharmacologic prophylaxis after cesarean delivery depends on the accurate determination of the true incidence of VTE. Retrospective data obtained from analysis of large databases may overestimate the incidence of VTE (up to 4% among women at high risk for VTE), resulting in a similar overestimation of the benefit of any intervention aimed at preventing it. By extrapolating from evidence in patients who have undergone general surgery, the ACCP suggests that the benefits of thromboprophylaxis outweigh potential harm when the absolute risk of VTE is 3% or higher [13]. However, other prospective studies have found that the incidence after cesarean delivery is significantly lower, being around 0.6 per 1000 deliveries for elective cesarean delivery and 0.8 per 1000 deliveries after emergency cesarean delivery [26]. The number needed to treat (NNT) to prevent 1 episode of VTE during the postpartum period therefore ranged from 1 in 640 to as high as 4000 among women at high risk for VTE who underwent cesarean delivery. On the other hand, the number needed to harm (NNH) with the use of pharmacologic VTE prophylaxis after cesarean delivery has been reported to be as low as 200 [13]. While precise estimations of the NNT and NNH are apparently not feasible based on the observational data currently in the literature, there is a strong suggestion that the NNH may be significantly lower than the NNT if the aggressive guidelines promoting universal or near universal pharmacologic VTE prophylaxis are followed, particularly in the absence of high risk factors or when only minor risk factors are present. As mentioned, after the implementation of prophylactic guidelines in the United Kingdom, a decrease in maternal mortality secondary to VTE was noted between 2004 and 2008. However, more recent data found that the reduction has not been sustained, with an increase in VTE-related maternal mortality after 2009 when compared with the initial reduction noticed in previous years [28]. As the RCOG protocol would increase the use of thromboprophylaxis in various clinical scenarios (including antenatally or after vaginal delivery) for women with risk factors, it became even more difficult to attribute any reduction in maternal mortality specifically to prophylaxis after cesarean delivery. A recent study reported only 1 maternal death from VTE among 465,880 women undergoing a cesarean delivery who received mechanical prophylaxis [29], so that the impact of VTE prophylaxis on maternal mortality and morbidity would indeed be hard to confirm statistically in any clinical trial due to the extremely low incidence of such events.

The Clinical Scenario of Thromboembolic Prophylaxis in Hong Kong

The occurrence of VTE in pregnant Chinese Women has been perceived to be rare [30] so VTE prophylaxis is often ignored in our local practice in Hong Kong. Nevertheless, from a 3-year study from January 1998 to December 2000 in an obstetric unit of a tertiary university teaching hospital in Hong

Kong, the incidence of VTE in pregnant Chinese Women (1.88 per 1000 deliveries) was not uncommon and was similar to that of the white population. The majority (75%) of cases were diagnosed in the postpartum period, mainly after caesarean section [27]. Advanced maternal age, obesity and caesarean section contributed most substantially to the rates of obstetric VTE [31]. These have also been identified as risk factors for VTE during pregnancy in Chinese [32] and the prevalence of these factors were apparently increasing in our locality. Women who underwent caesarean delivery would be at relatively high risk for thromboembolism postpartum if these additional risk factors were present [33]. We believe that the recommendations from the RCOG and ACOG which differed significantly between each other [14] were both unsuitable for Chinese populations. There is also a paucity of objective data as the efficacy of these protocols in the actual prevention of thromboembolism in targeted populations. Indeed, currently, most obstetric units in Hong Kong do not have specific protocols for VTE prophylaxis for caesarean section.

Different countries have their own guidelines of obstetric VTE prophylaxis. International guidelines recommendations were based on studies mostly carried out among white women and may not be applicable to us [30]. Asian is different from Caucasian like different BMI cut off for VTE risk [35]. A tertiary hospital in Italy derived its own risk score model for thromboprophylaxis following caesarean delivery [36], and although empirical, appeared to be clinically safe and effective. We therefore developed a modified risk score model adapted from the RCOG guidelines and formulated a guideline of VTE prophylaxis targeted for caesarean section for our local obstetric population. We then evaluated the application of this protocol in the prevention of caesarean delivery related VTE and to compare it with the RCOG and ACOG guidelines in terms of utilization rates for mechanical and pharmacologic prophylaxis. The incidence of VTE with our risk score model and the bleeding risks associated with LMWH usage were also assessed.

Our Hong Kong Scoring Model

From 1st May 2017 to 30th April 2018, a risk score model was implemented to assess the risk of VTE in all women undergoing either elective or emergency caesarean delivery in our unit (United Christian Hospital, Hong Kong), which is a regional tertiary referral obstetric centre in Hone Kong with around 4000 deliveries per year and a caesarean rate is about 22- 23% in the recent 5 years. Before the use of this risk score system, we had no specific protocols for VTE prophylaxis for caesarean sections, and high risk women such as those with morbid obesity were only empirically advised to have early mobilization after delivery.

Table 2. Local risk model of VTE prophylaxis for caesarean section

1) Patients who are on antenatal LMWH (such as previous DVT or high risk thrombo-embolism) or those who have already planned for LMWH for 6 weeks after delivery should have pneumatic cuff during CS and have LMWH after delivery as planned. Calculation of the VTE score will not be needed for these patients.
2) Patient who will undergo elective or emergency CS should have the following risk factors checked (each risk factor score one in VTE score unless specified): - Age ≥ 40 years - BMI (Pre-pregnant or early pregnancy BMI) ≥ 25 but < 30 kg/m2 - BMI ≥ 30 kg/m2 (Score as two in VTE score) - Parity ≥ 3 - Pre-eclampsia - Multiple pregnancy - Preterm gestation (<34 week) - Prolonged labour (>24 h) - Stillbirth in this pregnancy - Medical comorbidities e.g., cancer, heart failure, active SLE, IBD or inflammatory polyarthropathy, nephrotic syndrome, type I DM with nephropathy, sickle cell disease, current intravenous drug addict - Low-risk thrombophilia - Current smoker - Gross varicose veins - Current systemic infection - Immobility, e.g., paraplegia - Family history of VTE (1st degree relative) - Patient whose VTE score ≥ 2 should have pneumatic cuff during CS - Patient who has PPH ≥ 1000 ml or has blood transfusion during CS should add one score in VTE score - Patient whose VTE score ≥ 3 should have at least 10 days postnatal prophylactic LMWH Regimen: Maternal booking or early pregnancy body weight < 100 kg: enoxaparin subcutaneous 40 mg daily Maternal booking or early pregnancy body weight >= 100 kg: enoxaparin subcutaneous 60 mg daily

BMI = Body Mass Index; CS = caesarean section; DM = diabetes mellitus; IBD = inflammatory bowel disease; LMWH = low molecular weight heparin; PPH = postpartum haemorrhage; SLE = systemic lupus erythematous; VTE = venous thromboembolism.

Our model was based on demographic, obstetric and medical risk factors of each patient (Table 2). Before undergoing caesarean section, women received a risk score assessment based on the standardized VTE risk assessment form. The VTE risk score was then reviewed after caesarean section to look for additional factors present such as postpartum haemorrhage or blood transfusion during caesarean section. Women with increased risk (VTE score ≥ 2) would be prescribed mechanical prophylaxis in the form of pneumatic cuffs to the calves during caesarean section, and the application of the pneumatic cuffs would be continued post-operatively until the patients could fully mobilize. Those with high risk (VTE score ≥ 3) would be prescribed for pharmacological prophylaxis in the form of subcutaneous injection of LMWH for 10 days after delivery in addition to the pneumatic cuffs. The completed VTE risk assessment forms were collected after delivery. Demographic data, gestational age at delivery and postpartum complications were retrieved from the electronic obstetric database and individual medical records were reviewed manually when needed. The rates of mechanical and pharmacological prophylaxis for caesarean section using our risk score model was then compared with the model in the RCOG and the ACOG when their guidelines were applied on our patients.

There were a total of 3955 deliveries during the study period, of which 909 women (23%) underwent caesarean section. A total of 861 (94.7%) of the participants were Chinese and were included for analysis. Two patients were already on LMWH in antenatal period for specific medical indications, therefore pneumatic cuffs were prescribed during caesarean section and LMWH was continued after caesarean section, and they were excluded from the subsequent analysis. For the remaining 859 patients, their demographic, obstetric and medical characteristics are shown in Table 3. Overweight (15.3%), advanced maternal age > 40 years (9.7%), multiple pregnancy (5.1%), obesity (4.7%), and primary postpartum haemorrhage (4.1%) were the most common risk factors identified under our risk model. Within this cohort, 750 (87.3%) patients had VTE score ≤ 1 and were classified as low risk and were therefore only advised for early mobilization after caesarean section. Of the rest, 109 (12.7%) patients had VTE Score ≥ 2 and were given mechanical prophylaxis and 28 (3.3%) patients had VTE Score ≥ 3 and were prescribed pharmacological prophylaxis in addition to mechanical prophylaxis. If RCOG guidelines were applied to our cohort, 649 (75.6%) patients would receive LMWH for VTE prophylaxis after caesarean section. The main reason accounting for such a large difference was the recommendation in the RCOG guidelines that all cases of emergency caesarean section performed in labour should be given postnatal prophylactic LMWH, yet half of the caesarean sections (51.0%) in this cohort were performed emergently during labour. In contrast, no patient would receive LMWH under ACOG guidelines.

Nevertheless, all patients underwent caesarean sections would receive mechanical prophylaxis according to both RCOG and ACOG recommendations (Table 4). No patients during the study period had postpartum VTE events. No patients who had received LMWH prophylaxis after caesarean section had serious haemorrhage or complications. Only one patient who received LMWH after caesarean section had a 3 cm haematoma over the skin wound which was managed conservatively [37].

Table 3. Demographic, obstetric and medical characteristics of the patients undergoing the local risk model

Demographic factors	Number (%)
Maternal age in years, mean (SD)	32.9 (5.2)
Age ≥ 35	333 (38.8)
Age ≥ 40	83 (9.7)
Parity, mean (SD)	0.7 (0.7)
Multiparous > 3	17 (2.0)
Assisted reproductive technology	63 (7.3)
Pre-pregnant body mass index (BMI) in kg/m2, mean (SD)	22.5 (3.7)
Overweight BMI ≥ 25 but <30	131 (15.3)
Obesity BMI ≥ 30	40(4.7)
Obesity BMI ≥ 40	0 (0)
Gestational age at delivery, mean (SD)	38.2 (1.9)
Preterm delivery <37 weeks	78 (9.1)
Preterm delivery <34 weeks	28 (3.3)
Obstetric factors	
Pre-eclampsia	24 (2.8)
Multiple pregnancy	44 (5.1)
Prolonged labour >24 h	5 (0.6)
Stillbirth	0 (0)
PPH _ 1000 ml or required blood transfusion	35 (4.1)
Caesarean section in labour	438 (51.0)
Medical factors	
Medical comorbidities	7 (0.8)
Systemic lupus erythematous	4
Cancer	2
Crohn's disease	1
Heart failure	1
Low risk thrombophilia	0 (0)
Current smoker	8 (0.9)
Gross varicose veins	1 (0.1)
Current systemic infection	4 (0.5)
Immobility e.g., paraplegia	1 (0.1)
Family history of VTE (1st degree relative)	1 (0.1)

BMI = Body Mass Index; LMWH = low molecular weight heparin; PPH = postpartum haemorrhage; SD = standard deviation; VTE = venous thromboembolism.

Table 4. The rate of mechanical and pharmacological prophylaxis used under different models

	Mechanical	Pharmacological
Local risk model	12.7%	3.3%
RCOG	100%	75.6%
ACOG	100%	0%

ACOG = American Congress of Obstetricians;
RCOG = Royal College of Obstetricians and Gynaecologists.

Results of Our Scoring Model

The risk of VTE in pregnancy is estimated to be increased for women aged 35 years and older. In the postpartum period, women aged 35 and over had a 70% increase in risk compared to 25-34 year olds [2]. Advanced maternal age of ≥35 years constituted 33.8% of our study cases. Maternal overweight with BMI >25 and <30 kg/m2 (15.3%) and obesity with BMI ≥ 30 kg/m2 (4.7%) together also account for 20% of our cases. Obesity is associated with a higher risk of PE (adjusted OR [aOR] 14.9, 95% CI 3.0-74.8) and of DVT (aOR 4.4, 95% CI 1.6-11.9). Overweight, too, is a weak risk factor for pregnancy related VTE. A gradient of increasing VTE risk with increasing BMI had been demonstrated with ORs increasing from 1.4 in the 25-30 kg/m2 BMI group to 5.3 with BMI >30 kg/m2 [38]. The World Health Organization has recommended lower BMI cut off points for Asians when risk stratifying for diseases associated with obesity which may similarly apply to the risk stratification of VTE in the pregnant population [35]. We have therefore included overweight in addition to obesity as risk factors in our risk score model in contrast to the RCOG guidelines.

While our risk score model was modified from the RCOG, we adopted a less aggressive approach based on our overall estimation of a lower thromboembolic risk as compared to Western populations. For instance, we included women with older maternal age of 40 years old (as compared to 35 years old for RCOG) and preterm delivery of earlier gestation of 34 weeks (as compared to 37 weeks for RCOG). This has allowed us to drastically reduce the number of women requiring LMWH prophylaxis. If RCOG guidelines are followed, the clinical risks as well as costs of using LMWH in 75.6% of our cases (649 patients) is not inconsiderable. Our study did not demonstrate any additional risks of major bleeding with LMWH due to the small numbers involved. We did not identify any postpartum VTE incidence in our study cohort. This may be related to the limited sample size of our study in single centre, as well as the low overall absolute risks of VTE in pregnancy in our cohort. We did not screen for asymptomatic VTE after caesarean section and could theoretically miss these mild asymptomatic VTE cases. On the other hand, we were not aware of any of our patients who developed symptomatic VTE postnatally, nor any being diagnosed and managed by other units or hospitals. It could also be argued that asymptomatic mild VTE cases are likely to be clinically unimportant and should rapidly resolve spontaneously [13].

So far, we have not been able to directly demonstrate the efficacy of our risk model in VTE prevention with this current cohort, but by our latest audit of the three years after the initial study (from May 2018 till April 2021), we have not documented a single case of significant VTE post caesarean section. In the literature, studies of routine thromboprophylaxis for caesarean delivery have often been small, and similar to our situation were not adequately powered to assess a decrease in the risk of DVT or PE with anticoagulation therapy. The relative risks for symptomatic thromboembolic events post-caesarean with LMWH/UFH versus no heparin was 1.30 (95%CI 0.39 to 4.27) in four randomized controlled trials including 840 women [17]. It remains unproven whether women with risk factors would benefit from postpartum LMWH prophylaxis and there is insufficient evidence in the literature to allow us to define specific risk parameters. Large scale, high-quality randomized trials are warranted, but are obviously difficult to be conducted. We hope that further auditing of the performance of our protocol would yield more supportive evidence for its efficacy, at least among Chinese women in our locality.

Long Term Outcomes after Pregnancy Related Thromboembolism

There is limited knowledge of the long-term outcomes after pregnancy-related venous thrombosis. Cohort studies monitoring long-term complications have never been conducted in this population, and there is only limited evidence based on data from a few observational studies. Nevertheless, the risk of post-thrombotic syndrome (PTS) as a long-term complication after DVT in pregnancy appears considerable. It is most pronounced in women with a proximal DVT occurring postpartum. Quality of life is reduced, but limited to women who develop PTS. Mortality is higher than in the general population during the first year after acute thrombosis, but not thereafter, and the long-term risk of cancer does not seem to be increased. The long-term risk of recurrent venous thrombosis, subsequent arterial thrombosis, or chronic thromboembolic pulmonary hypertension is unknown and more research is highly warranted [39].

Conclusion

There is a need for post caesarean VTE prophylaxis guidelines due to the increasing prevalence of caesarean section, as well as the increasing prevalence of risk factors such as advances maternal age and obesity. The risk score model we have proposed, and its subsequent prophylactic measures appeared simple and easy to apply and avoids subjecting a large proportion of women to pharmacological prophylaxis under other authoritative guidelines. The rate of mechanical prophylaxis used in our cohort also appeared rational and practical. Further larger studies involving more hospitals will be needed to validate this risk assessment tool and evaluate and audit its safety and cost effectiveness in VTE prophylaxis.

References

[1] Heit JA, Kobbervig CE, James AH, Petterson TM, Bailey KR, Melton 3rd LJ. Trends in the incidence of venous thromboembolism during pregnancy or postpartum: a 30-year population-based study. *Ann Intern Med* 2005; 143: 697-706.

[2] Sultan AA, West J, Tata LJ, Fleming KM, Nelson-Piercy C, Grainge MJ. Risk of first venous thromboembolism in and around pregnancy: a population-based cohort study. *Br J Haematol* 2012; 156 366-73.

[3] Pomp ER, Lenselink AM, Rosendaal FR, Doggen CJ. Pregnancy, the postpartum period and prothrombotic defects: risk of venous thrombosis in the MEGA study. *J Thromb Haemost* 2008; 6: 632-7.

[4] Jackson E, Curtis KM, Gaffield ME. Risk of venous thromboembolism during the postpartum period: a systematic review. *Obstet Gynecol* 2011; 117: 691-703.

[5] Berg CJ, Callaghan WM, Syverson C, Henderson Z. Pregnancy related mortality in the United States, 1998 to 2005. *Obstet Gynecol* 2010; 116: 1302-9.

[6] Khan KS, Wojdyla D, Say L, Gulmezoglu AM, Van Look PF. Who analysis of causes of maternal death: a systematic review. *Lancet* 2006; 367: 1066-74.

[7] Cantwell R, Clutton-Brock T, Cooper G, Dawson A, Drife J, Garrod D, et al. Centre for maternal and child enquiries (CMACE). Saving mothers' lives: reviewing maternal deaths to make motherhood safer: 2006e2008. The eighth report of the confidential enquiries into maternal deaths in the United Kingdom. *BJOG* 2011; 118 (Suppl. 1):1- 203.

[8] Guimicheva Boriana, Czuprynska Julia, Arya Roopen. The prevention of pregnancy-related venous thromboembolism. *Br J Haematol* 2015; 168: 163-74.

[9] Friedman AM, Ananth CV, LU YS, D'Alton ME, Wright JD. Underuse of postcesarean thromboembolism prophylaxis. *Obstet Gynecol* 2013; 122: 1197-204.

[10] Bates SM, Greer IA, Middeldorp S, Veenstra DL, Prabulos AM, Vandvik PO, et al. VTE, thrombophilia, antithrombotic therapy, and pregnancy: antithrombotic therapy and prevention of thrombosis, 9th Edn. American College of Chest Physicians Evidence-Based Clinical Practice Guidelines. *Chest* 2012; 141 (Suppl. 2): E691s-736s.

[11] McLintock C, Brighton T, Chunilal S, Dekker G, McDonnell N, McRae S, et al. Recommendations for the prevention of pregnancy-associated venous thromboembolism. *Aust N Z J Obstet Gynaecol* 2012; 52: 3-13.

[12] Wu Pensee, Poole Tamsin C, Janet A, Pickett b, Bhat Ajit, Lees Christoph C. Current obstetric guidelines on thromboprophylaxis in the United Kingdom: evidence based medicine? *Eur J Obstet Gynecol Reprod Biol* 2013; 168: 7-11.

[13] Kotaska A. Postpartum venous thromboembolism prophylaxis may cause more harm than benefit: a critical analysis of international guidelines through an evidence-based lens. *BJOG* 2018; 125: 1109-16.

[14] Lussana Federico, Coppens Michiel, Cattaneo Marco, Middeldorp Saskia. Pregnancy-related venous thromboembolism: risk and the effect of thromboprophylaxis. *Thromb Res* 2012; 129: 673-80.

[15] Reducing the risk of venous thromboembolism during pregnancy and the puerperium. *Royal College of Obstetricians and Gynaecologists, green-top guideline No. 37a* April. 2015.

[16] Thromboembolism in pregnancy. ACOG practice bulletin No. 196. American College of Obstetricians and Gynaecologists. *Obstet Gynecol* 2018; 132: e1-17.

[17] Bain E, Wilson A, Tooher R, Gates S, Davis LJ, Middleton P. Prophylaxis for venous thromboembolic disease in pregnancy and the early postnatal period. *Cochrane Database Syst Rev* 2014;(2): CD001689.

[18] Lindqvist PG, Bremme K, Hellgren M. Swedish society of obstetrics and gynecology (SFOG) working group on hemostatic disorders (Hem-ARG). Efficacy of obstetric thromboprophylaxis and long-term risk of recurrence of venous thromboembolism. *Acta Obstet Gynecol Scand* 2011; 90: 648-53.

[19] Greer IA, Nelson-Piercy C. Low-molecular-weight heparins for thromboprophylaxis and treatment of venous thrombo-embolism in pregnancy: a systematic review of safety and efficacy. *Blood* 2005; 106: 401-7.

[20] Hayes-Ryan D, Byrne BM. Prevention of thrombosis in pregnancy: how practical are consensus derived clinical practice guidelines? *J Obstet Gynaecol* 2012; 32: 740-2.

[21] Fox NS, Laughon K, Bender SD, Saltzman DH, Rebarber A. Anti-factor Xa plasma levels in pregnant women receiving low molecular weight heparin thromboprophylaxis. *Obstet Gynecol* 2008; 112: 884-9.

[22] Cote-Poirier G, Bettache N, Cote AM, Mahone M, Morin F, Cumyn A, Bureau YA, Malick M, Sauve N. Evaulation of complications in postpartum women receiving therapeutic anticoagulation. *Obstet Gynecol* 2020; 136: 394-401.

[23] Seeho Sean KM, Nippita Tanya A, Roberts Christine L, Morris Jonathan M, Natasha Nassar. Venous thromboembolism prophylaxis during and following caesarean section: a survey of clinical practice. *Aust N Z J Obstet Gynaecol* 2016; 56: 54-9.

[24] Clark SL, Christmas JT, Frye DR, Meyers JA, Perlin JB. Maternal mortality in the United States: predictability and the impact of protocols on fatal post cesarean pulmonary embolism and hypertension-related intracranial hemorrhage. *Am J Obstet Gynecol* 2014; 211: 32.e1-9.

[25] Casele H, Grobman WA. Cost-effectiveness of thromboprophylaxis with intermittent pneumatic compression at cesarean delivery. *Obstet Gynecol* 2006; 108: 535-40.

[26] Society for Maternal-Fetal Medicine (SMFM), Pacheco LD, Saade G, Metz TD. Society for Maternal-Fetal Medicine Consult Series #51: Thromboembolism prophylaxis for cesarean delivery. *Am J Obstet Gynecol* 2020; 223: B11–17.

[27] Palmerola KL, D'Alton ME, Brock CO, Friedman AM. A comparison of recommendations for pharmacologic thromboembolism prophylaxis after caesarean delivery from three major guidelines. *BJOG* 2016; 123: 2157-62.

[28] Knight M, Kenyon S, Brocklehurst P, Neilson J, Shakespeare J, Kurinczuk JJ, eds. on behalf of MBRRACE-UK. *Saving Lives, Improving Mothers' Care - Lessons learned to inform future maternity care from the UK and Ireland Confidential Enquiries into Maternal Deaths and Morbidity*

2009e12. Oxford: National Perinatal Epidemiology Unit, University of Oxford; 2014.

[29] Clark SL, Christmas JT, Frye DR, Meyers JA, Perlin JB. Maternal mortality in the United States: predictability and the impact of protocols on fatal post cesarean pulmonary embolism and hypertension-related intracranial hemorrhage. *Am J Obstet Gynecol* 2014; 211: 32.e1–9.

[30] Blondon M, Harrington LB, Righini M, Boehlen F, Bounameaux H, Smith NL. Racial and ethnic differences in the risk of postpartum venous thromboembolism: a population-based, case-control study. *J Thromb Haemost* 2014; 12: 2002-2009.

[31] Chan LY, Tam WH, Lau TK. Venous thromboembolism in pregnant Chinese women. *Obstet Gynecol* 2001; 98: 471-5.

[32] Marik PE, Plante LA. Venous thromboembolic disease and pregnancy. *N Engl J Med* 2008; 359: 2025-33.

[33] Tam WH, Ng MHL, Yiu AKW, Lau KM, Cheng GYM, Li CY. Thrombophilia among Chinese women with venous thromboembolism during pregnancy. *Gynecol Obstet Invest* 2012; 73:183-8.

[34] Sultan AA, Tata LJ, West J, Fiaschi L, Fleming KM, Nelson-Piercy C, et al. Risk factors for first venous thromboembolism around pregnancy: a population based cohort study from the United Kingdom. *Blood* 2013; 121: 3953-61.

[35] Randhawa NK, Tan EK, Ashok SM. Effect of using population-specific body mass index cutoff points in the risk assessment of pregnant Asian women for venous thromboembolism. *Sing Med J* 2013; 54: 437-40.

[36] Stefania C, Pia RM, Adduci A, Gualtiero R. Thromboprophylaxis following cesarean delivery: one site prospective pilot study to evaluate the application of a risk score model. *Thromb Res* 2012; 129: 28-31.

[37] Lok WY, Kong CW, To WWK. A local risk score model or venous thromboprophylaxis for caesarean section in Chinese women and comparison with international guidelines. *Taiwanese J Obstet* Gynecol 2019; 58: 520-5.

[38] Larsen TB, Sorensen HT, Gislum M, Johnsen SP. Maternal smoking, obesity, and risk of venous thromboembolism during pregnancy and the puerperium: a population-based nested case-control study. *Thromb Res* 2007;120: 505-9.

[39] Wik HS, Jacobsen AF, Sandset PM. Long term outcome after pregnancy – related venous thrombosis. *Thromb Res* 2015; 135 Supp 1: S1-4.

Chapter 6

Caesarean Section for Placenta Praevia: Risk Factors for Severe Postpartum Haemorrhage

William W. K. To* and Choi Wah Kong
Department of Obstetrics and Gynaecology, United Christian Hospital, Hong Kong, China

Abstract

Placenta praevia is known to be one of the leading causes of severe postpartum haemorrhage (PPH). Many risk factors have been associated with severe bleeding during caesarean section (CS) for placenta praevia. However, the importance of individual factors in predicting pregnancy outcome remains controversial. Various predictive models to identify high risk cases for severe haemorrhage have been proposed in the literature. However, some of these models have been difficult to apply in practice as they require sophisticated ultrasound parameters, while other models involve a tedious scoring system. We have recently proposed a simple model based on three simple parameters, namely the presence of significant antepartum haemorrhage (APH) from the history, and anterior or posterior placenta and major or minor praevia from ultrasound findings, and found that it could predict up to 96.2% of all severe PPH. More importantly, the absence of APH, a posterior minor praevia, was associated with a negative predictive value (NPV) of 99.1% of severe PPH, implying that such cases could be treated as 'normal' low risk CSs.

Various conservative surgical treatment modalities have been proposed for the management of severe haemorrhage during CS for

* Corresponding Author's E-mail: towkw@ha.org.hk.

In: A Closer Look at Pregnancy and Childbirth
Editor: Louise J. Salgado
ISBN: 978-1-68507-658-0

placenta praevia, including intrauterine balloon tamponade systems, intrauterine gauge packing, various compression sutures, radiological uterine artery ligation or a combination of these methods. There is now emerging evidence that prophylactic use of balloon tamponade may reduce the incidence of severe PPH in placenta praevia.

The establishment of a differential protocol for placenta praevia based on a simple model of risks factors and meticulous planning to prepare for contingency measures are essential elements conducive to good outcomes in CS for placenta praevia.

Keywords: caesarean section, placenta praevia, risk factors, postpartum hemorrhage

Introduction

The incidence of postpartum haemorrhage (PPH) has been observed to be increasing worldwide [1, 2], and approximately 1-2% of deliveries in developed countries are associated with severe PPH [2]. Placenta praevia and morbidly adherent placenta was often the leading indication for peripartum hysterectomy due to increase in previous caesarean section (CS) [3, 4]. Placenta praevia is known to be one of the leading causes of severe PPH. Placenta praevia is diagnosed when there is partial or complete coverage of the internal cervical os by placental tissue in the third trimester. A classical series which included 127 women with placenta praevia found that no patients with placental edge greater than 2 cm from internal cervical os required CS for the indication of placenta praevia whereas 7 of 8 patients with placental edge <= 2 cm had CS because of antepartum haemorrhage (APH) [5]. This study established a rationale as guideline for allowing vaginal delivery if the placental edge was greater than 2 cm from cervical os.

The incidence of placenta praevia at the time of delivery was 2.54 and 0.44% in women with or without a previous history of CS [6] respectively. With an increasing CS rate in many countries in the past decades, an increased incidence of placenta praevia has been observed. PPH is often encountered in women with placenta praevia as the lower segment of the uterus, being anatomically as well as functionally different from the upper segment, is where the placental bed is located. In a recent cohort of 328 patients with placenta praevia from Austria, maternal morbidity was high, and included APH (42.3%), PPH (7.1%), maternal anemia (30%), comorbid adherent placentation (4%), and peripartum hysterectomy (5.2%). There was also a high incidence of neonatal complications including preterm birth (54.9%), low birth weight < 2500g (35.6%), low Apgar-score at five minutes <7 (5.8%), and fetal mortality (1.5%). The data confirmed a high overall adverse maternal (34.15%) and neonatal (60.06%) outcome [7] with placenta praevia.

Postpartum Haemorrhage Associated with Placenta Praevia

Major placenta praevia was found to have higher possibility of blood transfusion and emergency peripartum hysterectomy [8, 9]. Severe bleeding from placenta praevia was postulated to be due to bleeding from the less contractile lower uterine segment which is the site of placenta separation in praevia. Therefore, if a large portion of the lower segment is attached to the placenta, more bleeding would be expected [10, 11]. The management of PPH from placenta praevia tends to be different from that for uterine atony. A variety of techniques have been described to control bleeding associated with placenta praevia. The B-Lynch suture [12], multiple square suturing technique [13], intrauterine packing by pads, intrauterine balloon tamponade systems [14], or progressive devascularization of the uterus up to and including the internal iliac arteries have been used to achieve hemostasis. Radiological embolization of the uterine arteries has also been shown to be an effective treatment when such expertise is available. Other less conventional methods such as the application of TachoSil (Nycomed, Denmark), a collagen fleece coated with a mixture of human fibrinogen and thrombin, directly onto the bleeding surfaces of the lower uterine segment during CS have also been reported to be successful in small case series [15].

Intractable PPH from placenta praevia can also occur when the praevia is situated over a previous uterine scar, resulting in morbid adherence of the placenta. Abnormal invasion of the placenta or placenta accreta spectrum disorders refer to the penetration of the trophoblastic tissue through the decidua basalis into the underlying uterine myometrium, the uterine serosa or even extending beyond to adjacent pelvic organs. It is classified, depending on the degree of invasion, into placenta accreta (invasion <50% of the myometrium), increta (invasion >50% of the myometrium) and percreta (invading the serosa and adjacent pelvic organs). Clinical diagnosis is made intra-operatively, though often the confirmative diagnosis can only be made after a histopathological examination. The incidence of placenta accreta spectrum has increased in the recent decades, chiefly associated with the marked increase in CS rates. The ultimate treatment for massive haemorrhage from placenta praevia or praevia/accreta spectrum is hysterectomy. However, peripartum hysterectomy under such circumstances can be associated with further substantial blood loss and significant maternal morbidity, as well as the loss of future reproductive function. The average blood loss has been estimated to be 3000–5000 ml, and up to 90% of the patients would require a blood transfusion. Antenatal diagnosis using ultrasound or magnetic resonance imaging (MRI) is essential to allow adequate preparation for the possible major haemorrhage, and different approaches have been attempted to reduce complication rates, including leaving the placenta in-situ, partial myometrial excision, the 'Triple P procedure', or direct peripartum hysterectomy without attempting placenta separation [16].

A recent Australian study evaluated the association between APH and PPH and adverse outcomes in cases of placenta praevia in those delivered within a ten-year period from 2007 to 2017. There were 513 cases of placenta praevia, of which 67.3% delivered at term. APH was associated with an increased risk of blood transfusion (RR 3.29; 95% confidence interval (CI) 2.04–5.32), emergency CS (RR 1.38; 95% CI 1.18–1.62) and preterm delivery (RR 4.21; 95% CI 2.77–6.38). PPH was associated with more than doubled the risk of blood transfusion (RR 9.08 95% CI 5–16.44) and admission to the intensive care unit (RR 10.44; 95% CI 2.34–46.59), as well as increased the risk of peripartum hysterectomy (1.4%) [17].

A secondary cohort analysis of the NICHD Maternal-Fetal Medicine Units Network Caesarean Section Registry from the United States compared 496 women with placenta praevia without accreta to 24,201 women without praevia. It was found that maternal haemorrhagic morbidity (19 Vs 7%, adjusted relative risk (aRR) 2.6, 95% CI 1.9-3.5), atony requiring uterotonics (aRR 3.1, 95% CI 2.0-4.9), red blood cell transfusion (aRR 3.8, 95% CI 2.5-5.7) and hysterectomy (aRR 5.1, 95% CI 1.5-17.3) were more common with praevia. For women with praevia, factors associated with maternal hemorrhage were pre-delivery anemia, thrombocytopenia, diabetes, magnesium use, and general anesthesia [18].

When patient outcomes between planned and emergency caesarean deliveries for placenta praevia without morbidly adherent placenta were compared in a retrospective cohort of 304 patients, 10 (3.28%) had an intraoperative diagnosis of morbidly adherent placenta. Eighty (57.1%) underwent planned caesarean delivery, and 60 (42.8%) required emergency caesarean delivery due to uterine contractions and/or bleeding. Baseline characteristics were similar between the two groups except for the gestation at delivery being more advanced for the elective group (36.0 weeks Vs 34.0

weeks, p<.001). Composite maternal morbidity was not significantly different between two groups: 11 (18.3%) in the elective and 10 (12.5%) in emergency group (p=0.35). The authors concluded that in their referral tertiary centre, emergency and planned caesarean deliveries for placenta praevia without morbidly adherent placenta have similar maternal outcomes [19].

Ultrasound Signs to Predict Severe Haemorrhage

Placenta Accreta

The incidence of placenta accreta was increasing worldwide due to the increasing incidence of previous CS. It was reported that the risk of placenta accreta was 3% after the first CS but the risk rose to 40% after the third CSs [6]. Morbidly adherent placenta was found to be independent predictors for peripartum hysterectomy and severe maternal morbidity in placental praevia patients [9, 20]. Obstetricians should be aware of the possibility of placenta accreta in patients having placenta praevia with anterior-locating placenta and previous CS.

Lacunae had been suggested as the most predictive ultrasound sign for placenta accreta [21, 22]. A retrospective review of women with one or more prior caesarean delivery who received an ultrasound diagnosis of placenta praevia or low-lying placenta in the third trimester was done to establish a scoring system for diagnosing placenta accreta. Ultrasound parameters examined included loss of retroplacental clear zone, irregularity and width of uterine-bladder interface, smallest myometrial thickness, presence of lacunar spaces, and bridging vessels. Diagnosis of placental invasion was based on histologic confirmation. In a cohort of 184 gravidas, 54 (29%) had invasion confirmed on hysterectomy specimen. All sonographic parameters were associated with placental invasion (P < .001). Constructing a receiver operating characteristic (ROC) curve, the combination of smallest sagittal myometrial thickness, lacunae, and bridging vessels, in addition to number of caesarean deliveries and placental location, yielded an area under the curve (AUC) of 0.87 (95% CI 0.80-0.95). Using logistic regression, a predictive equation was generated and termed the "placenta accreta index." Each parameter was weighted to create a 9-point scale in which a score of 0-9 provided a probability of invasion [23]. The usefulness of this index remains to be confirmed by larger prospective studies.

Placental Edge

The clinical significance of the shape of the lower placental edge in 104 women with transvaginal sonographic diagnosis of placenta praevia before 32 weeks' gestation was evaluated. These were followed up by serial transvaginal sonographic examinations until delivery, with detailed recording of the placental location (anterior or posterior), the distance of its edge from the internal cervical os and its thickness. The clinical outcomes of those who had a thick-edge low-lying placenta were compared with those who had a thin-edge one. It was found that women having a low-lying placenta with a thick edge had a significantly higher rate of APH ($P = 0.0002$), abdominal delivery ($P = 0.02$), abnormally adherent placenta ($P = 0.012$) and low birth weight ($P = 0.006$) compared to those in whom the placental edge was thin. In the six patients requiring caesarean hysterectomy with complete placenta praevia because of severe peripartum hemorrhage, all of them had either central or thick-edge placenta [24]. It was proposed that abundant vasculature of the lower placental edge and the subplacental zone, as well as the interference of a thick-edge placenta with descent of the fetal head [25] would contribute to profuse haemorrhage. Another small prospective study including 54 women also showed that thick placenta was associated with significantly higher incidence of APH, emergency CS before 36 weeks and more peripartum blood transfusion and caesarean hysterectomy than thin placenta [26]. The results of these studies suggested that integrating the shape of the lower placental edge into transvaginal sonographic assessment of placenta praevia may improve the prediction of mode of delivery and clinical outcome.

Location of the Placenta Praevia

In placenta praevia, an anterior placenta, compared with posterior placenta, has been reported to more frequently cause massive hemorrhage during CS. Whether this is due to the high incidence of placenta accreta, previous CS, or a transplacental approach to deliver the fetus in anterior placenta is unclear. In a retrospective analysis of 205 women, it was found that patients with accreta, previous CS, total praevia, and anterior placentation bled significantly more than their counterparts. Multivariate logistic regression analysis showed that accreta (odds ratio (OR) 12.6), previous CS (OR 4.7), total praevia (OR 4.1), and anterior placentation (OR 3.5) were independent risk factors of massive hemorrhage >2400 ml. It was concluded that anterior placentation, namely, the placenta with a longer os-placental edge distance in the anterior wall than in the posterior wall, was a risk of massive hemorrhage during CS for placenta praevia [8].

One hypothesis for massive haemorrhage from anterior placenta praevia was that the uterus was incised more cephalad in anterior placenta patients than posterior patients in order to avoid transplacental delivery of the fetus. As the uterine wall would be thicker in uterine body than the lower segment, incisions other than low transverse incision, such as high transverse incisions or classical vertical incisions, would be expected to be associated with more bleeding. There would also be more blood vessels existing on the incision site for anterior located placenta than posterior located placenta. While transplacental approach to deliver the fetus will obviously increase bleeding, it is impractical to totally avoid transplacental approach to deliver the fetus in all the cases of placenta praevia. In addition, it is difficult for the surgeon to predict whether transplacental approach can be avoided before CS, as such decisions were usually only made on site at the operation. Therefore, it appears reasonable that anterior placenta location should be an independent overall risk factor to predict severe PPH, irrespective of the need for transplacental delivery of the fetus at CS.

Cervical Length

In a study to estimate the relationship between cervical length and hemorrhage leading to preterm delivery in women with placenta praevia, the transvaginal cervical-length measurements were obtained in all singleton pregnancies with placenta praevia identified at or beyond 24 weeks of gestation. Cervical length of 30 mm or less was considered short. Clinicians were blinded to cervical length measurements. Of 68 women confirmed to have placenta praevia at delivery, 29 (43%) of these had a short cervix. Women with praevia and a short cervix were more likely to require delivery for hemorrhage (79% Vs 28%), to deliver preterm (69% Vs 21%), both being statistically significant ($p < 0.001$). Tocodynamometer evidence of regular uterine contractions was more common with a short cervix than with a longer cervix (69% Vs 21% ($p <0.001$)). Conversely, 64% with a cervical length greater than 30 mm had no bleeding episodes and progressed to term. The authors concluded that in pregnancies with placenta praevia, a third-trimester cervical length of 30 mm or less is associated with increased risk for hemorrhage, uterine activity, and preterm birth [27].

In another study evaluating the effectiveness of cervical length and the lower placental edge thickness measurement in predicting the risk of APH and emergency preterm caesarean delivery in women with complete placenta praevia, the data yielded from transvaginal ultrasound assessment of 54 women in the third trimester were correlated to the clinical outcome. It was found that there was significantly more antepartum bleeding (53.3% vs. 20.8%) and emergency CS (46.6% Vs 16.6%) before 36 weeks due to massive bleeding in cases with thick lower placental edge or central placenta than cases with thin lower placental edge. By combining cervical length ($\leq$ 30 mm) with lower placental edge thickness measurements, sensitivity, specificity, positive predictive value (PPV) negative predictive value (NPV) and accuracy increased to 83.3, 78.4, 53.4, 79.8 and 89.7%, respectively for the prediction of antepartum bleeding and emergency CS before 36 weeks, with AUC being 0.882. The results appear to be consistent with the previous studies [26].

Another study evaluated whether serial changes in cervical length over time can be a predictor for emergency CS in patients with placenta praevia. In a retrospective cohort study of 93 patients with placenta praevia, serial measurement of cervical length by transvaginal ultrasound at 19 to 23 weeks, 24 to 28 weeks, 29 to 31 weeks, and 32 to 34 weeks were made. It was found that 31(33%) had emergency CS due to massive vaginal bleeding. The cervical length tended to decrease with advancing gestational age in all patients, but after the 29–31week measurement, the cervical length in those that had emergency CS decreased abruptly, but only continued to gradually decrease in those with elective CS. On multivariate analysis to determine risk factors, only admissions for bleeding (OR, 34.7; 95% CI, 5.2–229.9) and change in cervical length (OR 3.52; 95% CI, 1.2–10.2) were significantly associated with emergency CS. Analysis of the ROC characteristics showed that change in cervical length could be the predictor of emergency CS (AUC 0.734, $p < 0.001$), with optimal cutoff for predicting emergency delivery at 6.0 mm. The authors concluded that change in cervical length of more than 6 mm between the second and third trimester were at high risk of emergency CS in placenta praevia, while single measurements of short cervical length at the second or third trimester do not seem to be predictive [28].

Birth Weight Estimation

Apart from studying the direct ultrasound features of placenta praevia, an interesting study evaluated the association of birth weight deviation from the nationwide average with massive haemorrhage during delivery with a low-lying placenta in 40 women. An ROC curve analysis was used to determine the optimal birth weight deviation cut-off for predicting a massive haemorrhage, The ROC curve analysis indicated that the neonatal birth weight deviation from the nationwide average showed a good accuracy for the prediction of massive intrapartum haemorrhage (AUC 0.74). The best cut-off for predicting a massive haemorrhage was a birth weight deviation of +0.51

standard deviations from the nationwide average, with sensitivity 73.3%, specificity 68.0%, PPV 57.9% and NPV 80.9%. It was concluded that accurate risk stratification using the fetal weight as a marker for a predicting massive intrapartum haemorrhage may help in the management of patients with a low-lying placenta [29].

The Role of Magnetic Resonance Imaging

Many studies in the literature have focused on characterizing features on MRI to identify invasive placenta praevia and to differentiate placenta percreta from placenta accreta. In a series of 45 women with placenta praevia, and 93 women with accreta who underwent 1.5T placental MRI, it was found that placental bulge with distorted uterine outline and uterine serosal hypervascularity were independently associated with placenta percreta (OR = 48.6, P < 0.001; OR = 4.1, P = 0.018 respectively), and the combination of the two MRI features to distinguish percreta from accreta yielded an AUC of 0.92 for its predictive performance [30].

Another study developed a comprehensive severity score for morbidly adherent placenta by combining ultrasound and MRI. In a retrospective cohort of 41 women with placenta praevia (of which 16 had histologically confirmed accreta) who received both transvaginal ultrasound and MRI for suspicion for morbidly adherent placenta, ultrasound was scored for praevia, hypervascularity, loss of retroplacental clear space and lacunae, while MRI was evaluated for intraparenchymal vessels, abnormally dilated vessels, fibrin deposition, placental bulge and bladder dome irregularity. At the highest ultrasound score, the probability of accreta was 63.7%, while at the highest MRI score, the probability of adherent placentation was 90.5%. Combining the ultrasound and MRI findings had a sensitivity of 56% and a specificity of 92% [31].

Efforts have also been made to develop a scoring system for intraoperative massive hemorrhage combining MRI and clinical characteristics to predict the risk of massive hemorrhage in placenta praevia and accreta. In a retrospective cohort consisting of 259 patients with placenta praevia and accreta after previous CS as the derivation cohort and another 115 patients as the validation cohort, multivariable logistic regressions analysis was conducted to develop a scoring system for prediction of intraoperative massive bleeding > 2000 ml. Ten indicators, including clinically maternal age (1 point), preoperative hemoglobin level (1 point), gravidity number (1 point), number of CS (1 point), MRI T2 dark intraplacental bands (4 points), cervical canal length (3 points), placenta thickness on the uterine scar area (4 points), empty vascular shadow of the uterus (1 point), low signal discontinuity in the muscular layer of the posterior wall of the bladder (6 points) and attachment position of the placenta (1 point) were imputed. From the ROC analysis, a total score of 7 points was identified as the optimal cutoff value, allowing good differentiation of intraoperative massive bleeding in the derivation cohort (AUC, 0.863; 95% CI 0.811–0.916) and in the validation cohort (AUC, 0.933; 95% CI 0.885–0.980). This scoring system can potentially reduce the incidence of intraoperative massive bleeding by identifying patients at high risk [32].

The Prophylactic Use of Balloon Tamponade to Prevent Postpartum Haemorrhage

The effectiveness of routine rapid insertion of a Bakri balloon during CS for placenta praevia was evaluated in a retrospective control study. Among 266 women with singleton pregnancies who underwent CS for placenta praevia, 50 had routine balloon tamponade insertion during CS, while 216 had other hemostatic procedures except balloon tamponade. Bleeding was significantly less in the balloon group than in the non-balloon group: intraoperative bleeding (991 Vs 1250 g, $p<0.01$), postoperative bleeding (62 Vs 150 g, $p<0.01$), and total bleeding (1066 Vs1451 g, $p<0.01$). Furthermore, the mean surgical duration was shorter in the balloon group than the non-balloon group (30 Vs 50 min, $p<0.01$). In the balloon group, five patients suffered from increasing hemorrhage due to prolapse of the balloon from the uterus after the operation, but the hemorrhage was controlled by balloon re-insertion without additional hemostatic procedures. [33] In a later study, the same authors also reported that up to 13% of women would require additional procedures after CS for massive hemorrhage despite using prophylactic balloon tamponade, and these were defined as balloon failures. The total blood loss was 2409 g in the failure group Vs 971 g in the success group ($p < 0.01$). Two types of failures were encountered: balloon prolapse (89%) and accidental placental retention (11%). The hemorrhage was controlled in all patients with balloon prolapse by reinsertion and inflation of the balloon. The patient with placental retention required a uterine artery embolization. Although three patients required a blood transfusion, none required a hysterectomy. Logistic regression analysis for the risk of balloon failure showed that major praevia was the highest risk factor (Hazard Ratio; 19.1, 95% CI 3.17-367.9, $p < 0\ 01$) [34].

In a retrospective cohort of singleton pregnancies undergoing CS for placenta praevia, participants were divided into the balloon group who underwent routine prophylactic use (n=74) just after placenta removal and the non-balloon group (n=89), and into major and minor praevia groups. Intraoperative and perioperative blood losses for those with major praevia were significantly lower in the balloon group than the non-balloon group (1045 ml Vs 1553 ml, p= 0.016; and 1189 ml Vs 1810 ml, p=0.006). The frequency of massive postpartum hemorrhage with major praevia was also lower in the balloon group than in the non-balloon group (2.4% Vs 16.7%, p=0.027). The authors concluded that routine prophylactic use of Bakri balloon tamponade during and after CS is effective in controlling blood loss in major placenta praevia [35].

Another recent study also compared the effectiveness of routine Bakri balloon tamponade (n=98) and uterine gauze packing (n= 64) during CS in patients with placenta praevia. The estimated intraoperative blood loss was significantly lower in the balloon group (667 ± 358 Vs. 791 ± 360 ml, respectively). Additionally, the proportion of patients who required transfusion was significantly lower in the balloon than the gauge packing group (9/98 Vs 17/64 respectively). The operative duration (97.8 ± 17.7 Vs 108.2 ± 16.9 minutes) and the length of stay (3.79 ± 0.89 Vs 4.12 ± 0.85 days) were also significantly shorter in the balloon than gauge packing group. The authors concluded that prophylactic application of balloon tamponade was superior to uterine gauge packing for decreasing the intraoperative blood loss and transfusion rate and should be a more reliable technique to prevent and control postpartum hemorrhage [36].

Clinical Risks Scores to Predict Severe Haemorrhage from Placenta Praevia

Previous studies characterizing hemorrhage and morbidity due to placenta praevia have focused on those that are also complicated by morbidly adherent placenta, while data on the risks of severe haemorrhage from placenta praevia without accreta are less comprehensive. In a study to investigate predictors for massive hemorrhage during CS in patients with placenta praevia and adherence of the placenta, maternal history and antenatal ultrasound findings of the placenta, including location, presence of placental lacunae, lack of a clear zone, presence of spongelike findings of the cervix and presence of a marginal sinus in cases of placenta praevia were reviewed. Among 127 singleton pregnancies with placenta praevia, logistic regression analysis showed that advanced maternal age (OR 5.4; 95% CI 1.8–16.4), previous CS (OR 20.4; 95% CI 4.0–105.2) and sponge-like findings in the cervix (OR 5.6; 95% CI, 1.8–17.0) were associated with massive bleeding over >2500 ml, regardless of whether placental adherence was present. Placental adherence occurred in 5 cases and was more frequent where the placenta was located at the site of the scar of a previous CS (OR 123.1; 95% CI, 4.5–3395.2) and where there was lack of a clear zone (OR 48.0; 95% CI 3.8–604.7) [37].

In a Japanese study to generate a combined ultrasound and clinical model predictive for peripartum complications in pregnancies complicated by placenta praevia, 110 singleton pregnant women with placenta praevia delivered by CS were prospectively collected. A scoring model was formulated including type of praevia, presence of lacunae, uteroplacental hypervascularity, multiparity, history of CS and history of placenta praevia to predict the risk of peripartum complications. It was found that the risk of perioperative transfusion, uterine artery embolization, and caesarean hysterectomy were 26.4, 1.8 and 6.4%, respectively. The type of praevia, lacunae, uteroplacental hypervascularity, parity, history of CS, and history of placenta praevia were associated with complications in univariable analysis. However, due to the heterogeneous nature of the parameters analysed, no factor was independently predictive for any complication in logistic regression analysis. Using the scoring model, the total score significantly correlated with perioperative transfusion, caesarean hysterectomy and composite complication ($p < 0.0001$), with all patients requiring caesarean hysterectomy when total score was ≥ 7, and three-quarters of patients needing blood transfusions when total score was > 6. The authors concluded that the combined scoring model may provide useful information for prediction of peripartum complications in women with placenta praevia [38].

As mentioned earlier, in a retrospective cohort of 205 patients, placenta accreta, previous CS, major placenta praevia and anterior placenta were independent risk factor for massive haemorrhage during CS in patients with placenta praevia after multivariate logistic regression analysis [8].

A Local Risk Factor Analysis to Predict Severe Haemorrhage from Placenta Praevia in Hong Kong

It can be seen that different studies would identify different risk factors, and the importance of individual factors in predicting pregnancy outcome remains controversial. However, if a good predicting model for predicting PPH during CS of placenta praevia is established, better preparation with multi-disciplinary approach with involvement with experienced obstetricians, anaesthetists, haematologists and radiologists can improve the maternal outcomes. We therefore conducted a retrospective study on our local data from 2012-2016 to evaluate the value of clinical and ultrasound risk factors in predicting severe PPH (>1500 ml) in pregnancies undergoing CS for placenta praevia [39]. Both major and minor type of placenta praevia were recruited. According to our protocol. All the patients with placenta praevia undergoing either elective or emergency CS would have transabdominal and/or transvaginal ultrasound assessment one day before or on the day of the operation as pre-operative assessment. The shape of the placental edge was measured and defined according to the Ghourab categorization [24]. The lower placenta edge was assessed by measuring its maximum thickness within 1 cm of the meeting point of the basal and chorionic plates and an estimation of the angle between these plates. It was defined as 'thin' if the thickness was <=1 cm and/or the angle was < 45 degree; otherwise it was defined as 'thick'. The placental location, the distance of placental edge from internal os the presence of lacunae was documented prospectively in the medical notes and these data were then retrieved from the medical notes subsequently for analysis.

Within the 5-year study period, the incidence of CS for placenta praevia was 0.98% (n=215/21,908). Of these, 101 patients (46.9%) had PPH with blood loss >= 500 ml and 26 patients (12.1%) had severe PPH with blood loss >=1500 ml. There were 4 cases (1.85%) of peripartum hysterectomy and no cases of maternal death. There were 6 cases of placenta accreta (2.8%), in which 4 patients had severe PPH. For the other two patients without severe PPH, one had classical CS with the placenta left in situ followed by uterine artery embolization, and the final blood loss was 1330 ml. The other patient had classical section and direct hysterectomy with blood loss 920 ml. Univariate analysis showed that advanced maternal age, previous pregnancies with praevia or PPH, the type of praevia or distance of the placental edge from the os, occurrence of APH before delivery, anterior placenta, thick placental edge, and presence of accreta were all significantly associated with severe

PPH. A logistic regression model showed that major placenta praevia, APH before delivery and anterior placenta remained significant factors associated with severe PPH, whereas other factors were excluded (Table 1). Due to the differential treatment for accreta cases, placenta accreta was not a significant factor in the final equation. Based on the above model, taking the presence of either one of the three significant factors as being positive for high risk of severe PPH, 25 of the 26 patients in the cohort with severe PPH would be considered high risk, giving a sensitivity of 96.2%, while the specificity would be relatively low at 59.8% (113/189). On the other hand, of the 114 patients that would be considered low risk with this model, only 1 had severe PPH, giving a very high NPV of 99.1% (113/114), while the PPV would remain low at 24.8% (25/101).

Table 1. Logistic regression for indicators for severe PPH

Risk factors	**B**	**Standard error**	**Wald**	**Significance**	**Odds Ratio**	**95% Confidence interval**
Parameters in the equation						
Major Vs Minor praevia	1.33	0.675	3.88	0.049	3.78	1.007 to 14.18
Significant APH before C/S	2.248	0.657	11.71	0.001	9.47	2.61 to 34.3
Anterior or posterior placenta	1.59	0.64	6.12	0.013	4.91	1.39 to 17.29
Parameters excluded from equation						
Advanced Age	1.386	0.736	3.55	0.059	4.00	0.946 to 16.91
Hx of PPH in previous pregnancies	18.92	28384	0.001	0.99	16900	0.001 to 21.3
Ultrasound Sponge/lacunae features	2.81	1.87	2.31	0.13		
Thick/thin placental edge	0.832	0.68	1.48	0.22	17.32	0.44 to 683.5
Presence of Accreta	-1.14	2.13	0.288	0.59	0.32	0.005 to 20.65

Our data confirmed that while there was a high association between PPH and placenta praevia, severe PPH only occurred in 10-15% of these cases. The risk factors we have identified were compatible with most of the studies that available in the current literature. Due to the small proportion of patients with placenta accreta in our cohort, and the differential management in these cases, we were unable to draw any conclusion on the optimal management of accreta cases. However, the vigilant detection of lacunae and a high level of suspicion of accreta should be crucial to allow better pre-operative planning and to offer alternative management strategies to reduce severe haemorrhage. In our cohort, thick placenta was associated with higher incidence of severe PPH than thin placenta, but it did not reach statistically significant after logistic regression. One reason was that thick placental edge was also more often associated with major rather than minor placenta praevia, so that statistical significance was lost due to this confounding association.

Conclusion

Our simple risk scoring demonstrates that a predictive model can be constructed based on the various clinical features of the praevia to allow differential preparation and management of the caesarean delivery of these patients. Our final model with only 3 simple parameters, namely presence of significant APH from the history, and anterior or posterior placenta and major or minor praevia from ultrasound findings, could apparently already predict two thirds of all cases of severe PPH. More importantly, the absence of APH, a posterior minor praevia, was associated with a negative predictive value of 94% of severe PPH, implying that such cases could be treated as "normal" low risk CSs, and senior obstetricians would only need to be available for standby for contingencies. This simple model would allow differential pre-operative counselling of patients on risks and complications, planning and preparation of operation, allocation of staff as well as in contingency measures to be taken during operation. The application of such a model should be particularly useful for busy training and service units, as in our centre, when effective utilization of limited resources and manpower expertise are crucial. Improving the detection rate of placenta accreta before CS will also allow appropriate planning of surgical strategies to help to decrease the rate of severe PPH. Better liaison with blood bank before operation and adopting multi-disciplinary approach involving experienced obstetricians, anaesthetists and radiologists should improve the maternal morbidities and avoid mortalities in these cases.

References

[1] Kramer MS, Berg C, Abenhaim H, Dahhou, M, Rouleau J, Mehrabadi, A, Joseph KS. Incidence, risk factors, and temporal trends in severe postpartum hemorrhage. *Am J Obstet Gynecol* 2013; 209: 449. e1-7.

[2] Knight M, Callaghan WM, Berg C, Alexander S, Bouvier-Colle MH, Ford JB et al. Trends in postpartum hemorrhage in high resource countries: a review and recommendations from the International Postpartum Hemorrhage Collaborative Group. *BMC Pregnancy Childbirth* 2009; 9: 55.

[3] Jauniaux ERM, Alfirevic Z, Bhide AG, Belfort MA, Burton GJ, Collins SL, et al., on behalf of the Royal College of Obstetricians and Gynaecologists. 2019. Placenta Praevia and Placenta Accreta: Diagnosis and Management: Green-top Guideline No. 27a. *BJOG* 2018.

[4] Klar M, Michels KB. Caesarean section and placental disorders in subsequent pregnancies–a meta-analysis. *J Perinat Med* 2014; 42: 571–83.

[5] Oppenheimer LW, Farine D, Ritchie JW, Lewinsky RM, Telford J, Fairbanks LA. What is a low-lying placenta? *Am J Obstet Gynecol* 1991; 165:1036-8.

[6] Silver RM, Landon MB, Rouse DJ, Leveno KJ, Spong CY, Thom EA, et al. National Institute of Child Health and Human Development Maternal-Fetal Medicine Units Network. Maternal morbidity associated with multiple repeat caesarean deliveries. *Obstet Gynecol* 2006; 107:1226–32.

[7] Kollmann M, Gaulhofer J, Lang U, Klaritsch P. Placenta praevia: incidence, risk factors and outcome. *J Matern Fetal Neonatal Med* 2016; 29: 1395–8.

[8] Baba Y, Matsubara S, Ohkuchi A, Usui R, Kuwata T, Suzuki H. Anterior placentation as a risk factor for massive hemorrhage during caesarean section in patients with placenta praevia. *J Obstet Gynaecol Res* 2014; 40: 1243–8.

[9] Giambattista E, Ossola MW, Duiella SF, Crovetto F, Acaia B, Somigliana E, et al. Predicting factors for emergency peripartum hysterectomy in women with placenta praevia. *Arch Gynecol Obstet* 2012; 285: 901–6.

[10] Sekiguchi A, Nakai A, Kawabata I, Hayashi M, Takeshita T. Type and location of placenta praevia affect preterm delivery risk related to antepartum hemorrhage. *Int J Med Sci* 2013; 10: 1683–8.

[11] Tuzovic L. Complete versus incomplete placenta praevia and obstetric outcome. *Int J Gynaecol Obstet* 2006; 93: 1107.

[12] B-Lynch C, Coker A, Lawal AH, Abu J, Cowen MJ. The B-Lynch surgical technique for the control of massive postpartum haemorrhage: an alternative to hysterectomy. *Br J Obstet Gynaecol* 1997; 104: 372–5.

[13] Cho JH, Jun S, Lee CN. Hemostatic suturing technique for uterine bleeding after caesarean delivery. *Obstet Gynecol* 2000; 96: 129–31.

[14] Bakri YN, Amri A, Abdul JF. Tamponade – balloon for obstetrical bleeding. *Int J Gynaecol Obstet* 2001; 74: 139–42.

[15] Fuglsang K, Petersen LK. New local hemostatic treatment for postpartum hemorrhage caused by placenta praevia at caesarean section. *Acta Obstet Gynecol* 2010; 89: 1346–9.

[16] Carrillo AP, Chandraharan E. Placenta accreta spectrum: Risk factors, diagnosis and management with special reference to the Triple P procedure. *Womens Health* (Lond) 2019; 15: 1745506519878081.

[17] Balachandar K, Melov SJ, Nayyar R. The risk of adverse maternal outcomes in cases of placenta praevia in an Australian population between 2007 and 2017. *Aust N Z J Obstet Gynaecol* 2020; 60: 890–5.

[18] Gibbins KJ, Einerson BD, Varner MW, Silver RM. Placenta Praevia and Maternal Hemorrhagic Morbidity. *J Matern Fetal Neonatal Med* 2018; 31: 494–9.

[19] Erfani H, Kassir E, Fox KA, Clark SL, Karbasian N, Salmanian B, Shamshirsaz AA, Espinoza J, Nassr AA, Eppes CS, Belfort MA, Shamshirsaz AA. Placenta praevia without morbidly adherent placenta: comparison of characteristics and outcomes between planned and emergent deliveries in a tertiary center. *J Matern Fetal Neonatal Med* 2019; 32: 906-9.

[20] Coskun B, Akkurt I, Dur R, Akkurt MO, Ergani SY, Turan OT, et al. Prediction of maternal near-miss in placenta praevia: a retrospective analysis from a tertiary center in Ankara, Turkey. *J Matern Fetal Neonatal Med* 2018; 31: 370–5.

[21] Comstock CH, Love JJ, Jr, Bronsteen RA, Lee W, Vettraino IM, Huang RR, et al. Sonographic detection of placenta accreta in the second and third trimesters of pregnancy. *Am J Obstet Gynecol* 2004; 190: 1135–40.

[22] Hamada S, Hasegawa J, Nakamura M, Matsuoka R, Ichizuka K, Sekizawa A, Okai T. Ultrasonographic findings of placenta lacunae and a lack of a clear zone in cases with placenta praevia and normal placenta. *Prenat Diagn* 2011; 31: 1062–5.

[23] Rac MWF, Dashe JS, Wells CE, Moschos E, McIntire DD, Twickler DM. Ultrasound predictors of placental invasion: the Placenta Accreta Index. *Am J Obstet Gynecol* 2015; 212: 343. e1-7.

[24] Ghourab S. Third-trimester transvaginal ultrasonography in placenta praevia: does the shape of the lower placental edge predict clinical outcome? *Ultrasound Obstet Gynecol* 2001; 18: 103–8.

[25] Saitoh M, Ishihara K, Sekiya T, Araki T. Anticipation of uterine bleeding in placenta praevia based on vaginal sonographic evaluation. *Gynecol Obstet Invest* 2002: 54: 37–42.

[26] Zaitoun MM, El Behery MM, El Hameed AA, Soliman BS. Does cervical length and the lower placental edge thickness measurement correlates with clinical outcome in cases of complete placenta praevia? *Arch Gynecol Obstet* 2011; 284: 867–73.

[27] Stafford IA, Dashe JS, Shivvers SA, Alexander JM, McIntire DD, Leveno KJ. Ultrasonographic cervical length and risk of hemorrhage in pregnancies with placenta praevia. *Obstet Gynecol* 2010; 116: 595–600.

[28] Shin JE, Shin JC, Lee Y, Kim SJ. Serial change in cervical length for the prediction of emergency caesarean section in placenta praevia. *PLoS One* 2016; 1: e0149036.

[29] Shinohara S, Okuda Y, Hirata S. Association between birth weight and massive haemorrhage in pregnancy with a low-lying placenta: a 9-year single centre retrospective cohort study in Japan. *J Obstet Gynaecol* 2019; 39: 22-26.

[30] Chen X, Shan R, Zhao L, Song Q, Zuo C, Zhang X, Wang S, Shi H, Gao F, Qian T, Wang G, Limperopoulos C. Invasive placenta praevia: Placental bulge with distorted uterine outline and uterine serosal hypervascularity at 1.5T MRI – useful features for differentiating placenta percreta from placenta accreta. *Eur Radiol* 2018; 28: 708–17.

[31] Knight JC, Lehnert S, Shanks AL, Atasi L, Delaney LR, Marine MB, Ibrahim SA, Brown BP. A comprehensive severity score for the morbidly adherent placenta: combining ultrasound and magnetic resonance imaging. *Pediatr Radiol* 2018 48: 1945–54.

[32] Chen D, Xu JF, Ye PF, Li M, Duan X, Zhao F, Liu XH, Wang XD, Peng B. Risk scoring system with MRI for intraoperative massive hemorrhage

in placenta praevia and accreta. *J Magn Reason Imaging* 2020; 51: 947–58.

[33] Soyama H, Miyamoto M, Sasa H, Ishibashi H, Yoshida M, Nakatsuka M, Takano M, Furuya K. Effect of routine rapid insertion of Bakri balloon tamponade on reducing hemorrhage from placenta praevia during and after caesarean section. *Arch Gynecol Obstet* 2017; 296: 469–74.

[34] Soyama H, Miyamoto M, Ishibashi H, Nakatsuka M, Kawauchi H, Sakamoto T, et al. Analysis of prophylactic Bakri balloon tamponade failure in patients with placenta praevia. *Taiwanese J of Obstet Gynecol* 2019; 58; 159-63.

[35] Arakaki T, Takita AH, Oba T, Nakamura M, Sekizawa A.The routine use of prophylactic Bakri balloon tamponade contributes to blood loss control in major placenta praevia. *Inter J Gyecol Obstet* 2021; 154: 508-14.

[36] Lin B, Zhou B, Chen J, Yang J. Prophylactic application of Bakri balloon tamponade versus uterine gauze packing during caesarean section in patients with placenta praevia. *J Int Med Res* 2020; 48: 300060520910049.

[37] Hasegawa J, Matsuoka R, Ichizuka K, Mimura A, Sekizawa A, Farina A, Okai T. Predisposing factors for massive hemorrhage during Caesarean section in patients with placenta praevia. *Ultrasound Obstet Gynecol* 2009; 34: 80–4.

[38] Yoon SY, You JY, Choi SJ, Oh SY, Kim JH, Roh CR. A combined ultrasound and clinical scoring model for the prediction of peripartum complications in pregnancies complicated by placenta praevia. *Eur J Obstet Gynecol Reprod Biol* 2014; 180: 111-5.

[39] Kong CW, To WWK. Risk factors for severe postpartum haemorrhage during caesarean section for placenta praevia. *J Obstet Gynaecol* 2020; 40: 479-84.

Chapter 7

Tubal and Non-Tubal Ectopic Pregnancy: COVID-19 Pandemic Implications

Cristina de Miguel López[1,*], MD
Enrique Achiaga Sánchez[1], MD
María Teresa Gómez García[2,3], PhD
Lidia Gómez Muñoz[1], Gema Serrano García[1]
and Antonio Nicolás Amezcua Recover[2,3], PhD
[1]Obstetrics and Gynecology Department,
University and Hospital Complex of Albacete, Spain.
[2]Obstetrics and Gynecology Department of the University and Hospital Complex of Albacete, Spain
[3]Medical Science Department, School of Medicine of Albacete,
Universidad de Castilla-La Mancha, Spain

Abstract

Ectopic pregnancy is defined as an incorrect implantation of pregnancy implanted at a place other than the endometrial line of the uterine body mostly the fallopian tube (96%). In these days, EP remains the leading cause of early pregnancy related death. Diagnosis of this condition is usually made via transvaginal ultrasound. Serial serum beta-human chorionic gonadotrophin (β-hCG) measurement may help to differentiate normal from abnormal pregnancies and rise suspicion of an ectopic pregnancy. In earlier years, ectopic pregnancy was treated only by radical

* Corresponding Author's E-mail: cdmiguel@sescam.jccm.es.

In: A Closer Look at Pregnancy and Childbirth
Editor: Louise J. Salgado
ISBN: 978-1-68507-658-0

surgery, and a broad therapeutic armamentarium only became available in the late 20th century. This led directly to advances in diagnostic methods, specifically the advent of new techniques that allow uncomplicated ectopic pregnancy to be readily diagnosed with a high sensitivity and specificity.

At the beginning of the COVID-19 pandemic, questions concerning the best surgical approach for the treatment of an ectopic pregnancy aroused. During the first months, some international societies priorized open surgery to laparoscopy (LPS) because of the unknown effects of using pneumoperitoneum in an infected patient. Little was known, about the best surgical option in cases of EP. Nowadays, there is no scientific evidence supporting viral transmission through aerosol particles during LPS surgery. LPS indications remain unchanged. However, some authors recommend additional safety measures such as smoke evacuation or minimizing energy device.

We provide a detailed analysis of the various therapeutic options available for ectopic tubal and non-tubal pregnancy, and their indications, contraindications and special considerations during COVID-19 pandemic and patients affected with this disease.

In this chapter, our aim is to collect the latest evidence on treatment for tubal EP, focusing on the impact that drugs, expectant management and surgical techniques used for this purpose may have on contagion, morbidity and secondary effects derived from SARS-CoV-2.

Keywords: tubal ectopic pregnancy, COVID-19, methotrexate, laparoscopy, open surgery

Introduction

Ectopic pregnancy is defined as gestational sac implantation outside the uterine cavity and is estimated to account for 1.5% to 2% of all pregnancies (Chang et al. 2003). Tubal ectopic pregnancy is the most common of all blastocyst implantation disorders: at least 90% of all ectopic pregnancies occur in the fallopian tube, and 80% implant in the ampullary portion of the fallopian tube (Wong and Clark 1968). The condition has become more common in recent decades, mainly due to assisted-reproduction techniques (ART), although this rise has fortunately not been accompanied by higher rates of mortality or severe morbidity. Early diagnosis before fallopian tube rupture and greater treatment efficacy have lowered mortality (Chang et al. 2003), although tubal ectopic pregnancy still accounts for 4% of maternal deaths in the U.S. in the early 21st century (Noell et al. 2012).

The current therapeutic armamentarium includes expectant management of tubal ectopic pregnancy, medical treatment with methotrexate (MTX) at different doses and via different routes of administration, conservative surgery (salpingostomy), radical surgery (salpingectomy), and new medical strategies (mifepristone, gefitinib).

The spread of severe acute respiratory syndrome coronavirus (SARS-CoV-2) virus, also known as COVID-19, in December 2019, led the world to a pandemic of unprecedented dimensions. Reorganization of health care systems to protect patients and health care workers, the change in how and when population sought medical assistance as well as the implementation of strict lockdowns or social distancing altered how thousands of diseases have been handled. Ectopic pregnancy is no exception. In the upcoming chapter, we will review current literature about the effects, new insights, and recommendations on managing tubal and non-tubal ectopic pregnancy. Last but not least, the latest evidence regarding the different therapeutic options including surgical and medical treatment before and after the outbreak of the COVID-19 pandemic will be analysed.

COVID-19 Pandemic Implications

The first outbreak of COVID-19 started during December 2019 in a local market in the city of Wuhan, central-east China. Rapidly the spreading of the desease occurred and on March 11, 2020, the World Health Organization (WHO) classified COVID-19 outbreak as a pandemic. Fot the first time during 21st century, the WHO recommended strict restrictions worldwide regarding most aspects of our life including work, social, leisure time, and health care access. The clinical and pathological features of this infection have been extensively published, with a wide spectrum of disease seen, from asymptomatic infection, mild self-limiting symptoms to acute respiratory failure requiring invasive mechanical ventilation. The most common clinical findings are fever, cough and fatigue with some laboratory findings such as increased D dimers, serum ferritin, and C reactive protein (CRP). SARS-CoV-2 can spread through both direct means (droplet and human-to-human transmission) and by indirect contact (contaminated objects and airborne contagion). Person-to-person spread of SARS-CoV-2 is supposed to occur mainly via respiratory droplets, when a patient coughs, sneezes, or even talks or sings (Lotfi, Hamblin, and Rezaei 2020). Older age, obesity, inmunosuppresion and medical comorbidities increase the risk of developing a severe illness. Mortality rates around the world vary, secondary to their restriction measures, quarantines adheration rates, health care system's capacity, individual protection material availability and vaccination rates, among others. To date, United States of America, India are Brazil remain the countries were more confirmed deaths because of COVID-19 have been reported.

Depending on transmission levels, different stages of restrictions were followed by governments attempting to contain the rate of infections. At the beginning, some countries encouraged to limit social contacts whereas others implemented strict lockdowns to decrease virus spread. Fear of exposure to patients with COVID-19 led individuals to defer care for acute diseases. As a result, emergency department (ED) non-COVID-19 emergent conditions such as ischemic strokes, myocardial infarctions, appendicitis, nontraumatic subarachnoid haemorrhage and oncological complications declined dramatically, having a great impact in their mortality and morbidity that is still not yet fully quantified (Asokan, Rabadia, and Yang 2020; Zhao et al. 2020; De Rosa et al. 2020; Bhambhvani et al. 2021). Obstetrics-Gynaecology (OB-GYN) population was not an exception and so Spurlin et al. show in a retrospective study at a New York City Hospital, USA, reporting a 60% decrease of ED consults during the pandemic (Spurlin et al. 2020). Similar observations were reported in Haifa, Israel, but in lower proportions, reporting a 34,7% decrease in GYN triage and a 36,4% in OB population (Justman et al. 2020).

As previously mentioned in this chapter, a ruptured ectopic pregnancy is one of the most common GYN emergencies and accounts for 10% of all pregnancy related deaths (Ankum et al. 1996). Concerning ectopic pregnancy, pandemic-related modifications in access to health care centers revealed a change in clinical presentations and consequently in their treatment. Early diagnosis decreased dramatically, since patients suffering from mild symptoms such as light bleeding or mild abdominal pain hesitated to seek medical assistance due to fear of being exposed to the virus or to collapse hospitals by visiting them. Werner et al. reported during the height peak of incidence in New York City, between March 15th and May 17th, 2020, the same number (12) of ectopic pregnancies treated surgically as in the previous entire year (Werner and Katz 2021). 83% (10) of these cases were haemodynamically unstable, all of them only knowing they had a positive pregnancy test at home and being unaware of their diagnosis. Casadio et al. reported a higher proportion of ruptured EP during lockdown in comparison with pre-lockdown period in Italy (6/9; 66.7% vs. 52/201; 25.9%, Fisher's Exact Test P = 0.02) (Casadio et al. 2020). Similar results were reported in Israel (Dvash et al. 2021), even if the transmission rates and deaths due to COVID-19 were lower than in Italy. A significant difference was observed between the percentage of ruptured tubal ectopic pregnancy during the pandemic and in the previous years (58% vs. 17%, $P < 0.005$).

A very recent, multicenter observational, prospective study conducted in the UK threw out contrary results to the articles previously mentioned (Platts et al. 2021). It is to date, the largest study of these characteristics. The cohort consisted of two groups. The first one, included 162 ectopic pregnancy-diagnosed patients in the COVID-19 period and the second one, 179 in the paired pre COVID-19 period. A lower percentage of women presented haemodynamic instability and underwent surgical management in the first group compared to the second group (58.6% [95/162] vs. 72.6% [130/179]; P = 0.007). There was no difference in the 30-day complication rates between both groups.

The overload of health care systems, the need to expand their capacity to provide critical care and the desire to protect patients and health care workers from COVID-19 infection, forced hospital leaders to cancel all or almost all elective and non-urgent procedures when possible. Despite the attempt to limit surgeries, urgent and oncological procedures need to be performed when necessary, taking special caution measures that will be discussed further on in this chapter. Consequently, surgery distribution in GYN patients changed. Urgent surgeries, such as for ectopic pregnancy, went from a rate of 5,7% of all surgeries in the pre-COVID-19 era to a value of 18,8% during the COVID-19 era (Spurlin et al. 2020).

After a period of uncertainty, the RCOG (RCOG, Early Pregnancy 2020) issued a guideline for rationalizing early pregnancy services during the pandemic, which included ectopic pregnancy management recommendations. They emphasized the need of conservative management when possible and the need of a multidisciplinary team discussion in case of attending a severely unwell women with COVID-19 and ectopic pregnancy. The International Society of Ultrasound in Obstetrics and Gynaecology (ISUOG) (Bourne et al. 2020) also released a consensus statement on rationalization of early-pregnancy with similar recommendations to those of the RCOG.

During this pandemic, where sanitary resources remain scarce and only emergent or urgent surgical procedures should be held, if no contraindications are found, expectant or medical treatment of ectopic pregnancy are strongly recommended, whereas surgical treatment needs to be minimized. Numerous authors summarized their own experiences, re-organisation schemes and measures implemented to maintain GYN services during the pandemic (Alsharaydeh et al. 2020; Chiofalo et al. 2020; Rosa-E-Silva et al. 2020). All of them concluded that, even though health care centers and sanitary staff were hardly hit by this pandemic, the assistance given to patients diagnosed with ectopic pregnancy and their outcome slightly changed during and after the virus outbreak.

In the last section of this chapter, the following aspects will be discussed: the evidence available about each therapeutic approach of ectopic pregnancy during and after COVID 19 pandemic, changes in the management of this disease, and implications of the pandemic in diagnosing and treating ectopic pregnancy.

Expectant Management

As recommended by RCOG, follow-up protocols should be individualized. In order to minimize hospital attendance, β-hCG monitoring should be performed on a weekly basis. It therefore seems reasonable to use telemedicine to avoid hospital visits, when the patient's symptoms remain stable and β-hCG levels decrease as expected. As reported by Platts et al., there was a non-significant trend of less women managed by expectant management versus medical management comparing both cohorts, COVID-19 era with the non-COVID-19 era (57.1% [28/49] versus 73.1% [49/67]; $P = 0.0778$). As the authors discuss, clinitians may have tried to decrease the chances of failed expectant management's cases. Among those patients handled with expectant management, the COVID-19 cohort had a significantly lower median number of hospital visits compared to the pre-COVID cohort (3.0 [3, 5] versus 9.0 [5, 14], $P = <0.001$) (Platts et al. 2021). No difference in complications rates were reported.

A retrospective descriptive analysis of women diagnosed with an EP in London during 2019-2020, showed that there was a significant difference when comparing conservative and surgical intentions to treat, with 11% more planned conservative management and 13% less surgical treatment in 2020 compared with 2019 ($p=0.049$). However, the type of final EP management was similar, noting that there were more failed expectant management in the 2020 group (Kyriacou et al. 2021).

Medical Treatment

Metothrexate

As with many other drugs used in our daily practice, levels of worry started to grow around the safety of MTX used in patients in contact, infected or post infected with COVID-19 (Elito Júnior and Araujo Júnior 2020). As explained previously, MTX acts by destroying any rapidly dividing cells non-specifically. Cumulative doses of MTX can produce immunodeficiency since bone marrow cells may be affected. Doses of MTX used to treat ectopic pregnancy (either single 50mg/kg2 im, double or multiple) differ from doses used to reach anti-inflammatory and immunosuppressive response in disorders such as psoriasis, rheumatoid arthritis and other autoimmune diseases. Dermatologists reviewed the safety of systemic use of MTX in their daily practice, for example atopic dermatitis (Marko and Pawliczak 2021). As stated, they do not recommend discontinuation of MTX in non-infected patients but suggest discontinuation in cases of an active COVID-19 infection until clinical recovery. In addition to this minimal but existing immunosuppressive effect of MTX in ectopic pregnancy, COVID-19 infection typically produces leukopenia, which may worsen morbidity and mortality in infected patients. Although uncommon, another known adverse effect of MTX is a hypersensitivity-type pneumonitis, that may worsen previous or currently positive COVID-19 patient's symptoms.

The RCOG practice guideline (Bourne et al. 2020) states that the dose of MTX given for medical management of ectopic pregnancy is unlikely to increase vulnerability to COVID-19. Benefits include avoidance of hospital admission, high likelihood of resolution, and low probability of ending in surgery. On the other hand, as already mentioned, theoretical risk of immunosuppression needs to be discussed with the patient. Science evolves rapidly in these times, so it is feasible that in few months MTX could be used to prevent virus replication. A very recent study (Stegmann et al. 2021), raises the possibility that MTX diminishes the synthesis of the SARS-CoV-2 virus as observed in a cultured cell experiment. Until more conclusive studies are published, previous recommendations should be followed.

Usual criteria of MTX indication remain unchanged during this pandemic. Special care must be taken when evaluating an infected or previously infected COVID-19 patient. Some of the common complications that COVID-19 disease patients develop are absolute contraindications of MTX use (immunodeficiency, lymphopenia, pulmonary, renal, and hepatic dysfunction). In these situations, avoiding the use of MTX may seem reasonable.

Following RCOG issues, Platts et al. described a significant increase of non-surgical methods used for ectopic pregnancy during the pandemic (Platts et al. 2021). Examining this subgroup, a greater number of patients underwent medical management versus expectant management in the COVID-19 cohort compared with the pre-COVID-19 cohort (OR 3.46 [95% CI 1.29–9.24] P = 0.01). As authors discuss, clinicians may have tried to avoid failed expectant management. They also described a significantly lower median number of hospital visits among patients managed with MTX, comparing the COVID-19 cohort and the pre-COVID 19 cohort (6.0 [5, 8] vs. 9.0 [6, 10], P = 0.003). No different complication rates were detected in any of the two groups.

In September 2021, the first case report of a patient with an ectopic pregnancy and concomitant COVID-19 disease successfully treated with MTX was published. This patient had several comorbidities such as morbid obesity, asthma and chronic hypertension which worsened her COVID-19 symptoms. A multidisciplinary treatment planning is encouraged, and every change of patient status should previously be taken into account. In this clinical scenario, a tubal ectopic pregnancy was diagnosed and medical management of EP with a double dose MTX protocol was initiated. BHCG value pre-treatment was 4166,7 mIU/mL. The patient improved clinically and was discharged with low levels of BHCG by day 10. It is interesting, how the authors precluded surgical treatment due to increased risks of this option. On the other hand, given that BHCG serum levels were high and tubal rupture was likely, expectant management was also excluded (Millan et al. 2021).

Further case reports are needed, since detrimental pulmonary and inmunosuppresion effects secondary to MTX administration may be fatal in critically ill COVID-19 patients.

Mifepristone

Mifepristone selectively binds to endogenous progesterone receptors and competes with the hormone. Consequently, it destroys trophoblastic and decidual tissue, lowers luteinizing hormone levels, and blocks the corpora lutea, leading to embryo necrosis and abortion. In the case of ectopic pregnancy, trophoblastic tissue and a decidual reaction are present as well, but outside the uterus. This is why mifepristone has been proposed many times as an option in medical treatment of EP (Moore and Ariana 2014).

In our search for COVID-19 pandemic implications on the effects or uses of this drug, we were not able to find any. In response to the pandemic, Gambir et al. released a systematic review and meta-analysis that compared home-based and clinic-based administration of medical abortion in having a successful abortion. It included 3 RCTs and 16 non-randomized studies (NRS) with 11 576 women seeking abortion up to 9 weeks gestation. Neither the RCTs nor the NRS found any difference between home-based and clinic-based administration of medical abortion in having a successful abortion (RR 0.99, 95% CI 0.98 to 1.01, I2 = 0%; RR 0.99, 95% CI 0.97 to 1.01, I2 = 52%, respectively) (Gambir et al. 2020). This might reinforce the fact that the use of mifepristone as part of medical approach of EP does not increase the risk of SARS-COV-2 contagion as it can be conceived as a home-based treatment. What is more, some authors have explored and proposed the option of sending mifepristone through mail, in order to prevent the patients from contagion at medical centers (Moore and Ariana 2014).

We found no studies that analysed the use of mifepristone in patients with an active COVID-19 infection or patients that recovered from it. Given that mifepristone selectively attaches to progesterone receptors, we speculate that no secondary effects or worsening of COVID -19 symptoms are to be expected when using this drug in a positive patient. Likewise, we do not expect a decrease in the success rate of medical treatment of ectopic pregnancy. In conclusion, we believe mifepristone is a safe option and indications to use this pharmacologic agent should remain unchanged.

Other Pharmacologic Strategies

As seen in a previous chapter, *Tubal ectopic pregnancy: treatment update*, gefitinib would be indicated in hemodynamically stable patients with active ectopic pregnancies when the fallopian tube is not yet ruptured but the risk is high. This drug blocks EGF (epidermal growth factor) inducing cell death of ectopic trophoblastic tissue. Its main indication for use is as first-line treatment of patients with metastatic non-small cell lung cancer whose tumors have EGF receptors. As this indication is quite specific and nowadays gefitinib is rarely used in EP, no current studies have been published using gefitinib in COVID-19 patients. Theoretically, its mechanism of action should not interfere with COVID-19 pathogenic pathways.

Surgical Treatment

At the beginning of the COVID-19 pandemic, little was known about added perioperative morbidity and mortality and transmission rates in the surgery room when patients infected by COVID-19 were operated. Rapidly, significantly higher surgical complications (OR, 4.98; 95% CI, 1.81-16.07) and mortality (OR, 9.5; 95% CI, 1.77-96.53) were observed in a matched cohort study during a spike of the COVID-19 pandemic in Italy (Doglietto et al. 2020). Two main recommendations may arise from this article. First, health providers should contemplate these mentioned consequences at the moment of indicating a surgery. Regarding ectopic pregnancy urgent indications, such as haemodynamic instability, little controversy exists as they are life-threatening conditions that require surgical treatment. Secondly, multidisciplinary care should be taken if a woman with current or past COVID-19 infection is to be operated since intra and/or postoperative complications may arise. Therefore, preoperative COVID-19 testing with PCR is encouraged as well as checking clinical history of previous infection. It is not acceptable to delay urgent care until a PCR result is received, so universal precautions with use of PPE and patient isolation should be triggered in these cases. In August 2020, the American College of Surgeons, American Society of Anaesthesiologists and many other medical and nurse societies (American College of Surgeons 2020; Wright and Advincula 2020) developed a list of considerations to guide health care providers in need of essential surgery services. Some of the most important aspects are listed below.

Universal Precautions

- Careful and well stablished indication of surgical treatment
- Use of personal protective equipment (PPE) including N-95 respirator, eye protection, gloves, shoe covers, and gowns
- Preoperative COVID-19 testing, when possible
- Avoid presence of nonessential staff during surgery (especially during intubation and extubation)
- Multidisciplinary care (pre and postoperative)
- Special attention and re-evaluation in previously infected COVID-19 patients

As the risk of COVID – 19 infections dropped secondary to vaccination rates, inmunization, use of masks and self isolation, non-life threatening gynecologic diseases that required surgical treatment started to take place in hospitals. Still, ordering of severe conditions is needed, since surgery during a pandemic increases rate of morbimortality. The Society of Gynecologic

Surgeons (SGS) adapted a ranking list of gynecologic procedures made by the American College of Surgeons (ACS) to help health care providers decide who should undergo an operation. The most commonly performed gynecologic procedures including general gynecology, urogynecology and reproductive medicine are included, as well as the suggested location (outpatient, ambulatory surgery centers or hospital). The recommendation for scheduling patients should primarily be determined by the surgeon managing the patient. Secondary to this, a shared decision process between the surgeon and the patient should follow. Figure 1 shows a tiered system ranging from 1, "low acuity surgery/healthy patient" to 4, "emergent surgery". Concerning EP, as previously explained, the latter group includes a ruptured EP with haemodynamic instability. Since this classification does not mention other clinical spectrum EP, a discussion about their location in this ranking will be made. An asymptomatic EP with contraindications of medical treatment such as desire of early pregnancy, previous ipsilateral EP or high BHCG levels may belong to group 3. We believe this type of EP is similar to "Adnexal mass, complex, suspicious for torsion", as consequences of delaying surgery have a high potential for near future morbidity and mortality.

Updating this kind of rankings is necessary, based on the pandemic development taking special attention to surgical and nursing team availability, the incidence of oncological and life-threatening conditions, COVID-19 testing, personal protective equipment disposal and other local resource considerations.

Minimally Invasive Surgery

At the very beginning of the pandemic, April 2020, Pavan et al. reviewed the presence of virus such as Hepatitis B and Human Papiloma in the surgical smoke during laparoscopic surgeries (Pavan et al. 2020). Aerosol generating procedures such as minimaly invasive surgery may result in the aerosolization of viruses that are otherwise spread by droplets. Although these viruses studied by Pavan et al. were very different from the SARS-CoV-2 virus, concern regarding safety during laparoscopy procedures rapidly rose. As explained in an article by Chinese and Italian practitioners (Zheng, Boni, and Fingerhut 2020) leakage of artificial pneumoperitoneum as well as smoke and plume caused after burning or coagulating tissue, could generate aerosol exposure of the virus that might easily affect the operation team.

Therefore, surgical societies published guidelines, statements, and recommendations, not only to stop elective surgery but also to favor laparotomy over laparoscopy. In turn, Minimally Invasive Surgery societies including the European Society for Gynaecologycal Endoscopy (ESGE Recommendations, 2020) and the American Association of Gynecologic Laparoscopists challenged previous recommendations and issued practical recommendations to increase safety in the operating room. Some of these caution measures are hereby listed:

Tier	Definition	Gynecology Examples	Urogynecology Examples	Reproductive Examples	Suggested Location
Tier 1a	**Low acuity surgery/healthy patient** Not life-threatening illness	- Benign appearing adnexal mass, asymptomatic - Hysterectomy, without anemia, stable symptoms - Myomectomy, asymptomatic - Hysteroscopic metroplasty - Endometriosis, stable symptoms -Chronic pelvic pain requiring diagnosis (i.e. diagnostic laparoscopy) -AUB, without anemia, low suspicion malignancy -Bleeding requiring diagnosis (i.e. diagnostic/operative hysteroscopy) -Persistent PMB, low suspicion (neg EMB) -	-Stress urinary incontinence surgery -Surgery for symptomatic prolapse in patients without other significant sequelae. -Asymptomatic mesh exposure - Neuromodulation for urinary urgency incontinence, retention or fecal incontinence - Diverticulectomy	- Benign ovarian cyst aspiration	Outpatient ASC, or Hospital
Tier 1b*	**Low acuity surgery/unhealthy patient based on ASA or Charlson comorbidity index**				ASC or hospital
Tier 2a	**Intermediate acuity** surgery/healthy patient Not life threatening but potential for near future morbidity or mortality Significant impairment of QoL	-AUB with secondary anemia, stable -AUB age > 50y with inability to sample in office -Endometriosis, poorly controlled pain or fertility desired, low AMH/ovarian reserve -Endometrial polyps age > 50y - Symptomatic ovarian cyst - Myomectomy, symptomatic fibroid	-Fistula repair -Mesh-related complication (infection or severe pain) -Surgery for advanced prolapse in patients with significant sequelae (urinary retention, recurrent UTI, pain, etc)	- Missed abortion < 12 weeks	Outpatient or overnight hospitalization ASC or Hospital
Tier 2b*	**Intermediate acuity surgery/unhealthy patient**				ASC or hospital

Figure 1. (Continued)

Tier 3a	**High acuity surgery/healthy patient** High potential for near future morbidity or mortality Severe impairment of QoL	-Endometrial hyperplasia/EIN, highly suspicious for atypia/malignancy -Adnexal mass, complex, suspicious for torsion, malignancy -AUB, secondary anemia, unstable, worsening bleeding -Deeply infiltrating endometriosis with severe bowel/bladder symptoms, intractable/severe pain - CIN II, CIN III treatment -Symptomatic ovarian cyst, intractable, severe pain - Large fibroids, with hydronephrosis, debilitating pain, bulk symptoms or urinary retention -Other potential GYN malignancy cases -Sterilization procedures for women who are not LARC candidates	- Mesh in a viscus - Advanced stage prolapse with evidence of upper tract obstruction and unable to retain pessary - Obstructed voiding after MUS -incarcerated prolapse	-Myomectomy (for infertility) - Hysteroscopic metroplasty (for infertility) - -Transvaginal oocyte Aspiration in infertile woman; -Embryo transfer -Ovarian cyst that is affecting ability to do egg retrieval -Myomectomy, asymptomatic but affecting uterine cavity in infertile woman or affecting ability to monitor and perform egg retrieval -Hysteroscopic polypectomy/myomectomy infertility	Outpatient hospital with pathologist available ASC rare but possible
Tier 3b*	**High acuity surgery/unhealthy patient**				Hospital in-patient
Tier 4a	**Emergency Surgery/healthy patient**	-Ruptured ectopic with hemodynamic instability -Hemorrhage from SAB, incomplete -Ruptured TOA -Ovarian torsion -Perforated viscus or complete bowel obstruction -Delayed postoperative hemorrhage -Termination of pregnancy (6) -Wound dehiscence		-Prolapsing fibroid - Hematocolpos/Hematometra -Hemorrhage post-egg retrieval	ASC or Hospital

***Tier "b"** indicates patients with complicated medical conditions that, in the environment of COVID-19, may place them at high risk for ICU admission and increased perioperative morbidity and mortality. This will likely affect the order of prioritization of individuals for surgery.

AMH: anti-mullerian hormone; ASC: ambulatory surgery center; AUB: abnormal uterine bleeding; CPP Chronic pelvic pain; EIN: endometrial intra-epithelial neoplasm; LARC: long-acting reversible contraception; MUS: mid-urethral sling; SIS: saline infusion sonography; SAB: spontaneous abortion; TOA: tubo-ovarian abscess; TVUS: transvaginal ultrasonography; PMB: postmenopausal bleeding; UDS: urodynamics; EMB: Endometrial biopsy; UTI: urinary tract infection

Figure 1. Modified Elective Surgery Acuity Scale (mESAS) for Benign Gynecologic Indications and Surgeries. Taken from Joint Statement on Re-introduction of Hospital and Office-based Procedures in the COVID-19 Climate for the Practicing Gynecologist. SGS.

- Reduce surgery time
- Reduce leakage of carbon dioxide from any trocars (check seals or use
- disposable trocars)
- Minimize use of electrosurgery devices
- Reduce production of plume aerosol, and blood/fluid droplet spray or spread.
- Employ a smoke evacuation/filtration system with ultralow particulate air (ULPA) filter capability
- Avoid rapid desufflation or loss of pneumoperitoneum during instrument exchange or specimen extraction
- Use low intra-abdominal pressure (10-12 mmHg) without compromising visualization

With the ongoing of the pandemic, evidence showed contradictory results regarding this matter. In May 2020, Flemming et al., performed ascites, bile, liver gall bladder, as well as tracheal secretion PCR samples during an emergency cholecystectomy in a critically ill COVID-19 positive patient (Flemming et al. 2020). They observed negative SARS-CoV-2-RNA results in all abdominal samples but strongly positive results in the tracheal secretion, suggesting that the potential infectious risk for operating staff during surgery was lower than expected. On the other hand, a group of Italian authors reported SARS-CoV-2-RNA peritoneal fluid detection at a higher concentration than in the respiratory tract in a positive patient with bowel obstruction (Coccolini et al. 2020). A prospective study in a GYN oncology referral center in Italy was developed, in which they tested SARS-CoV-2 from 17 patients undergoing laparoscopy procedures in the endotracheal tube and the filter applied on the trocar valve (Bogani et al. 2020). All patients were previously screened with anamnestic data and CT scan of thorax, followed by RT-PCR nasopharyngeal swab whenever previous triage was positive. In 1 patient, RT-PCR analysis was positive in both swab tests showing a potential new method of transmission of COVID-19. A systematic review of case reports and multiple series of other cases, including 29 COVID-19 positive patients (Cheruiyot et al. 2021), concluded that current evidence does not support the hypothesis that SARS-COV2-2 could be aerosolized and transmitted through surgical smoke. However, as low-quality evidence is being discussed, it seems reasonable that practical measures to mitigate any theoretical risk should still be maintained until high quality evidence is available.

Platts et al. described a significantly lower percentage of women undergoing surgical management of ectopic pregnancy in the COVID-19 cohort versus non-COVID-19 cohort (58.6% [95/162] versus 72.6% [130/179]; P = 0.007). There were similar proportions of cases in each group documented as ruptured ectopic pregnancy and haemodynamically unstable (COVID-19 cohort 5/162 [3.1%] versus non-COVID-19 cohort 6/179 [3.4%], P = 1.000). There were no differerences in the median length of hospital stay, median volume of haemoperitoneum and number of surgical cases with haemoperitoneum greater than or equal to 500 ml. In light of these results, the main hypothesis of this study was rejected, as women with an ectopic pregnancy did not present with more complications during COVID-19 pandemic. (Platts et al. 2021)

Open Surgery. Laparotomic Approach

Early discussion in April 2020 about the safety of laparoscopic versus laparotomic procedures ended up with the conclusion that, when safety recommendations are followed, laparoscopy appears not to increase transmission rates in the operating room. It is true that theoretically, pneumoperitoneum in the abdominal cavity may be concentrated and if viral particles do exist, they could mean a high infectious transmitting via. On the other hand, filters may play an important role in this matter, as high percentage of this pneumoperitoneum is not released to the operating room. Whereas in laparotomy, even if there is no pneumoperitoneum, surgical smoke is freely released. In cases of EP that require laparotomy, it is basically unfeasible not to use electrocoagulation, since the risk of bleeding is high. Surgical team is then advised to use PPE (protective personal equipment).

Laparotomy should only be indicated in cases where no other medical/surgical approaches are safe, or surgeon's skills demand this option. Laparotomy has the disadvantage of increased hospital stay, higher morbidity, need for analgesia and slower recovery compared to laparoscopy. These disadvantages should be carefully taken into account, specially in countries where human and medical resources are scarce. Platts et al. proved no increase in the laparotomy rate for women who underwent surgical management (2.3% COVID-19 cohort versus 2.4% pre-COVID 19 cohort) (Platts et al. 2021).

Uterine Artery Embolization

Uterine artery embolization (UAE) is an effective minimally invasive treatment for the management of life-threatening gynecologic as well as obstetric hemorrhage. The technique of uterine artery embolization is basically the same as with other embolization procedures and it must be performed by a trained interventional radiologist. The main aim is to block the blood supply to a tumor or an abnormal area of tissue, such as a puerperal hemorrhagic uterous. Diagnostic angiography is initially performed. Then, the catheter is placed according to Seldinger technique (Seldinger 1953) under local anesthesia, generally lidocaine (Noel-Lamy et al. 2017). A small incision is made in the inner thigh and a thin catheter is inserted and guided into an artery near the abnormal tissue. A single dose of intravenous dexamethasone can be administered in order to reduce side effects (Kim et al. 2016). Embolization with gelfoam has proved to be an effective approach because the duration of occlusion is temporary (two to six weeks), but sufficient to reduce hemorrhage (Lipari and Badawy 2005).

According to our research, there are no studies describing the safety of UAE in patients with COVID-19. However, a similar procedure, bronchial artery embolization, has already been performed as part of the treatment of COVID-19 patients. A group of interventional radiologists in France, published a series of 25 cases of patients who presented with severe hemoptysis that were successfully treated with bronchial artery embolization (BAE) (Barral et al. 2020). Thirty-day mortality was 10% (2/21) in the non-COVID-19 group and 0% in the COVID-19 group. No complication related to BAE was reported. As no studies concerning UAE and COVID-19 safety are nowadays available, no reliable recommendations can be made. However, there is no reason to think UAE should increase the risk of SARS-COV-2 contagion or side effects. Besides, practice guidelines for the management of ectopic pregnancy have not changed their recommendations regarding UAE since the beginning of the pandemic.

References

Alsharaydeh, Ibrahim, Hasan Rawashdeh, Noura Saadeh, Basil Obeidat, & Nail Obeidat. (2020). “Challenges and Solutions for Maternity and Gynecology Services during the COVID-19 Crisis in Jordan.” *International Journal of Gynaecology and Obstetrics: The Official Organ of the International Federation of Gynaecology and Obstetrics*, *150* (2), 159–62. https://doi.org/10.1002/ijgo.13240.

American College of Surgeons. (2020). *Joint Statement: Roadmap for Maintaining Essential Surgery during COVID-19 Pandemic 1. Regional*

Cooperation Critical to Continuing to Provide Essential Surgery. August 10, 2020. https://www.facs.org/covid-19/clinical-guidance/roadmap-maintain-essential-surgery.

Ankum, W. M., Mol, B. W., Van der Veen, F. & Bossuyt, P. M. (1996). "Risk Factors for Ectopic Pregnancy: A Meta-Analysis." *Fertility and Sterility*, *65* (6), 1093–99.

Asokan, Ishan, Soniya V Rabadia. & Eric H Yang. (2020). "The COVID-19 Pandemic and Its Impact on the Cardio-Oncology Population." *Current Oncology Reports*, *22* (6), 60. https://doi.org/10.1007/s11912-020-00945-4.

Barral, Matthias, Marc Sirol, Mostafa El Hajjam, Norbert Zhang, Arthur Petit. & François H Cornelis. (2020). "Bronchial Artery Embolization Performed in COVID-19 Patients: Tolerance and Outcomes." *Cardiovascular and Interventional Radiology*. https://doi.org/10.1007/s00270-020-02621-3.

Bhambhvani, Hriday P., Adrian J Rodrigues, Jonathan S Yu, James B Carr II. & Melanie Hayden Gephart. (2021). "Hospital Volumes of 5 Medical Emergencies in the COVID-19 Pandemic in 2 US Medical Centers." *JAMA Internal Medicine*, *181* (2), 272–74. https://doi.org/10.1001/jamainternmed.2020.3982.

Bogani, Giorgio, Antonino Ditto, Loris De Cecco, Salvatore Lopez, Rocco Guerrisi, Federico Piccioni, Arianna Micali, Maria Grazia Daidone. & Francesco Raspagliesi. (2020). "Transmission of SARS-CoV-2 in Surgical Smoke during Laparoscopy: A Prospective, Proof-of-Concept Study." *Journal of Minimally Invasive Gynecology*, December, S1553-4650(20)31200-0. https://doi.org/10.1016/j.jmig.2020.12.026.

Bourne, T., Kyriacou, C., Coomarasamy, A., Al-Memar, M., Leonardi, E Kirk, M., Landolfo, C., et al. (2020). "ISUOG Consensus Statement on Rationalization of Early-Pregnancy Care and Provision of Ultrasonography in Context of SARS-CoV-2." *Ultrasound in Obstetrics & Gynecology : The Official Journal of the International Society of Ultrasound in Obstetrics and Gynecology*, *55* (6), 871–78. https://doi.org/10.1002/uog.22046.

Casadio, P., Youssef, A., Arena, A., Gamal, N., Pilu, G. & Seracchioli, R. (2020). "Increased Rate of Ruptured Ectopic Pregnancy in COVID-19 Pandemic: Analysis from the North of Italy." *Ultrasound in Obstetrics & Gynecology : The Official Journal of the International Society of Ultrasound in Obstetrics and Gynecology*. https://doi.org/10.1002/uog.22126.

Chang, Jeani, Laurie D Elam-Evans, Cynthia J Berg, Joy Herndon, Lisa Flowers, Kristi A Seed. & Carla J Syverson. (2003). "Pregnancy-Related Mortality Surveillance--United States, 1991--1999." *Morbidity and Mortality Weekly Report. Surveillance Summaries (Washington, D.C.: 2002)*, *52* (2), 1–8

Cheruiyot, Isaac, Prabjot Sehmi, Brian Ngure, Musa Misiani, Paul Karau, Beda Olabu, Brandon Michael Henry, Giuseppe Lippi, Roberto Cirocchi. & Julius

Ogeng'o. (2021). "Laparoscopic Surgery during the COVID-19 Pandemic: Detection of SARS-COV-2 in Abdominal Tissues, Fluids, and Surgical Smoke." *Langenbeck's Archives of Surgery, 406* (4), 1007–14. https://doi.org/10.1007/s00423-021-02142-8.

Chiofalo, Benito, Ermelinda Baiocco, Emanuela Mancini, Giuseppe Vocaturo, Giuseppe Cutillo, Cristina Vincenzoni, Simone Bruni, Valentina Bruno, Rosanna Mancari. & Enrico Vizza. (2020). "Practical Recommendations for Gynecologic Surgery during the COVID-19 Pandemic." *International Journal of Gynaecology and Obstetrics: The Official Organ of the International Federation of Gynaecology and Obstetrics, 150* (2), 146–50. https://doi.org/10.1002/ijgo.13248.

Coccolini, Federico, Dario Tartaglia, Adolfo Puglisi, Cesira Giordano, Mauro Pistello, Marianna Lodato. & Massimo Chiarugi. (2020). "SARS-CoV-2 Is Present in Peritoneal Fluid in COVID-19 Patients." *Annals of Surgery, 272* (3), e240–42. https://doi.org/10.1097/SLA.0000000000004030.

Doglietto, Francesco, Marika Vezzoli, Federico Gheza, Gian Luca Lussardi, Marco Domenicucci, Luca Vecchiarelli, Luca Zanin., et al. (2020). "Factors Associated With Surgical Mortality and Complications Among Patients With and Without Coronavirus Disease 2019 (COVID-19) in Italy." *JAMA Surgery, 155* (8), 691–702. https://doi.org/10.1001/jamasurg.2020.2713.

Dvash, Shira, Howard Cuckle, Noam Smorgick, Zvi Vaknin, Anna Padoa. & Ron Maymon. (2021). "Increase Rate of Ruptured Tubal Ectopic Pregnancy during the COVID-19 Pandemic." *European Journal of Obstetrics, Gynecology, and Reproductive Biology, 259* (April): 95–99. https://doi.org/10.1016/j.ejogrb.2021.01.054.

Elito Júnior, Júlio. & Edward Araujo Júnior. (2020). "Medical Treatment for Ectopic Pregnancy during the COVID-19 Pandemic." *Revista Brasileira de Ginecologia e Obstetricia : Revista Da Federacao Brasileira Das Sociedades de Ginecologia e Obstetricia*. Brazil. https://doi.org/10.1055/s-0040-1718438. [*Brazilian Journal of Gynecology and Obstetrics: Journal of the Brazilian Federation of Societies of Gynecology and Obstetrics*.]

"ESGE Recommendations for Gynaecological Endoscopic Surgery for COVID-19 Outbreak." (2020). *Facts, Views & Vision in ObGyn, 12* (1), 5.

Flemming, S., Hankir, M., Hering, I., Meybohm, P., Krone, M., Weissbrich, B., Germer, C. T. & Wiegering, A. (2020). "Abdominal Fluid Samples (Negative for SARS-CoV-2) from a Critically Unwell Patient with Respiratory COVID-19." *British Journal of Surgery, 107* (8), e259–60. https://doi.org/10.1002/bjs.11713.

Gambir, Katherine, Camille Garnsey, Kelly Ann Necastro. & Thoai D Ngo. (2020). "Effectiveness, Safety and Acceptability of Medical Abortion at Home versus in the Clinic: A Systematic Review and Meta-Analysis in

Response to COVID-19." *BMJ Global Health*, *5* (12). https://doi.org/10.1136/bmjgh-2020-003934.

Justman, Naftali, Gilad Shahak, Ola Gutzeit, Dikla Ben Zvi, Yuval Ginsberg, Ido Solt, Dana Vitner, Ron Beloosesky, Zeev Weiner. & Yaniv Zipori. (2020). "Lockdown with a Price: The Impact of the COVID-19 Pandemic on Prenatal Care and Perinatal Outcomes in a Tertiary Care Center." *The Israel Medical Association Journal : IMAJ*, 22 (9), 533–37.

Kim, S. Y., Koo, B. N., Shin, C. S.,Ban, M., Han, K. & Kim, M. D. (2016). "The Effects of Single-Dose Dexamethasone on Inflammatory Response and Pain after Uterine Artery Embolisation for Symptomatic Fibroids or Adenomyosis: A Randomised Controlled Study." *BJOG: An International Journal of Obstetrics and Gynaecology*, *123* (4), 580–87. https://doi.org/10.1111/1471-0528.13785.

Kyriacou, C., Cooper, N., Robinson, E., Parker, N., Barcroft, J., Kundu S., Letchworth, P., et al. (2021). "Ultrasound Characteristics, Serum Biochemistry and Outcomes for Ectopic Pregnancies Presenting during the SARS-CoV-2 Pandemic: Retrospective Analysis." *Ultrasound in Obstetrics & Gynecology: The Official Journal of the International Society of Ultrasound in Obstetrics and Gynecology*, October. https://doi.org/10.1002/uog.24793.

Lipari, Christopher W. & Shawky Z A Badawy. (2005). "Arteriovenous Malformation in a Bicornuate Uterus Leading to Recurrent Severe Uterine Bleeding: A Case Report." *The Journal of Reproductive Medicine*, *50* (1), 57–60.

Lotfi, Melika, Michael R Hamblin. & Nima Rezaei. (2020). "COVID-19: Transmission, Prevention, and Potential Therapeutic Opportunities." *Clinica Chimica Acta; International Journal of Clinical Chemistry*, *508* (September), 254–66. https://doi.org/10.1016/j.cca.2020.05.044.

Marko, Monika. & Rafał Pawliczak. (2021). "Can We Safely Use Systemic Treatment in Atopic Dermatitis during the COVID-19 Pandemic? Overview of Selected Conventional and Biologic Systemic Therapies." *Expert Review of Clinical Immunology*, April, 1–9. https://doi.org/10.1080/1744666X.2021.1919511.

Millan, N. M., Morano, J., Florez, L., Carugno, J. & Medina, C. A. (2021). "Management of Tubal Ectopic Pregnancy with Methotrexate in the Setting of Symptomatic Coronavirus Disease 2019 (COVID-19): A Case Report." *Facts, Views & Vision in ObGyn*, *13* (3), 277–81. https://doi.org/10.52054/FVVO.13.3.030.

Noel-Lamy, Maxime, Kong T Tan, Martin E Simons, Kenneth W Sniderman, Oleg Mironov. & Dheeraj K Rajan. (2017). "Intraarterial Lidocaine for Pain Control in Uterine Artery Embolization: A Prospective, Randomized Study."

Journal of Vascular and Interventional Radiology: JVIR, *28* (1), 16–22. https://doi.org/10.1016/j.jvir.2016.10.001.

Noell Dani, Isaac Delke, Washington C. Hill, Robert W. Yelverton, Donna L. Carden, Margaret H. Neal, Lindsay S. Womack, William M. Sappenfield, Deborah L. Burch, Leticia E. Hernandez, William M. Callaghan (2012) "Ectopic Pregnancy Mortality - Florida, 2009-2010." *MMWR. Morbidity and Mortality Weekly Report*, *61* (6), 106–9.

Pavan, Nicola, Alessandro Crestani, Alberto Abrate, Cosimo De Nunzio, Francesco Esperto, Gianluca Giannarini, Antonio Galfano., et al. (2020). "Risk of Virus Contamination Through Surgical Smoke During Minimally Invasive Surgery: A Systematic Review of the Literature on a Neglected Issue Revived in the COVID-19 Pandemic Era." *European Urology Focus*, *6* (5), 1058–69. https://doi.org/10.1016/j.euf.2020.05.021.

Platts, S., Ranawaka, J., Oliver, R., Patra-Das, S., Kotabagi, P., Neophytou, C., Shah, N., et al. (2021). "Impact of Severe Acute Respiratory Syndrome Coronavirus 2 on Ectopic Pregnancy Management in the United Kingdom: A Multicentre Observational Study." *BJOG: An International Journal of Obstetrics and Gynaecology*, May. https://doi.org/10.1111/1471-0528.16756.

Rosa-E-Silva, Julio Cesar, Paulo Ayroza Ribeiro, Luiz Gustavo Oliveira Brito, Mariano Tamura Vieira Gomes, Sergio Podgaec, Helizabet Salomão Abdalla Ayroza Ribeiro, Carlos Augusto Pires Costa Lino, Ricardo Quintairos, Walquiria Quida Salles Pereira Primo. & Agnaldo Lopes da Silva Filho. (2020). "Gynecological Surgery and COVID-19: What Is the Impact and How Should I Manage It?" *Revista Brasileira de Ginecologia e Obstetricia: Revista Da Federacao Brasileira Das Sociedades de Ginecologia e Obstetricia*, *42* (7), 415–19. https://doi.org/10.1055/s-0040-1715146.

Rosa, Salvatore De, Carmen Spaccarotella, Cristina Basso, Maria Pia Calabrò, Antonio Curcio, Pasquale Perrone Filardi, Massimo Mancone., et al. (2020). "Reduction of Hospitalizations for Myocardial Infarction in Italy in the COVID-19 Era." *European Heart Journal*, *41* (22), 2083–88. https://doi.org/10.1093/eurheartj/ehaa409.

Royal College of Obstetrician & Gynaecologist. (2020). "Guidance for Rationalising Early Pregnancy Services in the Evolving Coronavirus (COVID-19) Pandemic." *Royal College of Obstetrician & Gynaecologist*, no. May: 1–20. http://www.rcog.org.uk/globalassets/ documents/guidelines/ 2020-05-15-guidance-for-rationalising-early-pregnancy-services-in-the-evolving-coronavirus-covid-19-pandemic.pdf.

SELDINGER, S. I. (1953). "Catheter Replacement of the Needle in Percutaneous Arteriography; a New Technique." *Acta Radiologica*, *39* (5), 368–76. https://doi.org/10.3109/00016925309136722.

Spurlin, Emily E., Esther S Han, Elisabeth R Silver, Benjamin L May, Nicholas P Tatonetti, Myles A Ingram, Zhezhen Jin, Chin Hur, Arnold P Advincula. & Hye-Chun Hur. (2020). "Where Have All the Emergencies Gone? The Impact of the COVID-19 Pandemic on Obstetric and Gynecologic Procedures and Consults at a New York City Hospital." *Journal of Minimally Invasive Gynecology*, November. https://doi.org/10.1016/j.jmig.2020.11.012.

Stegmann, Kim M, Antje Dickmanns, Sabrina Gerber, Vella Nikolova, Luisa Klemke, Valentina Manzini, Denise Schlösser., et al. (2021). "The Folate Antagonist Methotrexate Diminishes Replication of the Coronavirus SARS-CoV-2 and Enhances the Antiviral Efficacy of Remdesivir in Cell Culture Models." *Virus Research*, *302* (June): 198469. https://doi.org/10.1016/j.virusres.2021.198469.

Werner, Sarah. & Adi Katz. (2021). "Change in Ectopic Pregnancy Presentations during the Covid-19 Pandemic." *International Journal of Clinical Practice*, *75* (5), e13925–e13925. https://doi.org/10.1111/ijcp.13925.

Wong, J. A. & Clark, J. F. (1968). "Correlation of Symptoms with Age and Location of Gestation in Tubal Pregnancy." *Journal of the National Medical Association*, *60* (3), 221–23.

Wright, Jason D. & Arnold P Advincula. (2020). "Gynecologic Surgical Considerations in the Era of COVID-19." *Seminars in Perinatology*, *44* (6), 151296. https://doi.org/10.1016/j.semperi.2020.151296.

Zhao, Jing, Hang Li, David Kung, Marc Fisher, Ying Shen, and Renyu Liu. (2020). "Impact of the COVID-19 Epidemic on Stroke Care and Potential Solutions." *Stroke*, *51* (7), 1996–2001. https://doi.org/10.1161/STROKEAHA.120.030225.

Zheng, Min Hua, Luigi Boni. & Abe Fingerhut. (2020). "Minimally Invasive Surgery and the Novel Coronavirus Outbreak: Lessons Learned in China and Italy." *Annals of Surgery*, *272* (1), e5–6. https://doi.org/10.1097/SLA.0000000000003924.

Chapter 8

Ectopic Pregnancy: Fertility Outcome

Enrique Achiaga Sánchez[1], MD, Cristina de Miguel López[1], MD, María Teresa Gómez García[1,2,*], PhD, José M. García Cebrián[1], MD, Sergio Rico Cardenal[1], MD, and Antonio Nicolás Amezcua Recover[1,2], PhD

[1]Department of Obstetrics and Gynecology,
Complejo Hospitalario Universitario de Albacete, Albacete, Spain
[2]School of Medicine, Universidad de Castilla La Mancha,
Albacete, Spain

Abstract

Ectopic pregnancy (EP) is defined as a pregnancy implanted at a place other than the endometrial line of the uterine body, mostly the fallopian tube (96%). However, EP can have other locations such as the ovary (3%), interstitial/cornual (2-3%), abdominal (1%), c-section scar (<1%) and cervical (<1%). These days, EP remains the leading cause of early pregnancy related death.

Choosing between expectant, medical or surgical treatment is based on clinical characteristics, medical conditions, radiologic and laboratory

* Corresponding Author's E-mail: tgomezg67@gmail.com.

In: A Closer Look at Pregnancy and Childbirth
Editor: Louise J. Salgado
ISBN: 978-1-68507-658-0

findings as well as patient-informed choice based on discussion of each approach. In this chapter, our aim is to address the impact of EP and these treatments on patients 'fertility.

Loss of fertility after an episode of tubal ectopic pregnancy (TEP) is obviously related to tubal lesions and, in some cases, tubal occlusion.

There is no clinical trial data available regarding post-treatment fertility after expectant management. However, authors have not found statistically significant differences when comparing this treatment line to others as far as subsequent intrauterine pregnancy is concerned.

As for methotrexate therapy, data suggests it does not affect fertility markers used in our daily practice, although conclusions are taken from small, observational studies. Further investigation concerning relevant fertility outcomes, like intrauterine pregnancy or live-birth rates, are needed.

When it comes to new drugs such as mifepristone, gefitinib or vinorelbine, data is extremely limited. However, only gefitinib appears to cause a significant impairment of female fertility due to its ovarian toxicity.

Surgical approach is usually addressed laparoscopically and it can be conservative (salpingotomy) or radical (salpingectomy). There is a meta-analysis which concludes there is no reason to believe salpingectomy harms fertility, although we should be cautious with the results.

There are two RCTs showing no difference in the outcomes between salpingectomy and salpingostomy for subsequent intrauterine pregnancy, while there are sixteen cohort studies which indicate that salpingectomy is approximately 50% less likely to result in a subsequent intrauterine pregnancy than it is with salpingostomy. However, surgical management should be individualized in each case.

Non-tubal ectopic pregnancy (NTEP) is a heterogeneous set of clinical presentations, so singling every case out will be crucial. This means it is very hard to determine an overall impact of treatment on our patients 'fertility.

Keywords: ectopic pregnancy, treatment, outcome, fertility

Introduction

Ectopic pregnancy (EP) is defined as a pregnancy implanted at a place other than the endometrial line of the uterine body. It occurs in the fallopian tube the vast majority of times -around 96%-, which is known as tubal ectopic pregnancy (TEP), but there are other places where the blastocyst can become implanted and this is known as non-tubal ectopic pregnancy (NTEP) [1].

The condition has become more common in recent decades, mainly due to assisted-reproduction techniques (ART), although this rise has fortunately not been accompanied by higher rates of mortality or severe morbidity [2]. Early diagnosis before fallopian tube rupture and greater treatment efficacy have lowered mortality [3], although tubal ectopic pregnancy still accounts for 4% of maternal deaths in the United States of America in the early 21st century [4].

The current therapeutic armamentarium includes expectant management of TEP, medical treatment with methotrexate (MTX) at different doses and via different routes of administration, conservative surgery (salpingostomy), radical surgery (salpingectomy), and new medical strategies (mifepristone, gefitinib, vinolerbine). All these are discussed in the chapter TUBAL ECTOPIC PREGNANCY: TREATMENT UPDATE. On the other hand, NTEP treatment depends on the location of the pregnancy and it will be necessary to individualize each case and approach, as it is detailed in the chapter NON-TUBAL ECTOPIC PREGNANCY: TREATMENT UPDATE.

As there are different treatment routes concerning EP, in this chapter our aim is to review the literature on fertility outcome after an episode of EP.

Expectant Management

Expectant management (EM) is a safe, acceptable, and effective treatment option of TEP in cases of very less active ectopic pregnancies that can be defined using the following criteria [5]:

- Clinical stability with no or minimal abdominal pain,
- No evidence of significant hemoperitoneum on ultrasound scan,
- Ectopic pregnancy measuring <30 mm in mean diameter with no evidence of embryonic cardiac activity,
- Serum β-human chorionic gonadotropin (β-hCG) > 1500 IU/L, and
- Patient consent

Regarding expectant management and the issue of tubal patency and subsequent fertility, the 2007 Cochrane Database System Review [6] showed that there was no clinical trial data at the time. Tubal patency is defined as the passage of contrast material through the ipsilateral fallopian tube in hysterosalpingography or tubal chromopertubation in laparoscopy. Future fertility will depend on whether spontaneous intrauterine pregnancy is achieved in patients who wish to have offspring.

In 2007, Burster and Krotz analyzed the data from previous studies to assess the impact of ectopic pregnancy treatment (laparoscopic salpingostomy, multiple-dose MTX, single-dose MTX, and expectant management) on subsequent fertility. They found no significant differences in reproductive results according to the treatment chosen. Among the 15 studies with expectant management, 76% (60/79) of patients showed tubal patency in hysterosalpingography. A total of 57% (388/681) of patients subsequently achieved intrauterine pregnancy, and 13% (90/681) experienced another ectopic pregnancy [7]. Shortly afterwards, Helmy et al. (2007) described a study that is the largest to date and included 444 patients (296 with salpingectomy; 134 with expectant management). Follow-up was possible in 173 (114 in the salpingectomy group; 59 in the expectant management group), and patients not desiring pregnancy were excluded. Spontaneous intrauterine pregnancy occurred in 41/49 (83.7%; 95% CI, 73.3%-94.2%) of patients managed expectantly and 62/97 (63.9%; 95% CI, 54.4-73.5%) in patients who underwent surgery (OR, 2.89; 95% CI, 1.22%-6.86%). There were no differences between the two groups in terms of the risk of a new ectopic pregnancy. These data showed that post-ectopic pregnancy fertility is similar between patients managed expectantly and patients treated by salpingectomy. However, the authors stated that the data should be interpreted with caution because the study was not a randomized trial [8].

Demirdag et al. (2017) compared the impact on reproductive outcomes of 3 different treatment options (expectant management, systemic MTX and surgical treatment, either salpingectomy or salpingostomy) in a retrospective study of 151 patients diagnosed with tubal ectopic pregnancy. After excluding 39 patients due to contraceptive use following initial treatment and extra tubal localization of pregnancy, 112 were followed-up between 24 to 72 months. 62.5% of all patients were pregnant after their initial diagnosis. There was no statistically significant difference in intrauterine pregnancy rates after ectopic pregnancy regarding treatment groups (expectant group 62,9%, MTX group 58,4%, surgery group 68,7%; $p = 0.867$). As no difference in terms of pregnancy rate outcome was seen, the authors concluded that choosing the less invasive and expensive treatment modality could be a good option in patients diagnosed with ectopic pregnancy desiring future offspring [9].

Loss of fertility after an episode of TEP is obviously related to tubal lesions and, in some cases, tubal occlusion. No data are available on hysterosalpingography findings after expectant management of ectopic pregnancy. However, according to the scientific literature to date, the effect of the various treatment strategies for ectopic pregnancy on subsequent fertility is still controversial. The main predictive factor for future fertility is the health of the contralateral fallopian tube. Hence, early diagnosis is essential for choosing the most conservative alternatives in the hope that tubal function and reproductive potential can be spared [10].

Methotrexate

At present, medical treatment of ectopic pregnancy is synonymous with methotrexate (MTX). MTX is a folic acid antagonist that selectively inhibits the enzyme dihydrofolate reductase, thus preventing folates from being reduced to tetrahydrofolates [11].

One of the key aspects in medical treatment for ectopic pregnancy is to identify the ideal candidate to receive MTX. An ideal patient for MTX would meet the following criteria [12, 13]:

- Hemodynamic stability and no severe or persistent abdominal pain
- Low initial β-hCG concentration (<5000 IU/l)
- Small mass (<4 cm) by transvaginal ultrasonography
- Unruptured mass
- No embryonic cardiac activity
- Certainty that there is no intrauterine pregnancy
- Willingness for follow-up
- No known sensitivity to MTX
- Normal baseline liver and renal function test results

When the candidate for treatment with MTX is adequately selected, the success rate has been reported as 63% to 96.7% of cases [14] and according to the Practice Committee of the American Society for Reproductive Medicine, MTX represents first-line therapy for unruptured ectopic pregnancy that is diagnosed early [15] (see chapter TUBAL ECTOPIC PREGNANCY: TREATMENT UPDATE).

Due to the antiproliferative effect of MTX, it has been speculated that the drug could act on the granulosa cells, preventing division and thus adversely affecting patients 'ovarian reserve and reproductive future. In addition, if women underwent a cycle of in vitro fertilization and experienced ectopic pregnancy as the result, then MTX administration could hypothetically lead to greater damage due to a gonadotropin-induced increase in ovarian blood flow, thus producing apoptosis in the granulosa cells and oocytes [16].

The DEMETER randomized trial designed in 2003 compared fertility in the first two years after ectopic pregnancy, according to the type of treatment received (medical, conservative surgery, or radical surgery). Patients were divided into two groups: the first (n = 207) included less active ectopic pregnancies and women were randomized to either conservative surgery plus MTX (n = 97) or to MTX treatment (1 mg/kg IM) alone (n = 110). After eliminating patients lost to follow-up, treatment failures, and patients not desiring pregnancy, the study saw no differences in the results. In the MTX treatment arm (87 women), 58 had intrauterine pregnancies and 8 had another ectopic pregnancy (12%). Among the conservative surgery group, 58/82 women had intrauterine pregnancies and 6/82 (9%) had another ectopic pregnancy. Based on these results, the authors concluded that post-ectopic pregnancy fertility did not vary according to the conservative treatment used [17].

Each year, the rate of infertile couples that require ART to achieve their goal to be parents increases. The incidence of ectopic pregnancy in women undergoing fertility treatments is approximately two to threefold higher. Therefore, specific concerns regarding future fertility outcomes appear in these patients when treatment options for ectopic pregnancy come to debate. Boots et al. (2013) specifically investigated these issues and concluded that MTX has no negative impact on later in vitro fertilization cycles, as patients treated with MTX have the same number of antral follicles, same FSH and retrieved oocyte levels, and overall good outcomes after treatment. The study was not free of limitations as it consisted of a retrospective design with a small sample (n = 66) and did not consider anti-müllerian hormone (AMH) levels to assess ovarian response [16]. Four previous studies also investigated this hypothesis, observing the same results, and most showed no significant differences in either in vitro fertilization cycle parameters or outcomes [18-21]. Shirazi et al. (2020) developed a prospective cohort study, in which 20 patients with ectopic pregnancy were treated with a single-dose MTX intramuscular injection. Several markers typically used in fertility assessment were tested before and after drug administration. AMH, FSH, E2 and AFC (antral follicle count) changes were not statistically significant, while increment of LH was significant (P = 0.02) 8 weeks post treatment [22].

Data suggests that MTX does not affect fertility markers used in our daily practice, although conclusions are taken from small, observational studies. Further investigation concerning relevant fertility outcomes, like intrauterine pregnancy or live-birth rates, are needed.

Mifepristone, Gefitinib and Vinorelbine

Within the past decades, much research has been done in pursuit of new drugs in order to increase the therapeutic armamentarium against tubal ectopic pregnancy. This has led to the use of two agents, mainly, which are mifepristone and gefitinib. However, some authors have postulated that other drugs could be useful due to their mechanism of action, such as vinorelbine.

Mifepristone is a selective progesterone receptor modulator (SPRM) which selectively occupies and competes with the endogenous progesterone receptor, thus destroying trophoblastic and decidual tissue, lowering luteinizing-hormone levels, and blocking the corpora lutea, which leads to embryo necrosis and abortion. It plays an important role as MTX co-adjuvant in the treatment of unruptured TEP in patients with elevated progesterone levels (>10ng/mL), given its luteolytic effect (see chapter TUBAL ECTOPIC PREGNANCY: TREATMENT UPDATE). Mifepristone is reported to be devoid of oestrogenic, anti-oestrogenic, mineralocorticoid and anti-mineralocorticoid properties [23].

It is hard to find published works evaluating mifepristone use's impact on fertility after treatment for TEP. This is probably due to the fact that this kind of treatment consists of a single dose of this drug administered alongside MTX. Some authors have studied the effect of oral mifepristone when used as a long term contraception method and have concluded it is able to suppress the LH surge and subsequently ovulation, providing contraception and inducing amenorrhoea [24]. What is more, it is also able to inhibit endometrial proliferation, but it sometimes causes unusual changes termed 'progesterone receptor modulator-associated endometrial changes '(PAECs) characterized by dilated, weakly secretory endometrial glands with few mitotic figures, and stromal effects ranging from compaction to non-uniform oedema [25]. However, we must insist on the fact that these effects are reversible and there is no reason to believe fertility should be compromised after the use of this drug. In addition, these authors have studied the effect of prolonged administration of mifepristone, not the long-term side effects of the single dose protocol.

Lastly, SPRMs could be a promising line of treatment when it comes to ovarian endometriosis, which is known to impair female fertility. Some authors have proposed the local injection of this group of drugs inside de endometrioma in order to suppress endometrial growth inside the cyst without damaging ovarian function [26]. Moreover, SPRMs have been studied as a uterus-sparing line of treatment against uterine fibroids in patients with desire of offspring with promising results which can lead us to think there should not be great damage on post-treatment fertility [27].

Gefitinib It is a small molecule that selectively inhibits tyrosine kinase in the epidermal growth factor receptor (EGFR). Placental tissue has been found to strongly express EGFR compared to other nonmalignant tissues. Moreover, its activation promotes cytotrophoblastic mobility, blocks programmed trophoblastic cell death, and rescues the placenta from apoptosis when exposed to hypoxia or toxic stimuli. By blocking EGF, gefitinib hypothetically induces cell death of ectopic trophoblastic tissue (see chapter TUBAL ECTOPIC PREGNANCY: TREATMENT UPDATE).

Gefitinib is also used as a therapeutic line for non-small cell lung cancer and some authors have done research on its side effects. Recently, Zhang et al. (2021) conducted a research project in order to determine the effect of gefitinib on mammalian oocytes in vitro. They used mouse oocytes and they observed this drug severely blocked oocyte meiotic progression which finally led to the generation of aneuploidy and early apoptosis of oocytes. Thus, they concluded there is evidence of gefitinib's reproductive toxicity [28]. However, further investigation should be performed in order to prove this toxicity in humans and other parameters should be investigated, such as live birth rate.

Vinorelbine is a semi-synthetic vinca-alkaloid derived from the Madagascar periwinkle. It induces cytotoxicity by binding to tubulin, which leads to an arrest of the cell cycle at the metaphase to anaphase transition. This ultimately leads to apoptosis of mitotic cells, which means it preferentially targets dividing and highly proliferative cells. It is currently approved to treat several types of cancer. Given the placenta is highly proliferative during the first trimester but the Fallopian tube is not, Hastie et al. (2018) postulated that it is plausible that vinorelbine could be efficacious in resolving an ectopic pregnancy whilst minimally affecting the surrounding tube [29]. In addition, these authors administered vinorelbine to several mice in order to determine this drug's impact on post-treatment fertility -four weeks after the last dose-

and they found out there were no differences between mice exposed to vinorelbine and controls in the number of pups per litter, pup or placental weight, crown to rump length, fetal placental ratio or gross fetal morphology. Maternal serum antimullerian hormone (AMH) is measured clinically as an indicator of ovarian reserve. Serum AMH concentrations in mice were no different in the vinorelbine treated group, compared to controls. However, we should be cautious with the interpretation of these results, as no clinical trials have been made when it comes to EP treatment in humans.

Salpingotomy

Surgical treatment is reserved for either ruptured or about to rupture ectopic pregnancies in hemodynamically unstable patients or if the use of medical treatment is not indicated [30]. The decision to perform conservative or radical surgery is usually made during the procedure and depends mainly on the patient's history (salpingectomy is indicated in the case of ipsilateral recurrence), the appearance and condition of the contralateral fallopian tube, and the presence of any bleeding (see chapter TUBAL ECTOPIC PREGNANCY: TREATMENT UPDATE).

It has classically been considered that organ-sparing requires conservative surgery, although this is not an absolute need in the case of paired organs. Conservative surgery (salpingotomy) is usually performed laparoscopically and its technique consists, briefly, of making a millimetric, longitudinal incision at the antimesenteric border of the fallopian tube. Afterwards, the trophoblast is aspirated through the salpingotomy. The intervention is completed with hemostasis control of the fallopian tube; slight pressure on the fallopian tube is simplest, as it is agreed that electrocoagulation (even when bipolar) should be avoided to prevent irreversible fallopian tube lesions. Salpingotomy suture is not necessary. Adequate lavage of the region is necessary to remove any trophoblastic residue in the abdominal cavity [31].

As far as the fertility outcome is concerned, its study is based on two variables:

- Probability of subsequent intrauterine pregnancy. The literature reports are inconsistent. Some classic studies apparently found no differences between conservative and radical techniques [32-34], whereas others report the rate of intrauterine pregnancies achieved was higher after salpingostomy [35-37]. However, these series were observational studies, and in 2009, the Cochrane Database System Review found no conclusive data related to subsequent fertility [6]. In 2012, the findings were presented for another observational study that included 164 patients from the Auvergne Registry who had been diagnosed with ectopic pregnancy between 1992 and 2008. The 24-month cumulative rate of intrauterine pregnancy was 67% after salpingectomy and 76% after salpingostomy. Intrauterine pregnancy was less likely to occur after radical treatment than after conservative treatments in univariate analyses. In multivariate analyses, however, the intrauterine pregnancy rate was significantly lower when patients were > 35 years old or had a history of infertility or tubal disease. In these patients, the intrauterine pregnancy rate was significantly more common after conservative treatment than after salpingectomy [38].

Consequently, these authors defend the use of conservative surgery whenever possible. Most recently, as stated earlier, two multicenter randomized clinical trials were conducted to compare fertility after ectopic pregnancy according to the type of treatment received. The first was called the DEMETER study and was designed in 2003; its second arm was proposed to compare conservative surgery plus MTX (101 patients) to radical surgery (98 patients). Once the analysis excluded patients lost to follow-up or who did not desire pregnancy, the rate of pregnancy was similar in both groups. The authors followed patients for 2 years after treatment (radical versus conservative), but found no significant differences in subsequent fertility [17]. The ESEP study was published the same year and showed that salpingotomy did not improve cumulative rates of ongoing pregnancy due to natural conception in women with a history of tubal pregnancy and a healthy contralateral tube. The median time to ongoing pregnancy by natural conception was 20 months (95% CI, 17-23) after salpingotomy and 26 months (95% CI, 15-37) after salpingectomy. The cumulative rate of ongoing pregnancy by natural conception after 36 months was 60.7% after salpingotomy and 56.2% after salpingectomy [39]. Therefore, both clinical trials had similar findings and conclusions, namely, that salpingectomy is preferable to salpingostomy in women with a healthy contralateral fallopian tube (the ESEP study excluded patients with contralateral tubal disease whereas the DEMETER study did not).

A very recent systematic review and meta-analysis released in October 2020, evaluated the fertility outcomes and rates of recurrence of salpingectomy compared to those of salpingostomy. The two aforementioned

RCTs and 16 cohort studies were included, with a mean follow-up time of 18 months. In the RCTs there is no difference in the outcomes between salpingectomy and salpingostomy for subsequent intrauterine pregnancy (OR 0,97, 95% CI 0.71 to 1.33). The cohort studies indicate that salpingectomy is approximately 50% less likely to result in a subsequent intrauterine pregnancy (IUP) than it is with salpingostomy (OR 0.45, 95% CI 0.39 to 0.52) [40].

- Risk of recurrence. The main argument for radical treatment is the need to eliminate recurrences, but the literature indicates that this is a false premise. Although this was already seen in previous observational studies, the DEMETER study showed that the recurrence rate in arm 2 (conservative surgery plus MTX versus radical surgery) was similar in both groups; in particular, recurrence was 8% (4/63) in the salpingostomy group and 12.5% (6/66) in the salpingectomy group. These results were also reported by the ESEP study (Femke Mol et al. 2014), which observed recurrence in 8% (18/215) of new ectopic pregnancies in the salpingotomy group and 5% (12/231) in the salpingectomy group (nonsignificant differences). Therefore, unilateral salpingectomy does not prevent the recurrence of ectopic pregnancy [17, 39].

In a recently published article, the difference observed between patients treated with salpingectomy vs. salpingostomy concerning a subsequent ectopic pregnancy was not significant (OR 0.77, 95% CI 0.41 to 1.47) in the RCTs. In the cohort study population, the overall OR was 0.732, with a 95% CI of 0.60 to 0.90, suggesting a lower risk of recurrence in women treated by salpingectomy. The authors analysed a subgroup of patients with various risk factors of infertility, namely: endometriosis, history of infertility, history of previous ovarian or tubal surgery, pregnancy conceived with IVF, known hydrosalpinx, known tubal occlusion, or intraoperative identification of contralateral tubal pathology. In this subgroup of women, salpingectomy still had a lower subsequent IUP rate and was associated with a higher recurrence. As the authors concluded, an even stronger recommendation for salpingostomy, if feasible, should be made for women with infertility risk factors [40].

Salpingectomy

Salpingectomy is the other surgical approach for tubal ectopic pregnancies and it is also referred to as radical surgery. The procedure is started by clamping the fallopian tube in place at its isthmic portion, thus achieving good exposure of the fallopian tube isthmus and mesosalpinx. Bipolar electrocoagulation is used to coagulate the mesosalpinx and its posterior cut. Once the fallopian tube is sectioned, the tube must be extracted (see chapter TUBAL ECTOPIC PREGNANCY: TREATMENT UPDATE).

Some authors have demonstrated that ipsilateral ovarian blood flow is compromised after salpingectomy due to the removal of the vascular arcade in the mesosalpynx and have postulated this may have a negative impact on ovarian function [41]. What is more, some authors have observed significant hormonal alterations in patients undergoing an IVF treatment the day of the BHCG injection [42]. This is why back in 2019, Luo et al. published a meta-analysis to provide a comparison of the ovarian reserve and ovarian response between pre and post salpingectomy in TEP patients. It consisted of 7 studies including 240 patients. The primary measured outcome was the ovarian reserve, including AMH, AFC, basal FSH, and basal E2. The second measured outcome was the ovarian response, including gonadotropin doses, gonadotropin stimulation days, E2 concentration on the hCG triggering day and the number of retrieved oocytes. The only statistically significant parameter was the amount of gonadotropin used in the IVF treatment, which was higher in the post-salpingectomy group, while other parameters in the present study were of little significant difference. That is the reason why authors believe salpingectomy does not harm ovarian function. However, this meta-analysis has several limitations because no other parameters were measured (such as subsequent pregnancy) and the interval between pre-salpingectomy and post-salpingectomy meant patients became older, which has a negative impact on ovarian reserve [43].

Non-Tubal Ectopic Pregnancy

Ectopic pregnancy occurs in the Fallopian tube the vast majority of times - around 96%-, but there are other places where the blastocyst can become implanted and this is known as non-tubal ectopic pregnancy (NTEP) [1]. A population-based study of 1800 surgically treated cases by Bouyer J (2002) showed that 3.2% of EP are located at the ovary, 2.4% at the uterine horn (also known as interstitial pregnancy) and 1,3% are abdominal pregnancies [44].

Up until now, we have got little solid evidence on NTEP treatment and the vast majority of published works consists of case reports and series of cases. Thus, many treatment routes have been described when it comes to NTEP approach, such as MTX, mifepristone, curettage, intra-amniotic potassium chloride (KCl) injection, uterine artery embolization (UAE), uterine arterial chemoembolization (UACE) or even hysteroscopic approach (see chapter NON-TUBAL ECTOPIC PREGNANCY: TREATMENT UPDATE).

There is not solid evidence against the performance of curettage for NTEP treatment due to its fertility outcome. However, we must not forget curettage may be a risk factor for infertility as it can lead to intrauterine adhesions (Asherman's syndrome) [45, 46].

Uterine artery embolization (UAE) is a technique used in selected cases of NTEP, but authors and clinicians have got more experience when used as a treatment route against leiomyomas. Thus, we found a review made by Keung et al. (2017) in which they explored UAE's impact on fertility in patients with uterine leiomyomata. They observed evidence is still controversial and interpretations of results must be extremely cautious [47, 48].

To sum up, NTEP is a heterogeneous set of clinical presentations, so individualization of each case will be crucial. This means it is very hard to determine an overall impact of treatment on our patients 'fertility.

References

[1] Hoffman, Barbara L, and J Whitridge Williams. 2016. *Williams Gynecology*. New York: Mcgraw-Hill Education. (Hoffman 2016, 161-176).

[2] Du, T., Chen, H., Fu, R., Chen, Q., Wang, Y., Mol, B., Kuang, Y. and Lyu, Q., 2017. Comparison of ectopic pregnancy risk among transfers of embryos vitrified on day 3, day 5, and day 6. *Fertility and Sterility*, 103(1), pp. 108-116.e1.

[3] Chang, Jeani, Laurie D Elam-Evans, Cynthia J Berg, Joy Herndon, Lisa Flowers, Kristi A Seed, and Carla J Syverson. 2003. "Pregnancy- Related Mortality Surveillance--United States, 1991--1999." *Morbidity and Mortality Weekly Report. Surveillance Summaries (Washington, D.C. : 2002)* 52 (2): 1–8.

[4] "Ectopic Pregnancy Mortality - Florida, 2009-2010." 2012. *MMWR. Morbidity and Mortality Weekly Report* 61 (6): 106–9.

[5] Mavrelos, D., Nicks, H., Jamil, A., Hoo, W., Jauniaux, E. and Jurkovic, D., 2013. Efficacy and safety of a clinical protocol for expectant management of selected women diagnosed with a tubal ectopic pregnancy. *Ultrasound in Obstetrics & Gynecology*, 42(1), pp.102-107.

[6] Hajenius, P J, F Mol, B W J Mol, P M M Bossuyt, W M Ankum, and F van der Veen. 2007. "Interventions for Tubal Ectopic Pregnancy." *The Cochrane Database of Systematic Reviews* 2007 (1): CD000324. https://doi.org/10.1002/14651858.CD000324.pub2.

[7] Buster, John E, and Stephan Krotz. 2007. "Reproductive Performance after Ectopic Pregnancy." *Seminars in Reproductive Medicine* 25 (2):131–33. https://doi.org/10.1055/s-2007-970052.

[8] Helmy, S, E Sawyer, D Ofili-Yebovi, J Yazbek, J Ben Nagi, and D Jurkovic. 2007. "Fertility Outcomes Following Expectant Management of Tubal Ectopic Pregnancy." *Ultrasound in Obstetrics&Gynecology : The Official Journal of the International Society of Ultrasound in Obstetrics and Gynecology* 30 (7): 988–93. https://doi.org/10.1002/uog.5186.

[9] Demirdag, E, I Guler, S Abay, Y Oguz, M Erdem, and A Erdem. 2017. "The Impact of Expectant Management, Systemic Methotrexate and Surgery on Subsequent Pregnancy Outcomes in Tubal Ectopic Pregnancy." *Irish Journal of Medical Science* 186 (2): 387–92. https://doi.org/10.1007/s11845-016-1419-5.

[10] Juneau, Caroline, and Gordon Wright Bates. 2012. "Reproductive Outcomes after Medical and Surgical Management of Ectopic Pregnancy." *Clinical Obstetrics and Gynecology* 55 (2): 455–60. https://doi.org/10.1097/GRF.0b013e3182510a88.

[11] Uptodate.com. 2021. *UpToDate*. [online] Available at: https://www.uptodate.com/contents/methotrexate-drug-information?search=methotrexate&topicRef=7509&source=see_link#F194514 [Accessed 16 November 2021].

[12] Bachman, Emelia Argyropoulos, and Kurt Barnhart. 2012. "Medical Management of Ectopic Pregnancy: A Comparison of Regimens." *Clinical Obstetrics and Gynecology* 55 (2): 440–47. https://doi.org/10.1097/GRF.0b013e3182510a73.

[13] Pfeifer S, Goldberg J, Lobo R, Thomas M, Widra E, Licht M, et al. Medical treatment of ectopic pregnancy: a committee opinion. Practice Committee of American Society for Reproductive Medicine. *Fertil. Steril.* 2013; 100(3): 638-44.

[14] Capmas, Perrine, Jean Bouyer, and Hervé Fernandez. 2014. "Treatment of Ectopic Pregnancies in 2014: New Answers to Some Old Questions."

Fertility and Sterility 101 (3): 615–20. https://doi. org/10.1016/ j.fertnstert.2014.01.029.

[15] "Medical Treatment of Ectopic Pregnancy: A Committee Opinion." 2013. *Fertility and Sterility* 100 (3): 638–44. https://doi.org/10. 1016/j.fertnstert. 2013.06.013.

[16] Boots, Christina E, Robert L Gustofson, and Eve C Feinberg. 2013. "Does Methotrexate Administration for Ectopic Pregnancy after in Vitro Fertilization Impact Ovarian Reserve or Ovarian Responsiveness?" *Fertility and Sterility* 100 (6): 1590–93. https://doi.org/10.1016/j.fertnstert. 2013.08.007.

[17] Fernandez, Hervé, Perrine Capmas, Jean Philippe Lucot, Benoit Resch, Pierre Panel, and Jean Bouyer. 2013. "Fertility after Ectopic Pregnancy: The DEMETER Randomized Trial." *Human Reproduction (Oxford, England)* 28 (5): 1247–53. https://doi.org/ 10.1093/humrep/det037.

[18] Orvieto, Raoul, Jenya Kruchkovich, Efraim Zohav, Jacob Rabinson, Eyal Y Anteby, and Simion Meltcer. 2007. "Does Methotrexate Treatment for Ectopic Pregnancy Influence the Patient's Performance during a Subsequent in Vitro Fertilization/Embryo Transfer Cycle?" *Fertility and Sterility* 88 (6): 1685–86. https://doi.org/10.1016/j.fertnstert.2007.01.064.

[19] Oriol, Bárbara, Ana Barrio, Alberto Pacheco, José Serna, José Luis Zuzuarregui, and Juan A Garcia-Velasco. 2008. "Systemic Methotrexate to Treat Ectopic Pregnancy Does Not Affect Ovarian Reserve." *Fertility and Sterility* 90 (5): 1579–82. https://doi.org/ 10.1016/j.fertnstert.2007.08.032.

[20] Provansal, M, A Agostini, O Lacroix, S Gerbeau, J-M Grillo, and M Gamerre. 2009. "Ultrasound Monitoring in Patients Undergoing In-Vitro Fertilization after Methotrexate Treatment for Ectopic Pregnancy." *Ultrasound in Obstetrics & Gynecology: The Official Journal of the International Society of Ultrasound in Obstetrics and Gynecology* 34 (6): 715–19. https://doi.org/10.1002/uog.7344.

[21] McLaren, Janet F, Richard O Burney, Amin A Milki, Lynn M Westphal, Michael H Dahan, and Ruth B Lathi. 2009. "Effect of Methotrexate Exposure on Subsequent Fertility in Women Undergoing Controlled Ovarian Stimulation." *Fertility and Sterility* 92 (2): 515–19. https://doi.org/10.1016/j.fertnstert.2008.07.009.

[22] Shirazi, Mahboobeh, Parichehr Pooransari, Neda Hajiha, Zeinab Shaker, Mohadeseh Ghazi, Fatemeh Davari Tanha, Batool Ghorbani Yekta, and Marjan Ghaemi. 2020. "Effect of Single-Dose Methotrexate Treatment on Ovarian Reserve in Women with Ectopic Pregnancy Undergoing Infertility Treatment: A Single-Center Experience." *International Journal of Fertility & Sterility* 14 (1): 23–26. https://doi.org/10.22074/ijfs.2020.5938.

[23] Critchley, H O D, and R R Chodankar. 2020. "90 YEARS OF PROGESTERONE: Selective Progesterone Receptor Modulators In Gynaecological Therapies." *Journal Of Molecular Endocrinology* 65 (1): T15-T33. doi:10.1530/jme-19-0238.

[24] Brown, Audrey, Linan Cheng, Suiqing Lin, and David T. Baird. 2002. "Daily Low-Dose Mifepristone Has Contraceptive Potential By Suppressing Ovulation And Menstruation: A Double-Blind Randomized Control Trial Of 2 And 5 Mg Per Day For 120 Days." *The Journal of Clinical Endocrinology & Metabolism* 87 (1): 63-70. doi:10.1210/ jcem.87.1.8140.

[25] Mutter, George L, Christine Bergeron, Liane Deligdisch, Alex Ferenczy, Mick Glant, Maria Merino, Alistair R W Williams, and Diana L Blithe. 2008. "The Spectrum of Endometrial Pathology Induced By Progesterone Receptor Modulators." *Modern Pathology* 21 (5): 591-598. doi:10.1038/ modpathol.2008.19.

[26] Benagiano, Giuseppe, Felice Petraglia, Stephan Gordts, and Ivo Brosens. 2016. "A New Approach To The Management Of Ovarian Endometrioma To Prevent Tissue Damage And Recurrence." *Reproductive Biomedicine Online* 32 (6): 556-562. doi:10.1016/j .rbmo.2016.03.001.

[27] Bartels, Chantal B., Kamaria C. Cayton, Farah S. Chuong, Kristine Holthouser, Sara A. Mehr, Tara Abraham, and James H. Segars. 2016. "An Evidence-Based Approach to the Medical Management of Fibroids." *Clinical Obstetrics & Gynecology* 59 (1): 30-52. doi:10.1097/ grf.0000000000000171.

[28] Zhang, Hong-Yong, Ying-Chun Ouyang, Jian Li, Chun-Hui Zhang, Wei Yue, Tie-Gang Meng, Heide Schatten, Qing-Yuan Sun, and Wei-Ping Qian. 2021. "Gefitinib Reduces Oocyte Quality By Disturbing Meiotic Progression." *Toxicology* 452: 152705. doi:10.1016/j.tox.2021.152705.

[29] Hastie, Roxanne, Elgene Lim, Pavel Sluka, Lisa Campbell, Andrew W. Horne, Lenore Ellett, Natalie J. Hannan, Fiona Brownfoot, Tu'uhevaha J. Kaitu'u-Lino, and Stephen Tong. 2018. "Vinorelbine Potentially Induces Placental Cell Death, Does Not Harm Fertility And Is A Potential Treatment For Ectopic Pregnancy." *Ebiomedicine* 29: 166-176. doi:10.1016 /j.ebiom.2018.01.041.

[30] "ACOG Practice Bulletin No. 193: Tubal Ectopic Pregnancy." 2018. *Obstetrics and Gynecology* 131 (3): e91–103. https://doi.org/ 10.1097/ AOG.0000000000002560.

[31] Hoffman, Barbara L, and J Whitridge Williams. 2016. *Williams Gynecology*. New York: Mcgraw-Hill Education. 1013-1014.

[32] Clausen, I. 1996. "Conservative versus Radical Surgery for Tubal Pregnancy. A Review." *Acta Obstetricia et Gynecologica Scandinavica* 75 (1): 8–12. https://doi.org/10.3109/00016349 609033276.

[33] Silva, P D, A M Schaper, and B Rooney. 1993. "Reproductive Outcome after 143 Laparoscopic Procedures for Ectopic Pregnancy." *Obstetrics and Gynecology* 81 (5 (Pt 1)): 710–15.

[34] Dubuisson, J B, F X Aubriot, H Foulot, D Bruel, J Bouquet de Jolinière, and L Mandelbrot. 1990. "Reproductive Outcome after Laparoscopic Salpingectomy for Tubal Pregnancy." *Fertility and Sterility* 53 (6): 1004–7. https://doi.org/10.1016/s0015-0282(16) 53575-4.

[35] Yao, M, and T Tulandi. 1997. "Current Status of Surgical and Nonsurgical Management of Ectopic Pregnancy." *Fertility and Sterility* 67 (3): 421–33. https://doi.org/10.1016/s0015-0282(97) 80064-7.

[36] Mol, B W, H C Matthijsse, D J Tinga, T Huynh, P J Hajenius, W M Ankum, P M Bossuyt, and F van der Veen. 1998. "Fertility after Conservative and Radical Surgery for Tubal Pregnancy." *Human Reproduction (Oxford, England)* 13 (7): 1804–9. https://doi.org/10. 1093/humrep/13.7.1804

[37] Bangsgaard, Nannie, Claus Otto Lund, Bent Ottesen, and Lisbeth Nilas. 2003. "Improved Fertility Following Conservative Surgical Treatment of Ectopic Pregnancy." *BJOG : An International Journal of Obstetrics and Gynaecology* 110 (8): 765–70.

[38] Bennetot, Marianne de, Benoît Rabischong, Bruno Aublet-Cuvelier, Fabien Belard, Hervé Fernandez, Jean Bouyer, Michel Canis, and Jean-Luc Pouly. 2012. "Fertility after Tubal Ectopic Pregnancy: Results of a Population-Based Study." *Fertility and Sterility* 98 (5): 1271–73. https://doi.org/10. 1016/j.fertnstert.2012.06.041.

[39] Mol, Femke, Norah M van Mello, Annika Strandell, Karin Strandell, Davor Jurkovic, Jackie Ross, Kurt T Barnhart, et al. 2014. "Salpingotomy versus Salpingectomy in Women with Tubal Pregnancy (ESEP Study): An Open-Label, Multicentre, Randomised Controlled Trial." *Lancet (London, England)* 383 (9927): 1483–89. https://doi.org/10.1016/S0140-6735(14) 60123-9.

[40] Ozcan, Meghan C H, Jeffrey R Wilson, and Gary N Frishman. 2021. "A Systematic Review and Meta-Analysis of Surgical Treatment of Ectopic Pregnancy with Salpingectomy versus Salpingostomy." *Journal of Minimally Invasive Gynecology* 28 (3): 656–67. https://doi.org/10.1016/ j.jmig.2020.10.014.

[41] Chan, C.C.W. 2003. "Impaired Ovarian Blood Flow And Reduced Antral Follicle Count Following Laparoscopic Salpingectomy For Ectopic Pregnancy." *Human Reproduction* 18 (10): 2175-2180. doi:10.1093/ humrep/deg411.

[42] Gelbaya, Tarek A., Luciano G. Nardo, Cheryl T. Fitzgerald, Greg Horne, Daniel R. Brison, and Brian A. Lieberman. 2006. "Ovarian Response To Gonadotropins After Laparoscopic Salpingectomy Or The Division Of Fallopian Tubes For Hydrosalpinges." *Fertility And Sterility* 85 (5): 1464-1468. Luo, Jiaqi, Yu Shi, Dan Liu, Danni Yang, Jiahui Wu, Lijuan Cao, Lan Geng, et al. 2019. "The Effect of Salpingectomy on the Ovarian Reserve and Ovarian Response in Ectopic Pregnancy: A Systematic Review and Meta-Analysis." *Medicine* 98 (47): e17901. https://doi.org/10.1097/MD.0000000000017901.

[43] Bouyer, J, Coste J, Fernandez H, Pouly JL, and Job-Spira N. 2002. "Sites of Ectopic Pregnancy: A 10 Year Population-Based Study of 1800 Cases." *Human Reproduction (Oxford, England)* 17 (12): 3224–30. https://doi.org/10.1093/HUMREP/17.12.3224.

[44] Deans, Rebecca, and Jason Abbott. 2010. "Review of Intrauterine Adhesions." *Journal Of Minimally Invasive Gynecology* 17 (5): 555-569. doi:10.1016/j.jmig.2010.04.016.

[45] Adoni A, Palti Z, Milwidsky A, Dolberg M. The incidence of intrauterine adhesions following spontaneous abortion. *Int J Fertil.* 1982;27(2):117-8. PMID: 6126446.

[46] Keung, Jonathan J., James B. Spies, and Theresa M. Caridi. 2018. "Uterine Artery Embolization: A Review Of Current Concepts." *Best Practice & Research Clinical Obstetrics & Gynaecology* 46: 66-73. doi:10.1016/j.bpobgyn.2017.09.003.

[47] Gupta, Janesh K, Anju Sinha, M.A Lumsden, and Martha Hickey. 2012. "Uterine Artery Embolization For Symptomatic Uterine Fibroids." *Cochrane Database Of Systematic Reviews*. doi:10.1002/14651858.cd005073.pub3.

Chapter 9

Ectopic Pregnancy: From Diagnosis to Treatment

Edip Aydın[*], MD
Health Sciences University,
Gazi Yaşargil Training and Research Hospital,
Diyarbakır, Turkey

Abstract

Ectopic pregnancy (EP) is defined as the implantation of a fertilized ovum anywhere outside of the endometrial cavity and constitutes 1% of all pregnancies.

Most common etiology is delayed transport of the fertilized ovum through the fallopian tube. EP mostly occurs in a fallopian tube (95-98%) and is rarely seen in ovaries, hysterectomy scar, cervical region, and abdomen.

Risk factors in ectopic pregnancy include previous ectopic pregnancy, history of pelvic (particularly fallopian tube surgery) or abdominal surgery, and pelvic inflammatory disease. Most common symptoms include abdominal pain and/or abnormal vaginal bleeding and menstrual delay. EP is diagnosed easily and promptly by a detailed pelvic examination, β-hCG test, and transvaginal ultrasound. There are two important notions to address in EP patients: prompt intervention following a rapid and accurate diagnosis and preservation of fertility. EP accounts for 4 - 10% of all pregnancy-related deaths. In the treatment of EP, laparoscopic techniques are used in the diagnosis and treatment to

[*] Corresponding Author's E-mail: dr_edip@msn.com.

In: A Closer Look at Pregnancy and Childbirth
Editor: Louise J. Salgado
ISBN: 978-1-68507-658-0

provide a correct and rapid intervention and conservative treatments (dilation and curettage [D&C] and methotrexate) can be used to preserve fertility.

Surgical treatment is performed in patients that are hemodynamically unstable, suspected of tubal rupture, contraindicated to methotrexate treatment, or who do not respond to methotrexate therapy.

Introductıon

Ectopic pregnancy occurs when a developing embryo implants at a site other than the endometrium of the uterine cavity, most commonly within the fallopian tube. Although the incidence of ectopic pregnancy is estimated to be approximately 2% of all pregnancies, it is one of the most common gynecologic emergencies encountered by community physicians [1].

Ruptured ectopic pregnancy can lead to severe hemorrhage and is a significant cause of pregnancy-related maternal mortality in the first trimester [2].

Thus, timely diagnosis of ectopic pregnancy is essential to prevent maternal mortality and improve treatment outcomes.

Maternal mortality related to ectopic pregnancy has plummeted over the last two decades due to the availability of quantitative beta-human chorionic gonadotropin (b-hCG) testing, transvaginal ultrasound, and laparoscopy, which allow for early diagnosis and intervention [1]. Despite this, ectopic pregnancy and its treatments remain a prevalent cause of morbidity among women and can affect long-term reproductive success. With a comprehensive understanding of ectopic pregnancy, community physicians can help women make informed decisions and thus provide personalized health care.

This review outlines the current practices, recent advances, and unresolved topics related to diagnosis, management, and prognosis of ectopic pregnancy.

Symptoms

Ectopic pregnancies may have no symptoms and are only detected through investigations. The most common features of ectopic pregnancy are irregular vaginal bleeding and lower abdominal pain. Later on, shoulder tip pain and rectal pain (pain in the bottom), may occur and these are usually suggestive of the condition worsening. Other symptoms include dizziness, collapse and diarrhoea. If you would like further explanation of these symptoms please ask your doctor or nurse.

Risk Factors

Only half of the women who are diagnosed with ectopic pregnancy have identifiable risk factors [2]. Thus, it is critical to maintain a high index of suspicion in all women of reproductive age who present with amenorrhea, abdominal pain, irregular vaginal bleeding, or a history of ectopic pregnancy [3]. The pretest probability of ectopic pregnancy is increased if multiple risk factors are elicited when taking a history, which can aid in making a prompt diagnosis.

The most well-documented risk factor for an ectopic pregnancy is a previous ectopic pregnancy [4, 5]. Women with a prior ectopic pregnancy have a 10-times higher risk of recurrence than the general population [6]. After one ectopic pregnancy, there is a 10% to 15% chance of recurrence, which increases to 25% in women who have had two or more ectopic pregnancies [6]. Recurrence can be attributed to congenital tubal dysfunction, acquired tubal damage from pelvic inflammatory disease, or previous tubal surgery—all of which may impede embryonic passage through the fallopian tube [4, 7]. Women with perihepatic adhesions (commonly known as Fitz-Hugh-Curtis syndrome), a complication of pelvic inflammatory disease, carry twice the risk of ectopic pregnancy recurrence compared to unaffected women [7].

Smoking, even "light" consumption of one to nine cigarettes per day, increases the risk of ectopic pregnancy by up to twofold [8]. Some other well-recognized risk factors for ectopic pregnancy are age over 35 years, history of infertility, prior tubal surgery, and laboratory/laparoscopy confirmed pelvic inflammatory disease [2]. Additionally, genital surgery, endometriosis, and dysmenorrhea have been recognized as significant risk factors [4]. Jacob and colleagues also described a 1.8-fold (95% CI 1.54 - 2.09) increase in the risk of ectopic pregnancy in women with a diagnosis of mental health disorders, including depression, anxiety, adjustment disorder, and somatoform disorder [4]. This finding might be limited to an association, confounded by increased rates of psychiatric disorders in women with a history of infertility, chronic pelvic pain, endometriosis, recurrent miscarriages, and so on. It is also possible that the medications used for treating such disorders disrupt embryo transport through the fallopian tube [4]. More studies are needed to understand the association between mental health and ectopic pregnancy before drawing definitive conclusions.

Older data associated intrauterine contraceptive devices (IUDs) with ectopic pregnancy [9]. And while it remains true that if pregnancy occurs with an IUD in situ the risk of ectopic pregnancy is high, all forms of contraception reduce the risk of pregnancy and ectopic pregnancy [6]. In vitro fertilization (IVF) was previously thought to be associated with increased risk of ectopic pregnancy due to possible underlying fallopian tube dysfunction in the infertile population and procedure-related factors [2]. The latter may not be relevant today because the IVF practices associated with increased rates of ectopic pregnancy, such as transfer of multiple embryos and day-3 embryo transfer, are less common in modern clinical practice.

As a result, the incidence of ectopic pregnancy after IVF has decreased significantly, and many physicians now suggest that IVF pregnancies may be at little or no increased risk of ectopic pregnancy compared to natural conceptions [6].

Diagnosis

History and Presentation

Ectopic pregnancies almost always occur in the fallopian tube (> 95%), particularly in the ampulla (distal portion) (70%) [7]. Fewer tubal pregnancies occur in the isthmus (middle portion) (12%) and fimbria (11%) [10]. Rarely, pregnancies may grow in the cervix (< 1%) or abdomen (1%), or on the ovary (3%) [10, 11]. It is important to obtain a full history, including menstrual and obstetrical history, to determine gestational age and evaluate for risk factors in all women of reproductive age. Women with an ectopic pregnancy most commonly present with abdominal pain, vaginal bleeding, or both [2]. However, these are also symptoms of miscarriage, which is, by far, the most common cause of failing pregnancy and/or abnormally rising b-hCG levels. An ectopic pregnancy may be intact or ruptured at presentation; the latter might present with hemodynamic instability and an acute abdomen that requires urgent surgical management to address ongoing hemorrhage [10]. Initial workup includes confirmation of pregnancy (through urine or serum b-hCG testing) and a transvaginal ultrasound to determine the location of the pregnancy [2].

Laboratory Investigations

Serial quantitative serum b-hCG testing can be helpful in determining if the current pregnancy is likely to be in an ectopic location. In a normal pregnancy, the b-hCG level rises steeply for the first 4 weeks, followed by a slower rise until 10 weeks gestational age, with an eventual plateauing [12]. In most normal intrauterine pregnancies, the b-hCG level will rise 65% to 100% every 48 hours, although even a short plateau in b-hCG can be normal in rare cases [2]. When performing serial b-hCG measurements, it is recommended that the same laboratory be used to minimize the risk of interassay variability, which can be 5% to 10% [10].

Decreasing b-hCG levels strongly suggest a failing pregnancy, but they do not indicate its location. If no intrauterine pregnancy has been confirmed, the woman should be closely monitored because it is possible for an ectopic pregnancy to rupture, even with very low b-hCG levels. The use of discriminatory b-hCG levels to determine when an intrauterine pregnancy should be visible on ultrasound is discouraged. Evidence from the 1980s suggested that b-hCG of 1000 to 2000 IU/L without a visible pregnancy could be assumed to be ectopic [13]. It is now widely acknowledged that b-hCG can be nonspecific, as many ectopic pregnancies will never reach a level of 2000 IU/L or might rupture before that threshold. Conversely, women who have had multiple gestations have higher b-hCG levels than women who have had a single gestation, and using 2000 IU/L as a discriminatory value might not be accurate for such pregnancies [2]. Historical use of a "threshold" has resulted in the treatment of intrauterine pregnancies with methotrexate, a chemotherapeutic agent; hence, newer studies have urged caution and patience when evaluating early pregnancies of uncertain viability [13].

Imaging

Transvaginal ultrasound is the optimal method for imaging pregnancies in the early first trimester. In a normal pregnancy, a gestational sac is visualized at 5 weeks gestation (3 weeks after conception), when it is 2 to 5mm in diameter

[13]. Following that, the yolk sac is the earliest structure to develop inside the gestational sac and is normally seen by 5 weeks and 5 days of pregnancy [10]. Presence of an intrauterine pregnancy (gestational sac plus a yolk sac or embryo) on transvaginal ultrasound effectively eliminates the diagnosis of an ectopic pregnancy other than the rare scenario of a heterotopic pregnancy (one embryo within the uterus and another extra-uterine) [10]. However, even with modern high-resolution ultrasound, it is rare that ultrasound alone is sufficient to be definitive. Without a yolk sac, an intrauterine pregnancy cannot be confirmed, and clinicians should be wary because it might represent a pseudosac—a fluid collection in the endometrial cavity caused by sloughing of the decidua [10]. To differentiate between a pseudosac and an early gestational sac, a follow-up ultrasound in 7 to 14 days should be arranged.

Transvaginal ultrasound can definitively diagnose an ectopic pregnancy if an extra-uterine gestational sac with yolk sac/embryo is visible [2] [Figure]. However, most ectopic pregnancies lack these definitive features on imaging and are often described as an inhomogeneous adnexal mass separate from the ovaries [10]. An adnexal mass might also represent a cyst, corpus luteum, or bowel [2]. The presence of hemoperitoneum (echogenic intraperitoneal fluid) and placental blood flow within the periphery of this mass ("ring of fire") on color doppler can aid in diagnosis [10].

Expectant Management

Sadly an ectopic pregnancy cannot lead to the birth of a baby, therefore all options must end the pregnancy in order to reduce the risks to your own health. Your options depend on:

- How many weeks pregnant you are.
- Your symptoms.
- If there has been a lot of bleeding inside your abdomen.
- The level of hCG.
- Your scan result.
- Your general health.
- Your personal views and preferences – this should involve a discussion about your future pregnancy plans.
- The options available at your local hospital.

Expectant management of ectopic pregnancy involves allowing the pregnancy to take its natural course with close physician follow-up until there is clinical resolution of symptoms, a negative urine pregnancy test, or negative serum b-hCG [14]. There is evidence that expectant management of ectopic pregnancy can be a safe option in a select population of women who are hemodynamically stable, asymptomatic, have a b-hCG value less than 2000 IU/L, with decreasing levels, and can reliably access regular physician follow-up [15]. These women can avoid the use of methotrexate and its possible side effects. It is worth noting, however, that a 5-year follow-up cohort study of 217 women who underwent expectant, medical, or surgical management of a first ectopic pregnancy suggested there was a 2.68 times higher risk of recurrent ectopic pregnancy in women who were managed expectantly [5]. A randomized study called ACTorNOT (ClinicalTrials.gov NCT02152696) has completed recruitment to compare expectant management versus uterine evacuation plus methotrexate versus methotrexate alone in women with ectopic pregnancy.

Medical Treatment

Methotrexate, the most common option for treating ectopic pregnancy, was first used for this purpose in 1982 [16]. It is a folate antagonist that prevents DNA replication and affects rapidly proliferating cells like that of a developing embryo [17]. A single dose of methotrexate is administered intramuscularly based on body surface area (50mg/m^2). Its effectiveness is assessed by serial b-hCG measurements on days 4 and 7 post-treatment, then weekly until resolution [2]. A reduction of less than 15% in b-hCG level between days 4 and 7 posttreatment may indicate that treatment is inadequate; therefore, a second dose of methotrexate might be required [2]. Close observation is required to ensure patient stability, declining b-hCG levels and normal liver function tests because methotrexate can affect liver function [2, 17].

The b-hCG level at presentation is strongly associated with treatment success of a single dose methotrexate injection. A systematic review that analyzed five observational studies determined that women with a baseline b-hCG level of more than 5000 IU/L were 4 times more likely to have treatment failure with single-dose methotrexate than those with a presenting baseline between 2000 and 4999 IU/L [18]. Thus, most guidelines suggest using methotrexate to treat ectopic pregnancy in women with a presenting b-hCG level less than 5000 IU/L. Other factors such as ectopic mass > 3.5 cm and presence of fetal heartbeat on transvaginal ultrasound are considered relative contraindications to the use of medical therapy because they might indicate a more developed embryo, which implies increased risk of ectopic rupture [2, 10]. However, few data are available to support these recommendations [10].

One in three women may experience mild, self-limited side effects of methotrexate, including nausea, diarrhea, stomatitis, and conjunctivitis [2]. Serious complications, including anaphylaxis, pulmonary damage, and myelosuppression, have also been reported [10]. Since methotrexate can cause temporary hepatic dysfunction, it is important to obtain a CBC and baseline liver and renal function laboratory results, and to monitor liver function if indicated. Patients should also be advised to stop their folate-containing supplements because they inhibit methotrexate function [10]. Nonsteroidal anti-inflammatory medications should also be avoided because they may reduce renal clearance of the drug by reducing renal blood flow [10]. Alcohol should be avoided during methotrexate treatment to prevent the combined effect of hepatotoxic drugs. Methotrexate should not be administered to patients with liver or renal dysfunction, lung disease, hematologic dysfunction, immunodeficiency, or peptic ulcer disease, or to those who are breastfeeding. Given that this is an outpatient treatment, and an ectopic pregnancy may rupture during therapy, it is important to alert patients to the symptoms of a ruptured ectopic pregnancy and to seek immediate medical attention if they occur.

Advances in medical treatment of ectopic pregnancy may be on the horizon. Researchers from the University of British Columbia have demonstrated that gonadotropin-releasing hormone (GnRH) and its receptor are expressed in trophoblast cells and fallopian tube epithelium at ectopic pregnancy implantation sites [19]. This presents the potential to use a targeted and less toxic agent for conservative treatment of ectopic pregnancies. A randomized controlled trial comparing GnRH agonist versus methotrexate was registered in March 2020 [20]. The trial is also planning to investigate the use of letrozole, an aromatase inhibitor that blocks the final step in estrogen synthesis, versus methotrexate to treat ectopic pregnancy, and is stated to conclude in 2022.

Surgical Management

With improved laparoscopic instruments and techniques, minimally invasive surgery has become the gold standard for treating ectopic pregnancy and has mostly replaced laparotomy. Laparoscopic surgery offers a safer, faster, cheaper, and more esthetic option [10, 21]. With improved operator experience, even stable but symptomatic ectopic pregnancies can be managed with laparoscopy, which can result in quicker hemostasis and better patient outcomes [21]. However, laparotomy is sometimes used for hemodynamically unstable cases because it might offer better field visualization when managing a large bleed [10].

Two laparoscopic techniques are available for treating tubal pregnancies: salpingectomy, where the fallopian tube containing the ectopic pregnancy is removed, and salpingotomy, where after removal of the ectopic mass, the affected fallopian tube is preserved. There is ongoing debate about treatment success, future fertility, and risk of repeat ectopic pregnancy after treatment with salpingotomy versus salpingectomy.

Salpingectomy versus Salpingotomy

Treatment Success and Future Fertility

Given that salpingotomy requires the surgeon to meticulously extract a small trophoblastic mass while preserving the fallopian tube, the method might be prone to trophoblastic tissue retention, which can necessitate a salpingectomy. Multiple retrospective studies report trophoblast persistence rates between 9.0% and 12.0% for salpingotomy and 1.8% for salpingectomy [22]. In an open-label, randomized control trial named European Surgery in Ectopic Pregnancy, women with ultrasound-confirmed ectopic pregnancy who were eligible for surgical management were randomly assigned to either salpingotomy or salpingectomy. The trial reported significantly higher postsurgical trophoblast persistence in the salpingotomy group (n = 215) than in the salpingectomy group (n = 231) (RR 15.0, $p = 0.01$) [23]. The trial also found no significant difference in rates of naturally conceived pregnancies 36 months postsurgery (fecundity ratio 1.06, $p = 0.687$) [23]. Thus, for women with tubal pregnancy and a healthy contralateral tube, salpingectomy is a reasonable treatment option because it minimizes risk of ectopic mass persistence and does not seem to reduce future fertility. However, for women with contralateral tubal pathology or no contralateral tube, conservative treatment with salpingotomy should be considered if they wish to maintain the potential for natural conception.

Risk of Recurrent Ectopic Pregnancy

Multiple studies have evaluated the risk of ectopic recurrence following salpingotomy versus salpingectomy, but no consensus has been reached.

A 12-year retrospective study found a recurrent ectopic pregnancy rate of 13% in the ipsilateral tube following salpingotomy, while in the salpingectomy group, there were no recorded recurrences [22]. These data might be confounded by the fact that women who choose to undergo salpingotomy are more likely intending to conceive and have higher pregnancy rates compared to those who choose to undergo salpingectomy. Multiple retrospective studies that have included only women who are actively wanting to conceive post-salpingotomy or post-salpingectomy have reported no difference in rates of ectopic pregnancy recurrence between the two groups [24, 25]. Thus, data on the rates of ectopic pregnancy recurrence after different surgical procedures are still conflicting.

References

[1] Creanga, A. A., Shapiro-Mendoza, C. K., Bish, C. L. et al. Trends in ectopic pregnancy mortality in the United States: 1980 - 2007. *Obstet. Gynecol.,* 2011; 117:837 - 843.

[2] Barnhart, K. T., Franasiak, J. ACOG Practice Bulletin No. 193: Tubal ectopic pregnancy. *Obstet. Gynecol.,* 2018; 131:e91 - e103.

[3] Ramakrishnan, K., Scheid, D. C. Ectopic pregnancy: Forget the "classical presentation" if you want to catch it sooner. *J. Fam. Pract.,* 2006; 55:388 - 395.

[4] Jacob, L., Kalder, M., Kostev, K. Risk factors for ectopic pregnancy in Germany: A retrospective study of 100,197 patients. *Ger. Med. Sci.*, 2017; 15:Doc19.

[5] Ellaithy, M., Asiri, M., Rateb, A. et al. Prediction of recurrent ectopic pregnancy: A five-year follow-up cohort study. *Eur. J. Obstet. Gynecol. Reprod. Biol.*, 2018; 225:70 - 78.

[6] Ectopic pregnancy. In: Taylor, H. S., Pal, L., Seli, E. *Speroff's clinical gynecologic endocrinology and infertility*. 9th ed. Philadelphia, PA: Wolters Kluwer; 2020. p. 1260 - 1288.

[7] Mullins, E., Agarwal, N., Oliver, R., Odejinmi, J. F. Implications of perihepatic adhesions in women undergoing laparoscopic surgery for ectopic pregnancy. *Int. J. Gynecol. Obstet.,* 2015; 130:247 - 249.

[8] Saraiya, M., Berg, C. J., Kendrick, J. S. et al. Cigarette smoking as a risk factor for ectopic pregnancy. *Am. J. Obstet. Gynecol.,* 1998; 178:493 - 498.

[9] Franks, A. L., Beral, V., Cates, Jr. W., Hogue, C. J. Contraception and ectopic pregnancy risk. *Am. J. Obstet. Gynecol.*, 1990; 163(4 Pt 1):1120 - 1123.

[10] Ectopic pregnancy. In: Hoffman, B. L., Schorge, J. O., Bradshaw, K. D. et al., editors. *Williams gynecology*. 3rd ed. New York: McGraw-Hill; 2016.

[11] Dunne, C., Havelock, J. C. Ovarian ectopic pregnancy after in vitro fertilization. *J. Obstet. Gynaecol. Can.,* 2012; 34:409.

[12] Morin, L., Cargill, Y. M., Glanc, P. Ultrasound evaluation of first trimester complications of pregnancy. *J. Obstet. Gynaecol. Can.,* 2016; 38:982 - 988.

[13] Doubilet, P. M., Benson, C. B. Further evidence against the reliability of the human chorionic gonadotropin discriminatory level. *J. Ultrasound Med.,* 2011; 30:1637 - 1642.

[14] Jurkovic, D., Memtsa, M., Sawyer, E. et al. Single-dose systemic methotrexate vs. expectant management for treatment of tubal ectopic pregnancy: A placebo–controlled randomized trial. *Ultrasound Obstet. Gynecol.,* 2017; 49:171 - 176.

[15] Odejinmi, F., Huff, K. O., Oliver, R. Individualisation of intervention for tubal ectopic pregnancy: Historical perspectives and the modern evidence based management of ectopic pregnancy. *Eur. J. Obstet. Gynecol. Reprod. Biol.,* 2017; 210:69 - 75.

[16] Tanaka, T., Hayashi, H., Kutsuzawa, T. et al. Treatment of interstitial ectopic pregnancy with methotrexate: Report of a successful case. *Fertil. Steril.,* 1982; 37:851 - 852.

[17] Olofsson, J. I., Poromaa, I. S., Ottander, U. et al. Clinical and pregnancy outcome following ectopic pregnancy; a prospective study comparing expectancy, surgery and systemic methotrexate treatment. *Acta. Obstet. Gynecol. Scand.,* 2001; 80:744 - 749.

[18] Menon, S., Colins, J., Barnhart, K. T. Establishing a human chorionic gonadotropin cutoff to guide methotrexate treatment of ectopic pregnancy: A systematic review. *Fertil. Steril.,* 2007; 87:481 - 484.

[19] Peng, B., Klausen, C., Campbell, L., Leung, P. C. K. Gonadotropin-releasing hormone and gonadotropin-releasing hormone receptor are

expressed at tubal ectopic pregnancy implantation sites. *Fertil. Steril.,* 2016; 105:1620 - 1627.e3.

[20] Ali, S. A. *The aromatase inhibitor and Gnrh antagonist versus methotrexate for management of undisturbed ectopic pregnancy.* NIH: U.S. National Library of Medicine 2020. Accessed 23 June 2020. https://clinicaltrials.gov/ct2/show/NCT04308343.

[21] Cohen, A., Almog, B., Satel, A. et al. Laparoscopy versus laparotomy in the management of ectopic pregnancy with massive hemoperitoneum. *Int. J. Gynecol. Obstet.,* 2013; 123:139 - 141.

[22] Lagana, A. S., Vitale, S. G., De Dominici, R. et al. Fertility outcome after laparoscopic salpingostomy or salpingectomy for tubal ectopic pregnancy A 12-years retrospective cohort study. *Ann. Ital. Chir.,* 2016; 87:461 - 465.

[23] Mol, F., van Mello, N. M., Strandell, A. et al. Salpingotomy versus salpingectomy in women with tubal pregnancy (ESEP study): An open-label, multicentre, randomised controlled trial. *Lancet,* 2014; 383(9927):1483 - 1489.

[24] Bangsgaard, N., Lund, C. O., Ottesen, B., Nilas, L. Improved fertility following conservative surgical treatment of ectopic pregnancy. *BJOG,* 2003; 110:765 - 770.

[25] Chen, L., Zhu, D., Wu, Q., Yu, Y. Fertility outcomes after laparoscopic salpingectomy or salpingotomy for tubal ectopic pregnancy: A retrospective cohort study of 95 patients. *Int. J. Surg.,* 2017; 48:59 - 63.

Index

D

E

F

G